Advanced Ureteroscopy

Scott G. Hubosky • Michael Grasso III
Olivier Traxer • Demetrius H. Bagley

Editors

Advanced Ureteroscopy

A Practitioner's Guide to Treating Difficult Problems

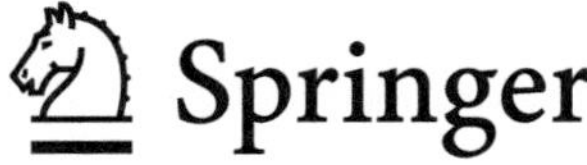

Editors
Scott G. Hubosky
Department of Urology
Sidney Kimmel Medical College at
Thomas Jefferson University Hospital
Philadelphia, PA
USA

Olivier Traxer
Sorbonne Université
GRC n°20, Groupe de Recherche Clinique
sur la Lithiase Urinaire, Hôpital Tenon
Paris, France

Michael Grasso III
Department of Urology
New York Medical College
Valhalla, NY
USA

Demetrius H. Bagley
Department of Urology and
Radiology, Sidney Kimmel Medical College
at Thomas Jefferson University Hospital
Philadelphia, PA
USA

ISBN 978-3-030-82353-5   ISBN 978-3-030-82351-1   (eBook)
https://doi.org/10.1007/978-3-030-82351-1

This Springer imprint is published by the registered company Springer Nature Switzerland AG
The registered company address is: Gewerbestrasse 11, 6330 Cham, Switzerland

"Advanced Ureteroscopy" is dedicated to our co-editor, senior colleague, mentor and friend: Demetrius H. Bagley.
His vision and tireless pursuit of excellence lit the path for the contemporary practice of semi-rigid and flexible ureteroscopy. Words cannot express our appreciation for his contributions and leadership in the field of endourology.

Scott G. Hubosky
Michael Grasso III
Olivier Traxer

Contents

1 Difficult Access to the Ureter 1
Demetrius H. Bagley and Scott G. Hubosky

2 Imaging of the Upper Urinary Tract 15
Wayne DeBeatham, Nicole M. Hindman, Andrew I. Fishman,
and Michael Grasso III

3 Instruments 29
Silvia Proietti, Vincent De Coninck, Olivier Traxer,
Salvatore Buttice, Jan Brachlow, Etienne Xavier Keller,
Kymora B. Scotland, Bree'ava Limbrick, Demetrius H. Bagley,
Scott G. Hubosky, and Thomas J. Hardacker

4 Basic Techniques 79
Steeve Doizi, Etienne Xavier Keller, Scott G. Hubosky, Olivier Traxer,
Nitin Sharma, Michael Grasso III, and Edward J. Kloniecke

5 Stones 105
Etienne Xavier Keller, Vincent De Coninck, Olivier Traxer,
Asaf Shvero, Nir Kleinmann, Scott G. Hubosky, Steeve Doizi,
Thomas J. Hardacker, Demetrius H. Bagley,
and Maryann Sonzogni-Cella

6 Upper Tract Urothelial Carcinoma 155
Benjamin H. Rudnik, Scott G. Hubosky, Kim HooKim,
Demetrius H. Bagley, María Rodríguez-Monsalve,
Etienne Xavier Keller, Vincent De Coninck, Olivier Traxer,
Michael Grasso III, Nitin Sharma, Andrew I. Fishman,
Joseph K. Izes, and Anna W. Komorowski

7 Ureteroscopic Management of Upper Urinary Tract Obstruction ... 209
Scott G. Hubosky and Demetrius H. Bagley

8   Ureteroscopic Treatment of Chronic Unilateral Hematuria 225
Abhay A. Singh, Scott G. Hubosky, Ryuta Tanimoto,
and Demetrius H. Bagley

9   Antegrade Ureteroscopy 235
Anthony T. Tokarski and Demetrius H. Bagley

10   Complications of Ureteroscopy 249
Scott G. Hubosky and Brian P. Calio

Index 275

Contributors

Demetrius H. Bagley, MD Department of Urology and Radiology, Sidney Kimmel Medical College at Thomas Jefferson University Hospital, Philadelphia, PA, USA

Jan Brachlow, MD, FEBU Sorbonne Université, Service d'Urologie, Assistance-Publique Hôpitaux de Paris, Hôpital Tenon, Paris, France

Sorbonne Université, GRC n°20, Groupe de Recherche Clinique sur la Lithiase Urinaire, Hôpital Tenon, Paris, France

Department of Urology, Kantonsspital Winterthur, Winterthur, Switzerland

Salvatore Buttice, MD Sorbonne Université, Service d'Urologie, Assistance-Publique Hôpitaux de Paris, Hôpital Tenon, Paris, France

Sorbonne Université, GRC n°20, Groupe de Recherche Clinique sur la Lithiase Urinaire, Hôpital Tenon, Paris, France

Department of Urology, San Giovanni di Dio Hospital, Agrigento, Italy

Brian P. Calio, MD Department of Urology, Sidney Kimmel Medical College at Thomas Jefferson University Hospital, Philadelphia, PA, USA

Vincent De Coninck, MD, FEBU Sorbonne Université, GRC n°20, Groupe de Recherche Clinique sur la Lithiase Urinaire, Hôpital Tenon, Paris, France

Wayne DeBeatham, MD Department of Urology, Phelps Hospital/Northwell Health, Sleepy Hollow, NY, USA

Steeve Doizi, MD, MSc Sorbonne Université, GRC n°20, Groupe de Recherche Clinique sur la Lithiase Urinaire, Hôpital Tenon, Paris, France

Andrew I. Fishman, MD Department of Urology, New York Medical College, Valhalla, NY, USA

Michael Grasso III, MD Department of Urology, New York Medical College, Valhalla, NY, USA

Thomas J. Hardacker, MD, MBA Department of Urology, Sidney Kimmel Medical College at Thomas Jefferson University Hospital, Philadelphia, PA, USA

Nicole M. Hindman, MD New York University, Grossman School of Medicine, New York, NY, USA

Kim HooKim, MD Department of Pathology, Anatomy and Cell Biology, Sidney Kimmel Medical College at Thomas Jefferson University Hospital, Philadelphia, PA, USA

Scott G. Hubosky, MD Department of Urology, Sidney Kimmel Medical College at Thomas Jefferson University Hospital, Philadelphia, PA, USA

Joseph K. Izes, MD Department of Urology, Sidney Kimmel Medical College at Thomas Jefferson University Hospital, Philadelphia, PA, USA

Etienne Xavier Keller, MD, FEBU Sorbonne Université, GRC n°20, Groupe de Recherche Clinique sur la Lithiase Urinaire, Hôpital Tenon, Paris, France

Nir Kleinmann, MD Department of Urology, Sheba Medical Center, Tel-Hashomer, Israel

Edward J. Kloniecke, MD, MPH Department of Urology, Sidney Kimmel Medical College at Thomas Jefferson University Hospital, Philadelphia, PA, USA

Anna W. Komorowski, MD Department of Medical Oncology, Donald and Barbara Zucker School of Medicine at Hofstra/Northwell, Hempstead, NY, USA

Bree'ava Limbrick, BS Department of Urology, David Geffen School of Medicine, University of California Los Angeles, Los Angeles, CA, USA

Silvia Proietti, MD, FEBU Sorbonne Université, Service d'Urologie, Assistance-Publique Hôpitaux de Paris, Hôpital Tenon, Paris, France

Sorbonne Université, GRC n°20, Groupe de Recherche Clinique sur la Lithiase Urinaire, Hôpital Tenon, Paris, France

Department of Urology, San Raffaele Hospital, Ville Turro Division, Milan, Italy

María Rodríguez-Monsalve, MD, FEBU Sorbonne Université, Service d'Urologie, AP-HP, Hôpital Tenon, Paris, France

Sorbonne Université, GRC n°20, Groupe de Recherche Clinique sur la Lithiase Urinaire, Hôpital Tenon, Paris, France

Department of Urology, Hospital universitario Puerta de Hierro, Majadahonda (Madrid), Spain

Benjamin H. Rudnik, MD Department of Urology, Sidney Kimmel Medical College at Thomas Jefferson University Hospital, Philadelphia, PA, USA

Kymora B. Scotland, MD, PhD Department of Urology, David Geffen School of Medicine, University of California Los Angeles, Los Angeles, CA, USA

Nitin Sharma, MD Phelps Memorial Hospital, Sleepy Hollow, NY, USA

Asaf Shvero, MD Department of Urology, Sidney Kimmel Medical College at Thomas Jefferson University Hospital, Philadelphia, PA, USA

Abhay A. Singh, MD Department of Urology, Sidney Kimmel Medical College at Thomas Jefferson University Hospital, Philadelphia, PA, USA

Maryann Sonzogni-Cella, BSN, RN, CPPS Department of Nursing, Thomas Jefferson University Hospital, Philadelphia, PA, USA

Ryuta Tanimoto, MD, PhD Department of Urology, Graduate School of Medicine, Dentistry & Pharmaceutical Sciences, Okayama University, Okayama, Japan

Anthony T. Tokarski, MD Department of Urology, Sidney Kimmel Medical College at Thomas Jefferson University Hospital, Philadelphia, PA, USA

Olivier Traxer, MD, PhD Sorbonne Université, GRC n°20, Groupe de Recherche Clinique sur la Lithiase Urinaire, Hôpital Tenon, Paris, France

Chapter 1
Difficult Access to the Ureter

Demetrius H. Bagley and Scott G. Hubosky

Introduction

Endoscopic treatment within the upper urinary tract clearly requires access for the endoscope to the point of interest. Although the techniques for basic access have been thoroughly studied and are well known, there are many difficulties, which can arise anywhere from the urethral meatus into areas within the kidney itself. Techniques to overcome these challenges can vary with the specific location and the clinical problem (Table 1.1).

Difficult Urethral Access

Obstacles to passage of an endoscope through the urethra can be encountered at any point from the meatus to the bladder neck. Difficult access is much more common in male than female patients. The solution to gain access will be related to the nature of the obstruction itself and to the purpose and, therefore, instruments needed for the upper tract endoscopy.

Meatal stenosis may be recognized on physical examination or may not be evident until one attempts to place an endoscope into the urethra. The obstructive narrowing can be evident quite distally, nearly on the glans penis, or may be located a few millimeters within the urethra. The latter may not be seen until the endoscope

D. H. Bagley
Department of Urology and Radiology, Sidney Kimmel Medical College at Thomas Jefferson University Hospital, Philadelphia, PA, USA

S. G. Hubosky (✉)
Department of Urology, Sidney Kimmel Medical College at Thomas Jefferson University Hospital, Philadelphia, PA, USA
e-mail: Scott.Hubosky@jefferson.edu

© Springer Nature Switzerland AG 2022
S. G. Hubosky et al. (eds.), *Advanced Ureteroscopy*,
https://doi.org/10.1007/978-3-030-82351-1_1

Table 1.1 Points of difficult access encountered during ureteroscopy

Urethra
Urethral meatal stenosis
Urethral stricture
Prostatic lobe hypertrophy
Pelvic prolapse (cystocele)
Ureteral orifice
Edematous ureteral orifice
Ureterocele
Heterotopic ureteral orifice
Impacted calculus at ureteral orifice
Primary ureteral pathology
Ureteral stone
Ureteral stricture
Ureteral neoplasm
Ureteropelvic junction (UPJ) obstruction
Ureteral tortuosity secondary to chronic obstruction
Intrarenal narrowing
Infundibular stenosis
Calyceal diverticulum

is introduced. Simple dilation of the stenotic segment is usually enough for endoscopic access. It may not be curative but can allow completion of the procedure with later follow-up and evaluation before a more definitive meatoplasty. Similarly, hypospadias may be accompanied by stenosis, either distally or more proximally within the urethra. Often there is no obstruction, and the endoscope can be introduced into the aberrant meatus.

Strictures more commonly occur proximally in the urethra. They can vary in length from a very short band to a longer stenotic segment. Again, dilation is the first choice to enlarge the lumen sufficiently for passage of an endoscope. A cystoscope is usually the first choice for inspection of the bladder and to place instruments or wires within the ureter. However, if access to the ureter is the only maneuver needed, a smaller diameter endoscope, such as a ureteroscope, can be adequate to navigate through most urethral narrowings on the way to the ureteral orifice.

Unique to the male are the difficulties presented by the prostate. The lumen may be visually obstructed from enlarged lateral prostatic lobes, but physical obstruction is much less common. Elevation of the bladder neck from prostatic enlargement is a more difficult problem. It may be impossible to elevate the tip of a rigid cystoscope enough to overcome the posterior prostate at the bladder neck. This same elevation can obscure visualization of the ureteral orifice. A flexible cystoscope can pass through the visually obstructed prostatic urethra into the bladder. Greater maneuverability allows visualization within the bladder and possibly deflection posteriorly and laterally to reach the ureteral orifice. The safest step at that point is to place a wire into the ureter and leave it to maintain access. An angled smooth coated wire will give the best chance of passing if the orifice is not located immediately in front of the cystoscope. Further angulation is achieved by placing an angled catheter through the lumen of the cystoscope and then the guidewire through that catheter.

If a rigid cystoscope has been placed into the bladder, visualization of the ureteral orifice may be even more difficult. It may be entirely hidden under the lobes of the prostate extending into the bladder. It may be impossible to angle the endoscope sufficiently to view the orifice with the 30° lens. There is a better chance to see the orifice with a 70° lens, but then it becomes nearly impossible to pass a wire or catheter into the ureter without additional attachments. An Albarran deflector is specifically designed to angle or deflect a catheter or other devices into the field of the 70° telescope (Fig. 1.1).

Ureteral Orifice

Unique difficulties in access to the ureter present at the ureteral orifice. It can be obscured by alterations in the bladder mucosa and by anatomic and inflammatory changes in the distal ureter. Within the bladder, trabeculation from outlet obstruction, generalized edema from infection or an indwelling balloon catheter, or localized edema from reaction to a distal ureteral calculus can obscure the ureteral orifice (Fig. 1.2). Tumor within the bladder overlying the orifice can also prevent visualization. In each case, the initial approach is the same.

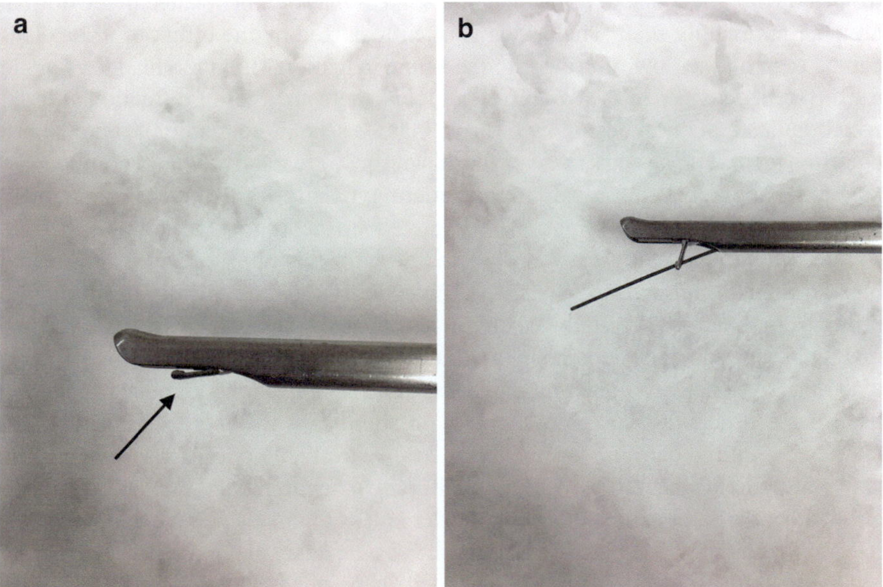

Fig. 1.1 (**a**) Side view of rigid cystoscope with Albarran deflector at near neutral position (black arrow). (**b**) The Albarran deflector can be adjusted to move wires or catheters with downward deflection into the field of view of the 70° lens

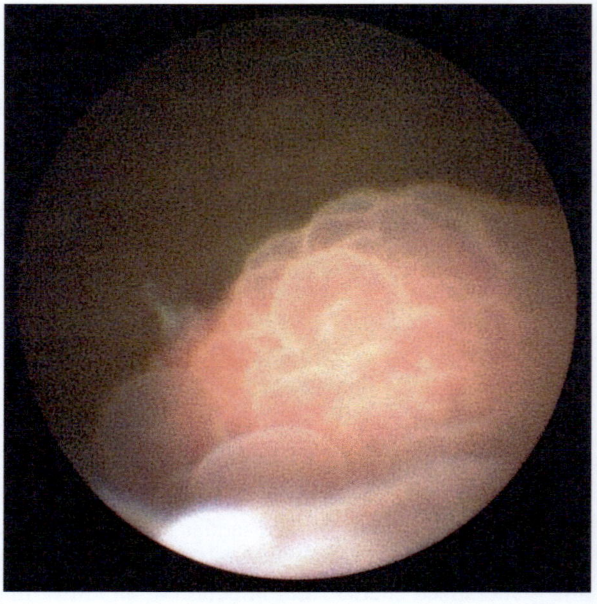

Fig. 1.2 Cystoscopic view of the left ureteral orifice in a patient with a left distal ureteral stone. The calculus has caused significant mucosal edema and has obscured the luminal opening of the left ureteral orifice

Each normal orifice is located on the floor of the bladder, each lateral to the midline along the interureteric ridge. The orifice is usually identifiable by its appearance, its location, and peristalsis with the efflux of urine. When the anatomy is distorted with trabeculation, scarring, or edema, it may still be located in the normal area but not readily seen. The orifice is often localized by the efflux of urine. This can be seen by the flow of urine into the saline irrigation filling the bladder. Due to the different densities of the two different fluids, there are lines of refraction of light, which indicate the flow. The flow of urine may be seen more readily if it contains a coloring agent. The best alternatives for this purpose are relatively inert compounds, able to be applied intravenously to the patient, typically while under general anesthesia, and after several minutes are excreted in the urine. Indigotindisulfonate sodium (indigo carmine) is a well-known agent for this purpose and is familiar to most urologists and gynecologists. After injection, it would typically result in blue efflux from the ureteral orifice, usually in less than 10 minutes in patients with normal renal function and adequate hydration. Reports of severe hypertension and bradycardia have been reported with indigo carmine [1, 2], and recommendations have been made to avoid its use in patients with significant cardiac disease [3]. More practically, indigo carmine has not been readily available due to a shortage in its active ingredient since 2014. Another well-known agent, methylene blue, has been utilized for the same purpose but is considered less reliable since it can be metabolized to leucomethylene blue, a colorless metabolite, even in the presence of normal renal function [4]. It also must be avoided in pregnant patients and those with glucose-6-phosphate dehydrogenase (G6PD) deficiency due to concern for methemoglobinemia. Due to these concerns, other agents have been studied for the purpose of ureteral orifice identification. Intravenous sodium fluorescein has been

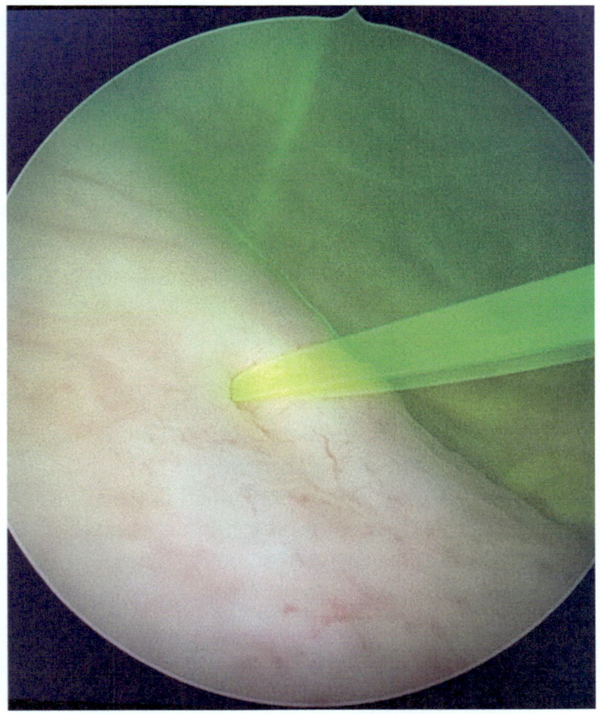

Fig. 1.3 Cystoscopic view of the right ureteral orifice following intravenous injection of sodium fluorescein. Note the efflux of greenish yellow-tinged urine from the orifice

utilized for retinal angiography and has since been studied for cystoscopic application [5, 6]. After intravenous injection, it results in a greenish yellow efflux of urine from the ureteral orifice (Fig. 1.3). Side effects include transient yellow sclera when used at higher does, as well as nausea, vomiting, and flushing. Independent of the intravenous agent selected, it is important to note that it may appear quickly or there may be a delay if there is diminished renal function or obstruction to the flow of urine. It is important to examine the area of the orifice carefully and steadily until the colored efflux is seen.

Ureteroceles or duplications are usually diagnosed preoperatively, but they can also be recognized endoscopically. There is always an orifice in the ureterocele, often, but not always, located medially and posteriorly. When visible, the orifice can be accessed endoscopically. With duplication the aberrant orifice is generally located endoscopically along the ureteric ridge. The edematous ureteral orifice is usually normally located with symmetrical mucosal edema obscuring the opening of the orifice. Again, it is essential to observe the area very closely for the efflux of urine before attempts at manipulation. If it is identified in this way, it should be entered immediately either with a guidewire or a small diameter semirigid ureteroscope. If either of these successfully enters the ureter, the guidewire is left in place and the cystoscope removed. Because of the difficulty finding and entering the ureter, this safety guidewire is always valuable in these cases to locate the orifice for reentry. If a coated guidewire has been used for access, it should be replaced with a more stable Teflon-coated wire, possibly a stiff design, to assure that the safety wire does not fall out of the ureter.

When careful observation and these maneuvers fail to locate the orifice, two other techniques can be helpful. Active irrigation in the suspected location can compress the mucosal edema and reveal the orifice itself. This effect can be emphasized or exaggerated by irrigating through the channel of a semirigid ureteroscope with syringe pressurization. The direct flow then compresses the edematous tissue more effectively. Only after these other techniques have clearly failed should one attempt to probe the expected location of the ureter. With excellent irrigation and visualization, the operator can place the straight, rounded tip of a coated guidewire very gently at the expected site. It should be used only as the last resort because it can be expected to cause bleeding.

Alternatively, when the orifice cannot be accessed, the ureterocele can be punctured. A series of adult patients with orthotopic ureteroceles and associated calculi has been described in which holmium laser incision of the ureterocele and laser lithotripsy of the calculi are performed in the same setting [7]. Although published clinical experience is not robust, this series of 16 patients reported complete stone clearance with transient vesicoureteral reflux (VUR) in a small subset of patients, which resolved after 6 months.

The Reimplanted Ureter

The location of the ureter after a ureteroneocystostomy can be difficult to anticipate and hard to find. There are numerous indications for reimplantation ranging from treatment of pediatric reflux to distal ureterectomy for tumor treatment or after damage to the distal ureter and, most commonly, after renal transplantation. Full, thorough, well-visualized cystoscopy is essential to locate the neo-orifice. We prefer initial endoscopy with a rigid cystoscope using both the 30° and the 70° telescopes. In some patients it may be necessary to use a flexible cystoscope to visualize the entire bladder since the orifice may be located almost anywhere.

Inspect the entire bladder thoroughly. Pay particular attention to the interureteric ridge. Some techniques for implantation involve advancement of the orifice medially along the ridge, but others result in a more lateral placement. Search for evidence of the orifice by seeing urine flowing into the bladder. This may be detected by observing the refraction lines caused by mixing of fluids of different densities.

The cross-trigonal reimplantation performed for reflux presents one of the most difficult positions for endoscopic access. It approaches the impossible to gain luminal access with a catheter or wire using a simple rigid cystoscope with a 30° telescope. There is some chance of gaining access with an angled hydromer-coated wire. Using an Albarran deflector with a 70° telescope to direct a wire or catheter gives a better chance for positioning into the lumen. Alternatively, a combination of angled glide wire placed through an angled glide catheter allows for passage of the wire at an angle of 120° from the axis of the rigid cystoscope and has been successful in achieving retrograde access in the cross-trigonal configuration [8].

Most reimplantations in adults result in the orifice being located more aberrantly. Most will be found laterally or even anteriorly along the lateral portion of the bladder. The neo-ureter commonly appears as a mucosal bud, a rounded protuberance formed by the end of the ureter itself. It has been described as appearing like a raspberry. The lumen is located within the center of this structure. Some surgical techniques place the neo-orifice posteriorly toward the floor of the bladder. Although these may be somewhat more technically difficult, they offer an excellent position for future endoscopic access [9].

In each case with such a difficult access, the first wire to be placed should be a straight hydromer-coated design. This will offer the best chance to pass through the orifice and throughout the lumen regardless of the specific anatomic difficulty. It may be necessary to exchange it for another specific wire design. For example, a long floppy-tipped wire like the Bentson or an angle-tipped wire can offer specific benefits to pass the curves in a very tortuous ureter. The ultimate wire for stability is the extra-stiff design, preferably with double-floppy tips. Any wire exchange should occur through a catheter. Our first choice is a 6 or rarely 5 Fr ureteral catheter. These usually offer enough stability to prevent coiling in the bladder with subsequent withdrawal of the wire from the ureter. An angled hydromer-coated catheter gives greater maneuverability within the ureter either to pass stones or to traverse tortuosities. When they are not adequate, greater stability to buttress the wire or catheter and wire combination can be provided with a ureteral access sheath or the sheath of the rigid cystoscope itself (Fig. 1.4).

Impacted Calculi

Urinary calculi can become impacted at any point in the ureter. They tend to occur in the distal ureter, in the mid-portion as it courses over the iliac vessels and in the upper ureter. Complicating factors can occur with calculi within the ureter at any level. There can be associated edema, in some cases with pseudopolyps, total obstruction, distortion of the course of the ureter, and infection proximal to the calculus. The approach to the calculus at the orifice noted above has similarities at other locations. When the stone is located at the ureterovesical junction, there may be relatively easy endoscopic access into the ureteral orifice. The lumen may lead directly to the calculus. It can be bypassed with a wire, pushed proximally into a more dilated portion of the ureter, or fragmented in situ. Although the anatomy can be distorted with alteration of the course of the lower ureter, it is less common than in more proximal locations. With hydronephrosis there is both dilation and lengthening of the ureter, but the distal portion is fixed to the bladder as a constant landmark.

Impaction in the mid-ureter presents additional problems. It usually occurs at, or just proximal to, the iliac vessels. As the ureter descends over the psoas muscle, it

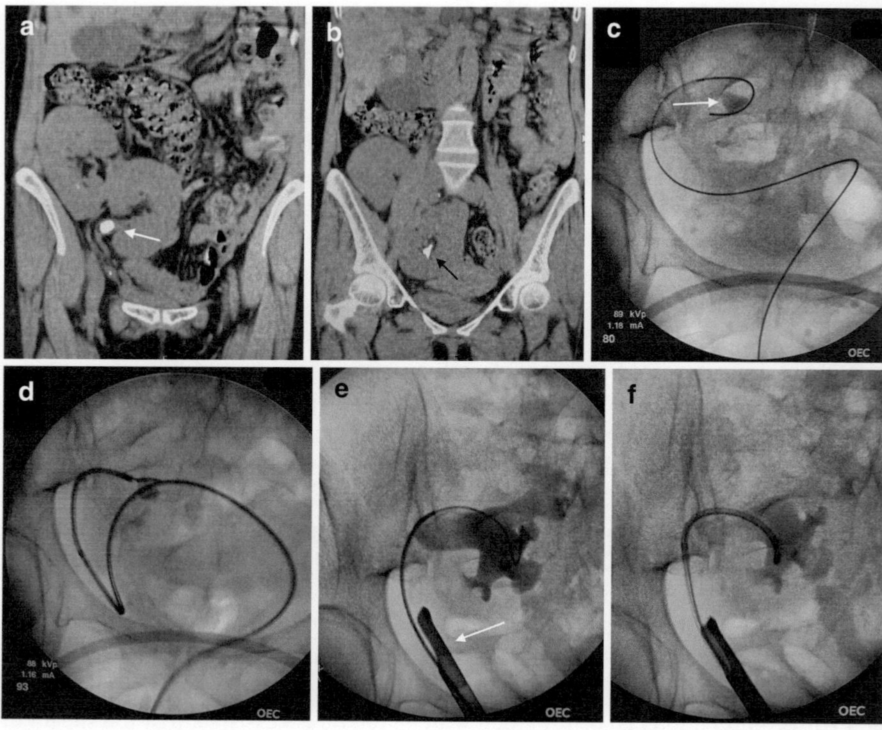

Fig. 1.4 (**a**) Coronal CT scan views of pediatric en bloc kidney transplant in an adult recipient with renal pelvic stone (white arrow) and (**b**) lower pole renal stone (black arrow). (**c**) Initial wire placement into transplant ureteral orifice along the right lateral bladder wall shows access is achieved but coiling of the wire has resulted. White arrow marks renal pelvic stone. (**d**) Flexible ureteroscopes can be placed over coiled wires, but this results in suboptimal maneuverability and potential damage to ureteroscope shaft. (**e**) Placement of wire and ureteral catheter combination through a rigid cystoscope sheath (white arrow) under fluoroscopy eliminates buckling of wire for most direct retrograde access. (**f**) Placement of flexible ureteroscope through the cystoscope sheath allows full access even to the transplant kidney lower pole without buckling

courses slightly posteriorly before moving anteriorly over the surface of the vessels before once again going posteriorly and laterally in the pelvis. This anatomy should be considered with any attempts to bypass the stone with a wire or to move it more proximally. If a highly or totally obstructing stone has been identified at the level of the vessels preoperatively or with the retrograde ureterogram, an angled hydromer-coated wire should be the first choice as an instrument to gain access beyond the stone. The wire can be rotated to position the tip at multiple different points where the stone and the ureteral wall meet. Placement of this wire through an angled cath-eter can give even more options in positioning. If these attempts at access fail, the flexible ureteroscope can be placed directly into the ureter to approach the calculus. From this position, the ureter will be coursing anteriorly over the vessels and then again posteriorly more proximal to the vessels. Placement of any wires or attempts to dislodge and move the stone should be in the expected direction of the course of the ureter. Under direct vision, the stone can often be seen even when there is surrounding edema. A wire is then placed at the edge of the stone adjacent to the least edematous portion of the ureter and directed toward the expected course of the lumen. When this is impossible, direct fragmentation of the stone can be initiated without first gaining access with a wire.

Obstructing stones in the proximal ureter more commonly cause tortuosity of the ureter along with hydronephrosis (Fig. 1.5). A similar approach to that used for more distal obstructing stones also can be used at this location. Additionally, techniques are needed to pass through the tortuous portion of the ureter to reach the renal pelvis for treatment of intrarenal stones or for drainage purposes. Both special guidewires and manipulation with the deflectable tip of the ureteroscope can be

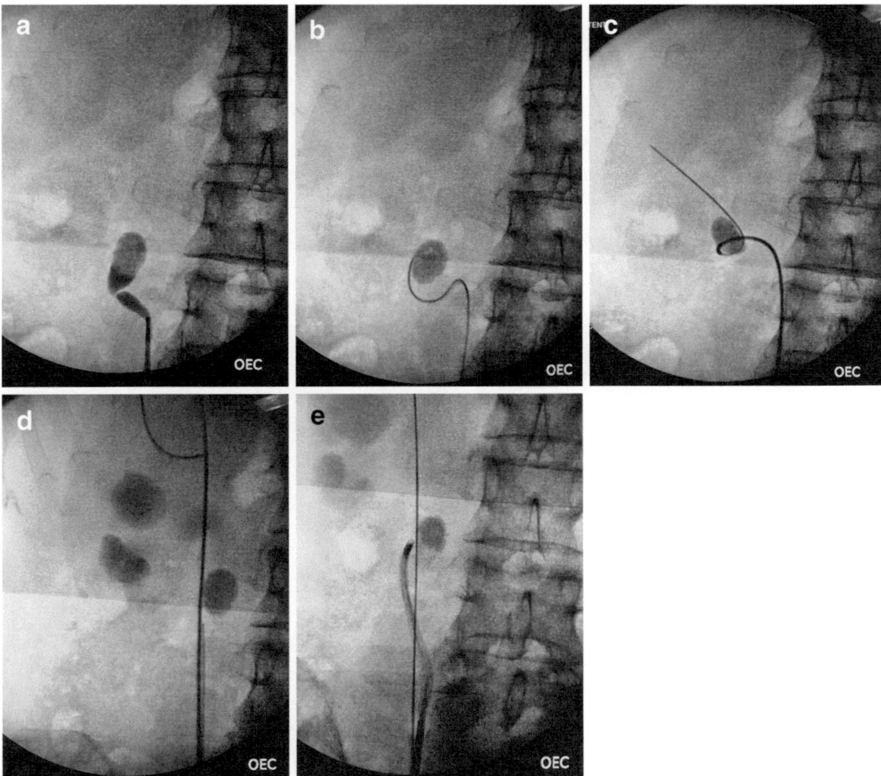

Fig. 1.5 (**a**) Retrograde pyelogram demonstrates a large right proximal ureteral stone with complete obstruction. (**b**) Resistance is met with initial placement of a guidewire. (**c**) Successful negotiation of the obstruction with an angled hydromer wire placed through a ureteral catheter under fluoroscopy. (**d**) Exchange of a super stiff wire through the ureteral catheter results in straightening of the ureteral tortuosity. Contrast can be seen in the dilated calyces of the right kidney. (**e**) Successful placement of flexible ureteroscope with reduction of stone burden with active laser lithotripsy

used to pass these tortuosities. Either an angled hydromer-coated wire or a Bentson wire with a long floppy tip will be useful in this maneuver.

Urinary sampling and subsequent internal drainage is usually necessary in these cases with highly obstructing calculi. After the proximal lumen of the ureter has been reached with a guidewire, a catheter should be placed over the wire to aspirate urine. If the encountered urine is very cloudy or malodorous, it should be sent to microbiology for formal culture. At that point, the system should be drained and the procedure terminated. If the aspirated urine happens to be clear, then the stone can be treated. Clearly, a stent should be left in place to drain the system in cases of high-grade obstruction.

Occlusive Ureteral Tumor

Ureteral tumors, even larger low-grade lesions, can cause ureteral obstruction and visual occlusion. It may be difficult to pass a wire beyond the neoplasm from the level of the bladder. Direct vision with ureteroscopy should demonstrate the margin between the tumor and the wall of the ureter (Fig. 1.6). The ureteroscope should be advanced with irrigation along that plane. If it does not pass because of an extensive base of the tumor or because of loss of vision from bleeding, a coated guidewire is passed along that same plane and advanced and rotated to pass. Once a guidewire

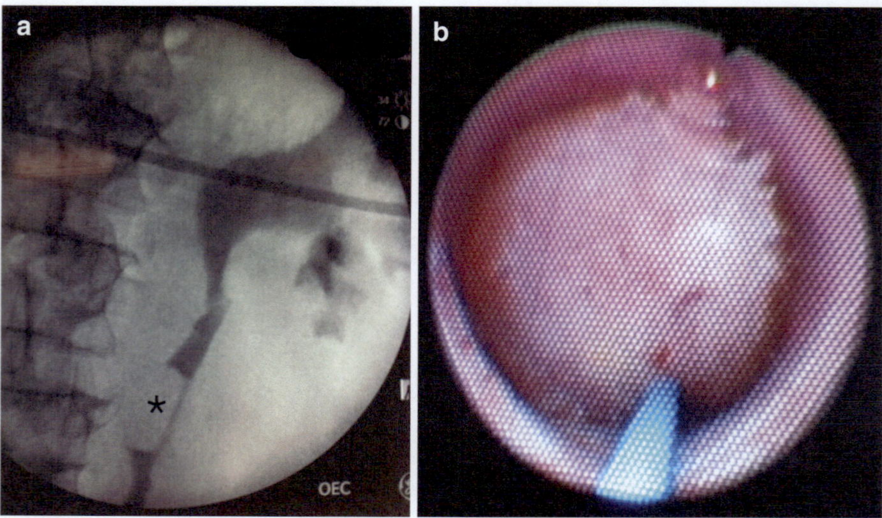

Fig. 1.6 (**a**) Retrograde pyelogram shows a large right proximal ureteral upper tract urothelial carcinoma with a very broad base (black asterisk). A small luminal narrowing exists as seen by contrast passage on the lateral aspect of the ureter. (**b**) Retrograde ureteral access between the tumor and the ureteral wall was possible by placing a wire under direct ureteroscopic visualization

has passed and the urine sampled, the tumor can be sampled or treated endoscopically.

Ureteral Narrowing or Stricture

Narrowing of the ureter itself may be unexpected or anticipated from preoperative contrast studies or the patient's history including previous radiation treatment or pelvic surgeries. A cone-tipped ureteropyelogram is particularly useful to define the anatomy and the lumen of the ureter (Fig. 1.7). A hydromer-coated wire should be used initially to gain access. The smallest diameter ureteroscope should be used. A very short stricture (1 mm or less) can be inspected endoscopically. Occasionally, these can be passed with the ureteroscope or can be successfully dilated with a balloon or a graduated dilator. Whenever there is severe dilation of the ureter proximal to the stricture, urine in that area should be sampled for inspection and culture. Strictures longer than a few millimeters can be more difficult to pass and to manage. If the stricture cannot be dilated quite easily to allow the endoscope to pass, an indwelling ureteral stent should be left in place to allow passive dilation. The endoscopic procedure can then be attempted again after several days.

Total occlusion of the ureter can also be grouped into very short or larger segments with the accompanying change in difficulty to treat and prognosis for success. If no contrast passes and no lumen can be seen with the ureteroscope, occasionally a symmetrical, usually central "dimple" can be seen. A straight-coated guidewire is placed against the dimple and advanced firmly and steadily. Often it

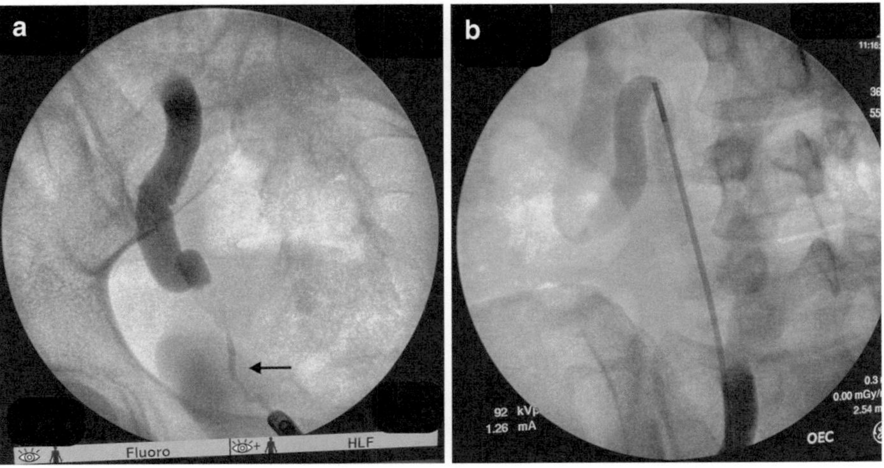

Fig. 1.7 (**a**) Retrograde pyelogram with a cone-tipped catheter shows a long distal ureteral stricture (black arrow) with severe ureteral dilation proximal to the obstruction. (**b**) View of the proximal ureter in the same patient. The hallmark of chronic ureteral obstruction is upstream ureteral dilation and tortuosity

will pass into the proximal lumen when this configuration is seen. If the ureteroscope will not pass through this area, it is removed, and an open-ended ureteral catheter is passed through the stricture to exchange the guidewire for a sturdier version. The short segment is then dilated. The endoscopic procedure can be continued if the proximal urine is clear.

When there is generalized scarring of the strictured segment as viewed endoscopically, distortion of the area, or evidence of a long obliterated area defined on preoperative imaging, then further procedures may be necessary. It is reasonable to attempt to place a wire as done for short segments, but the success will be lower. A smaller wire such as 0.025 inch may be helpful. If the obstruction cannot be passed, a combined antegrade and retrograde procedure can be useful. On completion of the ureteroscopic procedure, a ureteral catheter should be left in place for later administration of contrast when a nephrostomy tube has been placed. With contrast instilled proximally and distally, the length of the obstructed segment can be determined accurately radiographically. A decision can then be made on treatment. Either a laparoscopic repair or combined antegrade and retrograde endoscopy for recanalization may be indicated.

Ureteropelvic Junction Obstruction

Obstruction at the ureteropelvic junction (UPJ) can occur with various anatomic abnormalities. There may be a narrowing at the ureteropelvic junction, high insertion of the ureter into the renal pelvis, or a vessel crossing to cause obstruction. Although there is usually some distortion of the area, the greatest problem occurs when the distended renal pelvis angulates the junction of the ureter into the pelvis. It may lift the UPJ itself away from the ureter and form a very sharp angle into the pelvis. This deformity can be bypassed with techniques similar to those used for a tortuous ureter. An angled or a long floppy-tipped guidewire may enter it successfully. Alternatively, advancement with deflection and straightening of the flexible ureteroscope will often pass into the pelvis. It is very important to place a stiff guidewire through the UPJ to straighten it and maintain access.

Summary

Potential obstacles to upper urinary tract access exist within the luminal space from the urethral meatus all the way to the intrarenal collecting system. Successful access into the ureter in any circumstance requires the availability of rigid and flexible ureteroscopes as well as several different guidewires and ureteral catheters. When difficult access has been achieved, a stiff guidewire should be placed to maintain this access and allow for manipulations while minimizing the risk of buckling or creating ureteral perforations.

References

1. Naitoh J, Fox BM. Severe hypotension, bronchospasm, and urtricaria from intravenous indigo carmine. Urology. 1994;44:271–2.
2. Donaldson Craik J, Khan D, Afifi R. The safety of intravenous indigo carmine to assess ureteric patency during transvaginal uterosacral suspension of the vaginal vault. J Pelvic Med Surg. 2009;15(1):11–5.
3. Lee M, Sharifi R. Methylene blue versus indigo carmine. Urology. 1996;47:783–4.
4. Joel AB, Mueller D, Pahira JJ, Mordkin RM. Nonvisualization of intravenous methylene blue in patients with clincially normal renal function. Urology. 2001;58:607 vii.
5. Doyle PJ, Lipetskaia L, Duecy E, Buchsbaum G, Wood RW. Sodium fluorescein use during intraoperative cystoscopy. Obstet Gyn. 2015;125:548–50.
6. Grimes CL, Patankar S, Ryntz T, Philip N, Simpson K, Truong M, et al. Evaluating ureteral patency in the post-indigo carmine era: a randomized controlled trial. Am J Obstet Gynecol. 2017;217:601.e1–10.
7. Shah HN, Sodha H, Khandkar AA, Kharodawala S, Hegde SS, Bansal M. Endoscopic management of adult orthotopic ureterocele and associated calculi with holmium laser: experience with 16 patients over 4 years and review of the literature. J Endourol. 2008;22(3):489–95.
8. Wallis MC, Brown DH, Jayanthi VR, Koff SA. A novel technique for ureteral catheterization and/or retrograde ureteroscopy after cross-trigonal ureteral reimplantation. J Urol. 2003;170:1664–6.
9. Krambeck AE, Gettman MT, BaniHani AH, Husmann DA, Kramer SA, Segura JW. Management of nephrolithiasis after Cohen cross-trigonal and Glenn-Anderson advancement ureteroneocystotomy. J Urol. 2007;177:174–8.

Chapter 2
Imaging of the Upper Urinary Tract

Wayne DeBeatham, Nicole M. Hindman, Andrew I. Fishman,
and Michael Grasso III

Introduction

The overall prevalence of upper urinary tract stones is on the rise [1, 2], making accurate and efficient diagnosis of this problem more important than ever. Imaging plays a central role in defining the extent of stone burden, therapeutic planning, and follow-up of patients with urolithiasis. Imaging techniques include conventional radiography (abdominal X-ray of the kidneys, ureter, and bladder or KUB), intravenous urography (IVU), ultrasound (US), magnetic resonance urography (MRU), and computed tomography (CT) scans; each of these modalities is associated with advantages and limitations. Plain film radiographs and intravenous pyelographic techniques were replaced in emergency rooms and office clinics by sonography and single-slice CT, beginning in the early 1990s [3–5].

Additional advances in imaging, including multidetector CT scanning, dual-energy CT scanning, improved sonographic equipment, and scanning techniques, have further refined the use of imaging in stone disease. Imaging in suspected stone disease helps confirm the diagnosis and exclude other pathologies (such as acute appendicitis, diverticulitis, ovarian torsion, etc.) with high accuracy [6, 7]. Once the diagnosis of urolithiasis has been made, imaging provides anatomical, functional,

W. DeBeatham
Department of Urology, Phelps Hospital/Northwell Health, Sleepy Hollow, NY, USA

N. M. Hindman
New York University, Grossman School of Medicine, New York, NY, USA
e-mail: Nicole.hindman@nyumc.org

A. I. Fishman · M. Grasso III (✉)
Department of Urology, New York Medical College, Valhalla, NY, USA

© Springer Nature Switzerland AG 2022
S. G. Hubosky et al. (eds.), *Advanced Ureteroscopy*,
https://doi.org/10.1007/978-3-030-82351-1_2

and physiological information about the stone and the collecting system, factors that help in implementing therapeutic strategies.

Stones in the renal pelvis above the ureteropelvic junction are more often treated with shock wave lithotripsy (SWL), ureteroscopy, or percutaneous nephrolithotomy (PCNL). Larger stones and staghorn calculi are removed with PCNL. PCNL requires percutaneous ultrasonography (US) or fluoroscopically guided puncture of a renal calyx, tract dilation, and stone fragmentation-extraction. Stones in the ureter are usually treated via medical expulsive therapy, hydration, and pain control. Larger ureteral stones may require intervention with SWL or ureteroscopy with fragmentation-extraction. Imaging is therefore important both in the initial diagnosis of these stones in terms of location and size and in follow-up of therapies to assess for resolution/complication.

Upper tract urothelial carcinoma (UTUC) is relatively rare. Bladder tumors account for 90–95% of urothelial carcinomas. Upper tract lesions account for 5–10% of urothelial carcinomas, with an estimated incidence of two cases per 100,000 inhabitants in the Western world [8]. Within the upper tract, tumors of the renal pelvis are twice as common as tumors of the ureter, and both can present with simultaneous bladder tumors in about 17% of initial cases [9]. UTUC can spread locally by way of mucosal extension and systemically by either hematogenous or lymphatic pathways. Metastatic sites most frequently involve retroperitoneal and/or pelvic lymph nodes, the liver, lungs, and bone [10].

Patients with UTUC often have non-specific and variable presentations. While hematuria is the most common presenting symptom (70–80%) [8], this finding is non-specific and can, in fact, be attributable to other causes, such as renal stones, prostatic hyperplasia, or urinary tract infections. Patients may also present with symptoms of urinary obstruction or, less frequently, with evidence of metastatic spread. In this light, non-invasive imaging plays an appreciable role in the diagnosis, workup, and follow-up of UTUC.

Conventional Radiography/Abdominal Plain Film

Traditionally, diagnosis of suspected renal stones was made via a plain film radiograph, termed a radiograph of the kidneys, ureters, and bladder (KUB). Since the majority of urinary tract stones contain calcium, most stones that are sufficiently large (at least 2.6 mm in size) [11] should be visible on plain radiography. However, certain stone compositions, particularly radiolucent stones (such as uric acid or matrix stones), are not visible on KUB. The advantages of a KUB include its wide availability, minimal radiation exposure, and low cost. However, visualization of stones is limited by small stone size, overlying bowel gas/fecal retention in the colon, body habitus of the patient, and overlying bony structures.

The sensitivity and specificity of KUB for detecting urinary tract calculi (when utilizing CT as the gold standard) have been reported as 45–59% and 71–77%, respectively [12]. Another limitation of plain film radiography is the lack of soft tissue detail of the viscera, limiting evaluation of the kidney, ureter, and associated fascial planes. Thus, it is not typically used for preoperative planning for percutaneous nephrolithotomy or extirpative renal procedures. Rather, it is primarily used in planning fluoroscopically guided SWL, in follow-up of known radiopaque calculi (for patients who have elected for surveillance of their calculi), and for monitoring the status of stone fragments after SWL, ureteroscopy, and PCNL [13].

Ultrasound

Ultrasound (US) is a popular modality for evaluation of the urinary tract. It does not utilize ionizing radiation and is thus a procedure of choice for children and pregnant patients with suspected urolithiasis (Fig. 2.1). US is also the preferred imaging modality to detect hydronephrosis and hydroureter, although it often does not reveal the cause of the obstruction [14].

In the setting of acute renal colic, measurement of the resistive index of the kidney may provide information about the true presence of obstruction, but the exact threshold for the resistive index (usually defined as greater than 0.7) is not precise. As background, in urinary tract obstruction, pathophysiological changes affecting the pressure in the collecting system and kidney perfusion occur. Ultrasound is very sensitive for the detection of collecting system dilation, but the collecting system may be dilated without obstruction. To differentiate these conditions, color Doppler sonography can be performed with measurement of the resistive index (RI) in the intrarenal arteries. True obstruction (except in the hyperacute stage) leads to intrarenal vasoconstriction with a consecutive increase of the RI above the upper limit of 0.7, whereas non-obstructive dilation does not cause an increase in the RI. Unfortunately, there is crossover between other physiological conditions besides obstruction that may lead to an elevated RI, so that this measure in isolation has a relatively high variability between readers [15, 16].

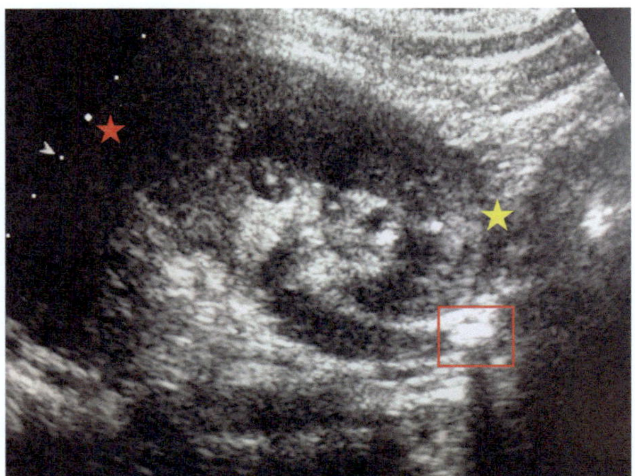

Fig. 2.1 Renal ultrasound with sagittal view of the left kidney demonstrates mild hydronephrosis and a proximal ureteral stone with shadowing (red box). By convention, the upper pole is marked with a red star and lower pole marked with a yellow star

It is important to recognize the limitations of US in the diagnosis of renal and ureteral stones, which are limited sensitivity for stone detection and the overestimation of stone size. Many well-designed studies, by multiple groups, have compared the performance of non-contrast computed tomography (NCCT) to US for the detection of renal and ureteral stones. On the whole, these studies demonstrate US is not as sensitive for stone detection and tends to overestimate the size of stones, especially for smaller-sized calculi. In a prospective study, Sheafor et al. reported 96% sensitivity for NCCT to detect ureteral stones compared to only 61% with US [17]. A review of the literature performed by Ray et al. reported a pooled sensitivity of only 45% for US in the detection of ureteral and renal stones compared to NCCT [18]. Another more contemporary study comparing NCCT to US done within 24 hours of each other for patients with nephrolithiasis reported that US missed 37% of the stones detected by NCCT, with the average size of the missed stones noted to be 4.5 mm [19]. The same study made note of the common overestimation of stone size by US. For stones measuring ≤ 5 mm on NCCT, but seen on both NCCT and US, overestimation in size was made by US in 82% by an average of 3.3 mm. In another study, stones ≤ 4 mm on NCCT were overestimated by US in 33% [20]. Overestimation of stone size by US must be appreciated as a limitation since it could potentially alter management, and it is for this reason that KUB X-rays are often ordered together with US for follow-up of nephrolithiasis in lieu of NCCT, in an effort to limit patient radiation exposure. It is important to relay the limitations of US with patients in order to properly manage expectations.

Ultrasound has some limited use in the assessment of upper tract urothelial cancer. Renal pelvic lesions may appear as a soft tissue mass within an echogenic renal sinus. These lesions are typically hyperechoic relative to normal renal parenchyma. Lesions within an infundibulum may cause focal calyceal dilation. As ultrasound rarely visualizes ureters, it is limited in the assessment of ureteral lesions [10].

Intravenous Urography/Intravenous Pyelography

Intravenous pyelography (IVP) previously served as the gold standard for the diagnosis and follow-up of urinary stones. This modality involves taking successive plain films targeted at the depth of the kidneys, after a bowel preparation has been administered, first with a scout radiograph and then at predetermined time points after the administration of hypertonic radiopaque contrast intravenously. The resultant high-resolution images demonstrate the kidneys in various stages of contrast enhancement and demonstrate the excretion of the contrast into the collecting system of the kidney, thereby providing excellent anatomical detail of the minor and major calyces, infundibula, renal pelvises, and ureters. A renal or ureteral stone is seen as a filling defect within the collecting system in this modality.

Advantages of IVP include its availability, its ability to estimate renal function, degree of obstruction, and its superior depiction of fine anatomy due to its high resolution (excellent demonstration of the cystic tubular ectasia of medullary sponge kidney, subtle calyceal diverticula, and subtle contrast extravasation) [21].

The disadvantages of IVP include its requirement for a bowel preparation for improved visualization of the kidneys, its requirement for intravenous contrast administration, the requirement for radiation, its poor depiction of intra-abdominal and pelvic organs, and its variable acquisition times (up to 108 min in one study) [22]. Furthermore, the sensitivity of IVP for detecting ureteral calculi varies from 59.1% to 64% in the literature, with a specificity of 92% [22, 23]. Additionally, a meta-analysis of four studies involving 296 patients concluded that non-contrast helical CT was significantly better than IVP at diagnosing and excluding stones (pooled positive likelihood ratios for non-contrast CT and IVP were 23.15 and 9.32, respectively) [24]. Due to the better sensitivity and specificity of non-contrast (unenhanced) helical CT scans relative to IVP, this modality has been largely replaced by CT scans for the diagnosis of urolithiasis. Limited contemporary indications for IVP include situations in which immediate evaluation of the upper urinary tract is necessary, such as in the operating room during trauma cases or to rule out iatrogenic injury [25]. IVP is also uniquely useful in the diagnosis of renal ptosis, a rare condition in which there is renal descent when moving from the supine to the upright or erect position (Fig. 2.2), which causes renal colic when the patient is upright, but is relieved when they are recumbent. Once diagnosed, this condition is effectively treated with nephropexy.

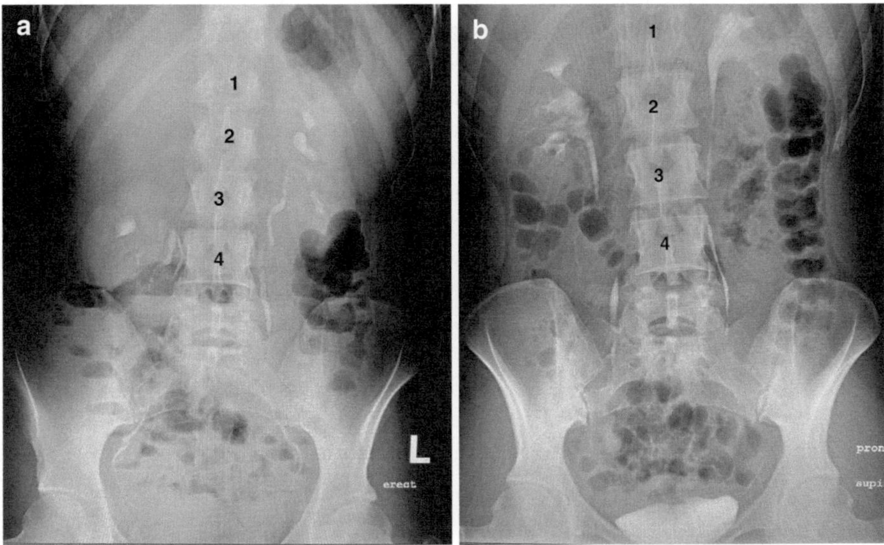

Fig. 2.2 (**a**) Intravenous pyelogram in the erect position with lumbar vertebra numbered. Note significant kinking of the right proximal ureter at the level of the L4 vertebra. (**b**) Same patient in the supine position, showing significant upward migration of the right kidney with straightening of the right ureter. This patient had right renal ptosis successfully treated with robotic nephropexy

Renal UTUC may present as a filling defect within the contrast-enhanced collecting system. Irregular or stippled appearance reflects the tracking of contrast material into the interstices of a papillary lesion. This appearance, however, is non-specific and may reflect the presence of clot or fungal lesions. This modality is also limited in the presence of hydronephrosis or poor contrast excretion [10].

Computed Tomography

Background

Non-contrast helical CT is currently viewed as the optimal initial study for investigating patients with suspected urolithiasis [26, 27]. Non-contrast CT was first described as useful in the investigation of stones in 1995, since when it has been repeatedly proven to have unrivaled accuracy in the diagnosis of urinary tract stones, with a reported sensitivity of 95–98% and a specificity of 96–100% [3, 4, 28–32].

Initially, all CT scans were performed utilizing single-slice, point, and shoot technology (these are non-helical, non-spiral CT scanners). However, since 1998, when the first multidetector (also termed helical or spiral) CT scanners were introduced, almost all single-slice scanners have been replaced by multidetector scanners, ranging from 2 detectors to 128 detectors. These advances have allowed the resolution of CT scanners to dramatically improve, by acquiring data of sub-centimeter slice thickness, allowing isotropic volume acquisition such that three-dimensional datasets can be generated by a single 1-min axial acquisition. Additionally, there have been advances in the post-processing algorithms and workstations, which generate multi-planar datasets. These advances have improved the diagnostic image quality of CT, such that the depiction of renal and ureteral stones, including the number, size, and location of the stones; skin-to-stone distance; and distance to the ureterovesical junction, is easily made. Additionally, when axial images are reviewed in conjunction with high-resolution coronal reformatted images (generated from the isotropic thin slice axial acquisition), there is improved detection of stones [33, 34].

With these advances in the depiction of small stones, there is also an improved ability of multidetector CT to assess the attenuation measurements and internal structure of stones, which again helps predict response to treatment. Although determination of exact stone composition is not reliably achievable with CT, given the overlap of Hounsfield units (HU) range for various stone types and combinations [35–37], response to therapy can be predicted. Multiple groups have shown more effective treatment response using SWL when the stone attenuation is less than 900–1000 HU [38, 39]. CT also provides skin-to-stone distance, which has also been shown to affect SWL success with the best outcomes in patients with skin-to-stone distance of ≤ 10 cm [38, 40, 41].

Dual-energy CT has evolved and can better characterize stone type relative to conventional multidetector CT [42]. Dual-energy CT is performed with either one (with rapid kilovolt peak switching between the low and high energy) or two X-ray tubes of low and high energy, with two corresponding 64-detector arrays in opposition at 90° angles [43, 44]. The dual X-ray tubes allow for scanning at two different energies (typically 80 and 140 kVp), which allows the obtained data to be characterized for tissue content [45]. The tissue has variable X-ray attenuation at the low and high kVp energies, which the dual-energy software utilizes to determine the material being scanned. Thus, with dual-energy CT, it is possible to differentiate between pure uric acid, mixed uric acid, and calcified stones [46].

Tumor Assessment

As a part of a hematuria workup, three-phase (non-contrast, contrast/nephrogenic, and excretory/post-contrast phase) CT imaging (commonly referred to as CT urogram in most centers) can be helpful in identifying sources of hematuria that non-contrast imaging alone may miss. CT urography involves multiphasic helical imaging of the abdomen and pelvis without and with intravenous contrast. The pre-contrast phase evaluates for renal or ureteral stones and provides a baseline set of images to assess for any possible renal mass, to be compared to contrast-enhanced images derived later. The nephrogenic phase, usually 80–140 seconds after contrast infusion, allows for assessment of the renal parenchyma, and an excretory phase, typically 4–8 minutes after infusion, allows for assessment of the urothelium. Reconstructions allow for assessment of the entire luminal space of the upper urinary tract.

CT urography has the highest diagnostic accuracy of available imaging techniques, sensitivity of 0.67–1.0, and a specificity of 0.93–0.99, although it is less effective in assessment of flat or particularly small (less than 5 mm) lesions [8]. It is generally the preferred imaging modality for initial diagnosis and clinical staging of UTUC.

The appearance of UTUC on CT is variable. It frequently appears as an enhancing soft tissue mass within the collecting system or ureter. Depending on the phase of the imaging, UTUC may appear somewhat hyperdense on pre-contrast images and may demonstrate early enhancement with washout on post-contrast phases. Urothelial lesions are typically seen as filling defects during the excretory phase (Fig. 2.3) or may present as an irregularity, mural thickening, or an obstructed calyx. Advanced lesions may demonstrate infiltration into renal parenchyma (Fig. 2.4) with distortion of normal architecture. An additional benefit of CT urography is for the purposes of staging of the tumor, as it allows for concurrent imaging of the most common sites of metastatic spread – lymph nodes, liver, bones, and lungs. The overall accuracy of prediction pathologic stage however ranges between 36 and 83% [10].

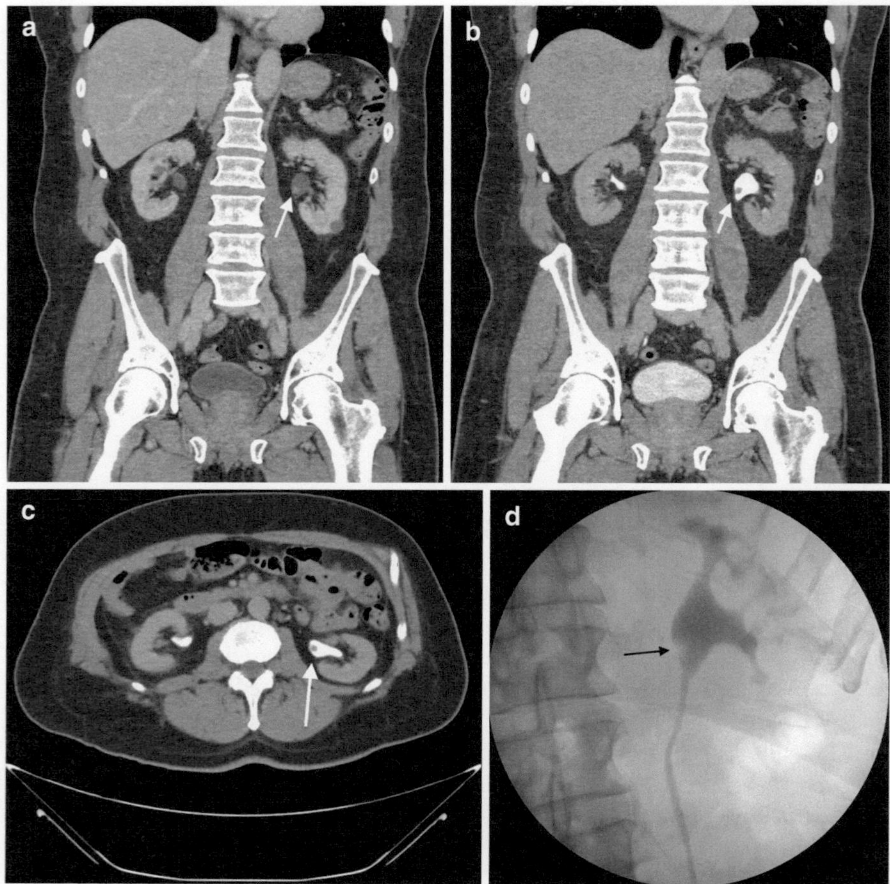

Fig. 2.3 (**a**) Coronal view of CT urogram during nephrogenic phase. White arrow points toward enhancing luminal tumor in the left renal pelvis. (**b**) Same patient with coronal view during delayed, urogram phase clearly shows a filling defect worrisome for upper tract urothelial carcinoma (white arrow). (**c**) Same patient with axial view during urogram phase with white arrow showing left renal pelvis filling defect. (**d**) Retrograde pyelogram performed in the operating room shows the lesion as a filling defect (black arrow), which was later identified as upper tract urothelial carcinoma

Limitations

There are disadvantages of CT scanning, predominantly related to the increased radiation dose of this modality relative to standard plain films and IVP (or ultrasound/MRI, which do not use ionizing radiation). While the long-term effects of repeated CT scans for patients who are habitual stone formers are not established, there is a concern about the potential for increased malignancy (e.g., leukemia and thyroid cancer). The radiation dose delivered to a patient for a routine CT scan is approximately 8–16 millisieverts (mSV) compared with 0.5–0.9 mSV for a plain

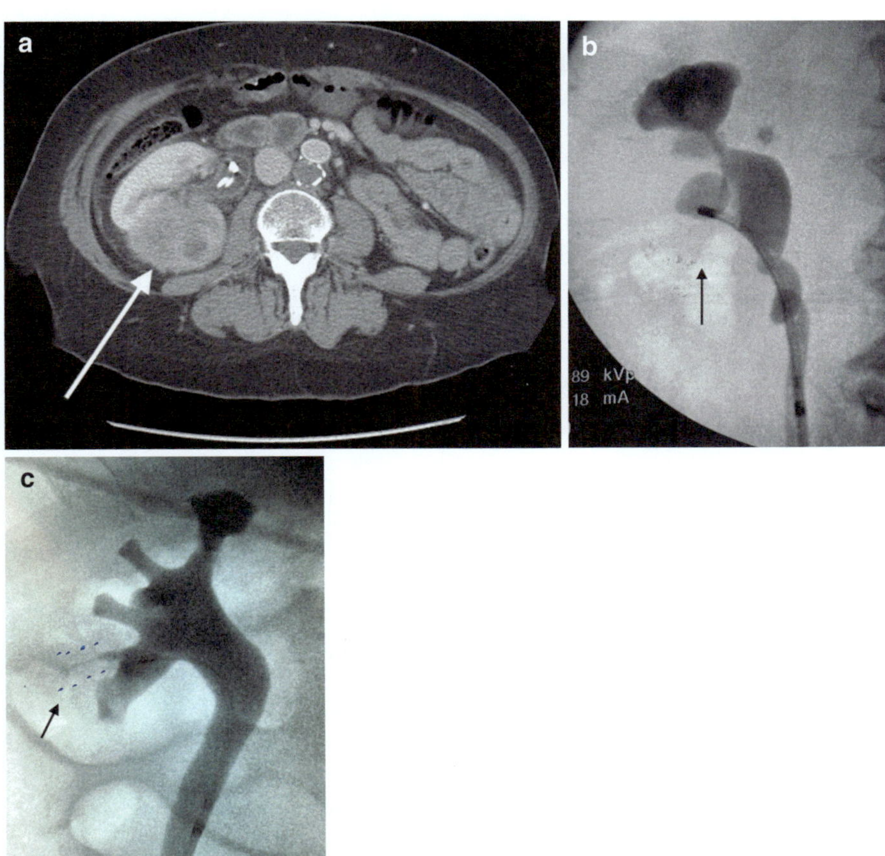

Fig. 2.4 (**a**) CT urogram axial view during nephrogenic phase shows infiltrating upper tract urothelial carcinoma (white arrow) in the posterior lower pole of the right kidney, consistent with parenchymal invasion. (**b**) Retrograde pyelogram in the same patient demonstrating missing lower pole portions of the collecting system, an ominous finding frequently seen with locally advanced upper tract urothelial lesions. (**c**) Retrograde pyelogram of a different patient showing infundibular narrowing (black arrow and blue dashes). When associated with upper tract urothelial carcinoma, this is also a finding often seen with locally advanced disease

film of the abdomen and 1.3–3.5 mSV for an IVP [47]. Reports with lower-dose CT scans deliver radiation similar to that of abdominal plain films (0.5–2 mSV), and these studies have shown no change in accuracy in detecting stones compared with standard CT, with a sensitivity of 98% and specificity of 95% in the low-dose cohort [47, 48]. One important caveat is that sensitivity and specificity for ureteral stone detection using low-dose CT are diminished in patients with BMI over 30 kg/m^2. This is reflected in contemporary protocols which call for low-dose CT in patients suspected to have ureteral stones with BMI $\leq$ 30 kg/m^2, while conventional CT is used for patients with BMI > 30 kg/m^2, in order to maintain diagnostic effectiveness [49].

CT imaging requires the administration of intravenous contrast, which can result in contrast-induced nephropathy or allergic reactions to the contrast medium. This concern has, in recent times, been addressed by protocols established by the American College of Radiology regarding pre-medication for interventions and protocols advocating for reduced dosage intravenous contrast and optimization with intravenous volume expansion with normal saline or bicarbonate [50].

Another shortcoming of CT imaging can result from incomplete opacification of the ureters from peristalsis. Some techniques to remedy this have included the administration of IV saline or furosemide to facilitate distention of the collecting system and ureters [51]. Additionally, in patients with ureteral obstruction, contrast excretion may be inhibited, impeding adequate evaluation of the collecting system and ureter, rendering this study less effective for this population of patient.

Magnetic Resonance Imaging

Background

Magnetic resonance imaging (MRI) has gained popularity, and its current use is mixed, given the respective benefits and limitations of the technology. As it is not sensitive for the detection of calcifications, MRI is of limited value in the direct evaluation or diagnosis of renal stone disease but is of utility in the staging and surveillance of upper tract urothelial carcinoma. However, in patients for whom radiation should be avoided (e.g., young patients, pregnant patients), MRI has utility in the diagnosis of obstructive stone disease, where it is usually used as an adjunct to sonography, and has utility in the initial workup of UTUC for similar reasons. Furthermore, the use of gadolinium as a contrast agent makes MRI beneficial to patients with a history of allergy to iodinated contrast or those with impaired renal function. Newer techniques involving chelation of gadolinium have further improved the safety profile of this agent. As with CT imaging, MRI is capable of assessing the ureters, renal parenchyma, perinephric tissues, and distant anatomy. MRI's utility is limited by the fact that it is time-consuming and costly and had decreased spatial resolution relative to CT imaging. Increased acquisition time may lead to motion artifact introduced by breathing or peristalsis.

Stone Management

Diagnosis of an obstructing stone on non-contrast MRI is usually seen on fluid-sensitive sequences as a dilated collecting system with increased signal (edema) surrounding the kidney/ureter; the stone (although usually not seen) may occasionally present as a signal void [52]. Regan et al. evaluated the efficacy of MR urography in the diagnosis of stone disease and concluded that it is highly accurate in identifying the level and degree of ureteric obstruction when compared with IVP [53].

Tumor Management

Urothelial cancers have lower signal intensity than urine on T2-weighted images, allowing for presentation of tumors in a dilated system [10]. However, since it is isointense to parenchyma, gadolinium is of benefit to assess the extent. Static MR urography performed by using heavily T2-weighted sequences can permit accurate localization of ureteric obstruction.

Positron Emission Tomography (PET)

18-Fluorodeoxyglucose (18-FDG) PET/CT is an imaging modality of utility in staging and surveillance of a host of metabolically active malignancies. As a result, it is effective at detection of metastatic disease in lymph nodes, with a greater sensitivity and specificity compared to CT imaging alone [54]. The sensitivity and specificity of PET CT for nodal disease in untreated patients is 77% and 97%, respectively, with an attendant drop to as low as 50% in patients who have previously received chemotherapy [55]. The marked uptake and excretion of the tracer in the urinary tract often limit direct assessment of UTUC. Other compounds, like ^{11}C choline and ^{11}C acetate, may help identify urothelial lesions on fusion CT imaging; however, these agents are currently not readily available [55].

Conclusion

Radiographic imaging is indispensable to the urologist as a part of diagnosis, planning, and surveillance for stones and upper tract urothelial lesions. As the resolution and cost of newer modalities have improved, so too has their relative utility. Imaging of renal stones in the future may allow detailed and accurate identification of the stone composition, which has the potential to further refine management. Furthermore, as these and future technologies improve, our capacity to diagnose UTUC earlier and stage the disease more effectively will lead to improved outcomes for patients.

References

1. Scales CD Jr, Curtis LH, Norris RD, Springhart WP, Sur RL, Schulman KA, et al. Changing gender prevalence of stone disease. J Urol. 2007;177:979–82.
2. Pearle MS, Calhoun EA, Curhan GC, Urologic Diseases of America Project. Urologic Diseases of America project: urolithiasis. J Urol. 2005;173:848–57.
3. Smith RC, Verga M, McCarthy S, Rosenfield AT. Diagnosis of acute flank pain: value of unenhanced helical CT. Am J Roentgenol. 1996;166:97–101.

4. Smith RC, Rosenfield AT, Choe KA, Essenmacher KR, Verga M, Glickman MG, et al. Acute flank pain: comparison of non- contrast-enhanced CT and intravenous urography. Radiology. 1995;194:789–94.

5. Saw KC, McAteer JA, Monga AG, Chua GT, Lingeman JE, Williams JC Jr. Helical CT of urinary calculi: effect of stone composition, stone size, and scan collimation. Am J Roentgenol. 2000;175:329–32.

6. Rosen MP, Siewert B, Sands DZ, Bromberg R, Edlow J, Raptopoulos V. Value of abdominal CT in the emergency department for patients with abdominal pain. Eur Radiol. 2003;13:418–24.

7. Dalrymple NC, Verga M, Anderson KR, Bove P, Covey AM, Rosenfield AT, et al. The value of unenhanced helical computerized tomography in the management of acute flank pain. J Urol. 1998;159:735–40.

8. Roupret M, Babjuk M, Burger M, Capoun O, Cohen D, Comperat E, et al. European Association of Urology guidelines on upper urinary tract urothelial carcinomas: 2020 update. Eur Urol. 2021;79:62–79.

9. Cosentino M, Palou J, Gaya JM, Breda A, Rodriguez-Faba O, Villavicencio-Mavrich H. Upper urinary tract urothelial carcinoma : location as a predictive factor for concomitant bladder carcinoma. World J Urol. 2013;31:141–5.

10. Browne RFJ, Meehan CP, Colville J, Power R, Torreggiani WC. Transitional cell carcinoma of the upper urinary tract: spectrum of imaging findings. Radiographics. 2005;25:1609–27.

11. Katz D, McGahan JP, Gerscovich EO, Troxel SA, Low RK. Correlation of ureteral stone measurements by CT and plain film radiography: utility of the KUB. J Endourol. 2003;17:847–50.

12. Levine JA, Neitlich J, Verga M, Dalrymple N, Smith RC. Ureteral calculi in patients with flank pain: correlation of plain radiography with unenhanced helical CT. Radiology. 1997;204:27–31.

13. Nelson WK, Houghton SG, Milliner DS, Lieske JC, Sarr MG. Enteric hyperoxaluria, nephrolithiasis, and oxalate nephropathy: potentially serious and unappreciated complications of Roux-en-Y gastric bypass. Surg Obes Relat Dis. 2005;1:481–5.

14. Ripolles T, Errando J, Agramunt M, Martinez MJ. Ureteral colic: US versus CT. Abdom Imaging. 2004;29:263–6.

15. Mostbeck GH, Zontsich T, Turetschek K. Ultrasound of the kidney: obstruction and medical diseases. Eur Radiol. 2001;11:1878–89.

16. Rud O, Moersler J, Peter J, et al. Prospective evaluation of interobserver variability of the hydronephrosis index and the renal resistive index as sonographic examination methods for the evaluation of acute hydronephrosis. BJU Int. 2012;110(8 Pt B):E350–6.

17. Sheafor DH, Hertzberg BS, Freed KS, Carroll BA, Keogan MT, Paulson EK, et al. Nonenhanced helical CT and US in the emergency evaluation of patients with renal colic: prospective comparison. Radiology. 2000;217:792–7.

18. Ray AA, Ghiculete D, Pace KT, Honey RJ. Limitations to ultrasound in the detection and measurement of urinary tract calculi. Urology. 2010;76:295–300.

19. Sternberg KM, Eisner B, Larson T, Hernandez N, Han J, Pais VM. Ultrasound significantly overestimates stone size when compared to low-dose non-contrast computed tomography. Urology. 2016;95:67–71.

20. Viprakasit DP, Sawyer MD, Herrell SD, Miller NL. Limitations of ultrasonography in the evaluation of urolithiasis: a correlation with computed tomography. J Endourol. 2012;26:209–13.

21. Niall O, Russell J, MacGregor R, Duncan H, Mullins J. A comparison of non- contrast computerized tomography with excretory urography in the assessment of acute flank pain. J Urol. 1999;161:534–7.

22. Wang JH, Shen SH, Huang SS, Chang CY. Prospective comparison of unenhanced spiral computed tomography and intravenous urography in the evaluation of acute renal colic. J Chinese Med Assoc. 2008;71:30–6.

23. Sandhu C, Anson KM, Patel U. Urinary tract stones – part I: role of radiological imaging in diagnosis and treatment planning. Clin Radiol. 2003;58:415–21.

24. Worster A, Preyra I, Weaver B, Haines T. The accuracy of noncontrast helical computed tomography versus intravenous pyelography in the diagnosis of suspected acute urolithiasis: a meta-analysis. Ann Emerg Med. 2002;40:280–6.
25. Hale Z, Hanna E, Miyake M, Rosser CJ. Imaging the urologic patient: the utility of intravenous pyelogram in the CT scan era. World J Urol. 2014;32:137–42.
26. Ege G, Akman H, Kuzucu K, Yildiz S. Acute ureterolithiasis: incidence of secondary signs on unenhanced helical CT and influence on patient management. Clin Radiol. 2003;58:990–4.
27. Heneghan JP, McGuire KA, Leder RA, DeLong DM, Yoshizumi T, Nelson RC. Helical CT for nephrolithiasis and ureterolithiasis: comparison of conventional and reduced radiation-dose techniques. Radiology. 2003;229:575–80.
28. Boulay I, Holtz P, Foley WD, White B, Begun FP. Ureteral calculi: diagnostic efficacy of helical CT and implications for treatment of patients. Am J Roentgenol. 1999;172:1485–90.
29. Fielding JR, Silverman SG, Samuel S, Zou KH, Loughlin KR. Unenhanced helical CT of ureteral stones: a replacement for excretory urography in planning treatment. Am J Roentgenol. 1998;171:1051–3.
30. Fielding JR, Fox LA, Heller H, Seltzer SE, Tempany CM, Silverman SG, et al. Spiral CT in the evaluation of flank pain: overall accuracy and feature analysis. J Comput Assist Tomogr. 1997;21:635–8.
31. Katz DS, Lane MJ, Sommer FG. Unenhanced helical CT of ureteral stones: incidence of associated urinary tract findings. Am J Roentgenol. 1996;166:1319–22.
32. Hamm M, Wawroschek F, Weckermann D, et al. Unenhanced helical computed tomography in the evaluation of acute flank pain. Eur Radiol. 2001;39:460–5.
33. Lin WC, Uppot RN, Li CS, Hahn PF, Sahani DV. Value of automated coronal reformations from 64-section multidetector row computerized tomography in the diagnosis of urinary stone disease. J Urol. 2007;178(3 Pt 1):907–11. discussion 911
34. Metser U, Ghai S, Ong YY, Lockwood G, Radomski SB. Assessment of urinary tract calculi with 64-MDCT: the axial versus coronal plane. Am J Roentgenol. 2009;192:1509–13.
35. Mitcheson HD, Zamenhof RG, Bankoff MS, Prien EL. Determination of the chemical composition of urinary calculi by computerized tomography. J Urol. 1983;130:814–9.
36. Motley G, Dalrymple N, Keesling C, Fischer J, Harmon W. Hounsfield unit density in the determination of urinary stone composition. Urology. 2001;58:170–3.
37. Sheir KZ, Mansour O, Madbouly K, Elsobky E, Abdel-Khalek M. Determination of the chemical composition of urinary calculi by noncontrast spiral computerized tomography. Urol Res. 2005;33(2):99–104.
38. Perks AE, Schuler TD, Lee J, Ghiculete D, Chung DG, D'A Honey RJ, et al. Stone attenuation and skin-to-stone distance on computed tomography predicts for stone fragmentation by shock wave lithotripsy. Urology. 2008;72:765–9.
39. El-Nahas A, El-Assmy AM, Mansour O, Sheir KZ. A prospective multivariate analysis of factors predicting stone disintegration by extracorporeal shock wave lithotripsy: the value of high-resolution noncontrast computed tomography. Eur Urol. 2007;51:1688–94.
40. Pareek G, Hedican SP, Lee FT, Nakada SY. Shock wave lithotripsy success determined by skin-to-stone distance on computed tomography. Urology. 2005;66:941–4.
41. Patel T, Kozakowski K, Hruby G, Gupta M. Skin to stone distance is an independent predictor of stone-free status following shockwave lithotripsy. J Endourol. 2009;23:1383–5.
42. Matlaga BR, Kawamoto S, Fishman E. Dual source computed tomography: a novel technique to determine stone composition. Urology. 2008;72:1164–8.
43. Fletcher JG, Takahashi N, Hartman R, Guimaraes L, Huprich JE, Hough DM, et al. Dual-energy and dual-source CT: is there a role in the abdomen and pelvis? Radiol Clin N Am. 2009;47:41–57.
44. Flohr TG, McCollough CH, Bruder H, Petersilka M, Gruber K, Suss C, et al. First performance evaluation of a dual-source CT (DSCT) system. Eur Radiol. 2006;16:256–68.
45. Johnson TR, Krauss B, Sedlmair M, Grasruck M, Bruder H, Morhard D, et al. Material differentiation by dual energy CT: initial experience. Eur Radiol. 2007;17:1510–7.

46. Primak AN, Fletcher JG, Vrtiska TJ, Dzyubak OP, Lieske JC, Jackson ME, et al. Noninvasive differentiation of uric acid versus non-uric acid kidney stones using dual-energy CT. Acad Radiol. 2007;14:1441–7.
47. Kluner C, Hein PA, Gralla O, Hein E, Hamm B, Romano V, et al. Does ultra-low-dose CT with a radiation dose equivalent to that of KUB suffice to detect renal and ureteral calculi? J Comput Assist Tomogr. 2006;30:44–50.
48. Mulkens TH, Daineffe S, de Wijngaert R, Bellinck P, Leonard A, Smet G, et al. Urinary stone disease: comparison of standard-dose and low-dose with 4D MDCT tube current modulation. Am J Roentgenol. 2007;188:553–62.
49. Fulgham PF, Assimos DG, Pearle MS, Preminger GM. Clinical effectiveness protocols for imaging in the management of ureteral calculous disease : AUA technology assessment. J Urol. 2013;189:1203–13.
50. Davenport MS, Perazella MA, Yee J, Dillman JR, Fine D, McDonald RJ, et al. Use of intravenous iodinated contrast media in patients with kidney disease: consensus statements from the American College of Radiology and the National Kidney Foundation. Radiology. 2020;294:660–8.
51. Silverman SG, Akbar SA, Mortele KJ, Tuncali K, Bhagwat JG, Seifter JL. Multi- detector row CT urography of normal urinary collecting system: furosemide versus saline as adjunct to contrast medium. Radiology. 2006;240:749–55.
52. Lubarsky M, Kalb B, Sharma P, Keim SM, Martin DR. MR imaging for acute nontraumatic abdominopelvic pain: rationale and practical considerations. Radiographics. 2013;33:313–37.
53. Regan F, Bohlman ME, Khazan R, Rodriguez R, Schultze-Haakh H. MR urography using HASTE imaging in the assessment of ureteric obstruction. Am J Roentgenol. 1996;167:1115–20.
54. Palou J, Carrio I, Villaviciencio H. Urothelial cell carcinoma in upper urinary tract – role of PET imaging. In: Rosette J, Manyak M, Harisinghani M, Wijkstra H, editors. Imaging in oncologic urology. London: Springer; 2009. p. 155–60.
55. Patil VV, Wang ZJ, Sollitto RA, Chuang KW, Konety BR, Hawkins RA, et al. 18F-FDG PET/CT of transitional cell carcinoma. Am J Roentgenol. 2009;193:497–504.

Chapter 3
Instruments

Silvia Proietti, Vincent De Coninck, Olivier Traxer, Salvatore Buttice, Jan Brachlow, Etienne Xavier Keller, Kymora B. Scotland, Bree'ava Limbrick, Demetrius H. Bagley, Scott G. Hubosky, and Thomas J. Hardacker

S. Proietti
Sorbonne Université, Service d'Urologie, Assistance-Publique Hôpitaux de Paris, Hôpital Tenon, Paris, France

Sorbonne Université, GRC n°20, Groupe de Recherche Clinique sur la Lithiase Urinaire, Hôpital Tenon, Paris, France

Department of Urology, San Raffaele Hospital, Ville Turro Division, Milan, Italy

V. De Coninck · O. Traxer (✉) · E. X. Keller
Sorbonne Université, GRC n°20, Groupe de Recherche Clinique sur la Lithiase Urinaire, Hôpital Tenon, Paris, France
e-mail: olivier.traxer@aphp.fr

S. Buttice
Sorbonne Université, Service d'Urologie, Assistance-Publique Hôpitaux de Paris, Hôpital Tenon, Paris, France

Sorbonne Université, GRC n°20, Groupe de Recherche Clinique sur la Lithiase Urinaire, Hôpital Tenon, Paris, France

Department of Urology, San Giovanni di Dio Hospital, Agrigento, Italy

J. Brachlow
Sorbonne Université, Service d'Urologie, Assistance-Publique Hôpitaux de Paris, Hôpital Tenon, Paris, France

Sorbonne Université, GRC n°20, Groupe de Recherche Clinique sur la Lithiase Urinaire, Hôpital Tenon, Paris, France

Department of Urology, Kantonsspital Winterthur, Winterthur, Switzerland

© Springer Nature Switzerland AG 2022
S. G. Hubosky et al. (eds.), *Advanced Ureteroscopy*,
https://doi.org/10.1007/978-3-030-82351-1_3

K. B. Scotland · B. Limbrick
Department of Urology, David Geffen School of Medicine, University of California Los
Angeles, Los Angeles, CA, USA
e-mail: KScotland@mednet.ucla.edu; blimbrick@mednet.ucla.edu

D. H. Bagley
Department of Urology and Radiology, Sidney Kimmel Medical College at Thomas Jefferson
University Hospital, Philadelphia, PA, USA
e-mail: Demetrius.BagleyJr@jefferson.edu

S. G. Hubosky · T. J. Hardacker
Department of Urology, Sidney Kimmel Medical College at Thomas Jefferson University
Hospital, Philadelphia, PA, USA
e-mail: Scott.Hubosky@jefferson.edu; Thomas.hardacker@jefferson.edu

Ureteroscope Specifications: Flexible, Semi-rigid, and Single Use

Silvia Proietti, Vincent De Coninck, and Olivier Traxer

Historical Background of Ureteroscopy

Historically, ureteroscopic surgery has evolved from a mere diagnostic procedure with several limitations to an accurate, complex, and technologically advanced surgical procedure able to navigate the entire upper urinary tract, allowing for treatment of different stones and tumors of the collecting system.

The first ureteroscopy was inadvertently performed by Hugh Hampton Young in 1912. He was able to visualize the renal pelvis and calyces endoscopically with a cystoscope as the patient had dilated ureters [1]. The introduction of the rod lens system by Hopkins in 1956 allowed for a brighter and more superior image relative to older models. It also helped in reduction of the diameter of the endoscope [2]. The first ureteroscope used in clinical practice was developed by Richard Wolf Company with a sheath design available in 13, 14.5, 16 Fr, and 30 cm in length. In 1978, Lyon et al. reported its first use by performing a diagnostic ureteroscopy [3]. Surpassing the sole diagnostic purpose of ureteroscopy, Pérez-Castro and Martinez-Piniero in 1980 described the first ureteroscopy for stone treatment [4]. They used an 11 Fr rigid ureteroscope manufactured by Karl Storz Company.

The real breakthrough in ureteroscopy was made by the introduction of fiberoptic technology that allowed the development of flexible ureteroscopes. In 1964, Marshall described the first application of flexible ureteroscopy [5], and Takagi in 1971 reported the first clinical use of a flexible ureteroscope with an active deflectable tip [6]. The drawback of this instrument was that it had poor image resolution and lacked a working and irrigation channel. Subsequently, developments were made in terms of design, which included secondary passive deflection, greater degrees of active deflection, and integration of a working channel.

The next major development was application of groundbreaking fiberoptic technology to rigid ureteroscopes. The first semi-rigid ureteroscope was introduced in 1989 [7]; since then, the manufactures have been able to reduce the size of semi-rigid ureteroscopes and increase the diameter of the working channel thanks to the use of fiberoptics. The flexibility of the shaft induced by the fiberoptic bundles compared to rigid endoscopes, without any image distortion, has resulted in the use of term "semi-rigid."

Another real breakthrough in endourology was with the introduction of digital technology in an effort to improve the limitations of fiberoptic image, characterized by the honeycomb pattern due to the spaces between the fiberoptic strands. Digital technology was introduced in the 1960s and 1970s, initially in military uses. The first digital flexible ureteroscope was the Gyrus ACMI Invisio DUR D.

Rigid and Semi-rigid Ureteroscopes

Rigid ureteroscopes are available in many sheath sizes and eyepiece designs to facilitate the negotiation of the ureteral orifice and the navigation along the ureter. The real step forward in ureteroscopy was the introduction of fiberoptic technology and the development of semi-rigid ureteroscopes. These endoscopes are characterized by high-density fiberoptic bundles inside a semi-rigid metal sheath. The use of fiberoptics reduces the space requirements for the optical component within the endoscope, allowing for a larger working channel. The semi-rigid ureteroscopes can be made smaller without sacrificing the size of the working channel. More recently, ultra-thin semi-rigid ureteroscopes have been developed by different manufacturers, with their shaft ranging between 4.5/6.5 and 6.5/9.9 Fr (Table 3.1).

The large working channel of semi-rigid ureteroscopes is an important feature for allowing simultaneous instrument passage and irrigation, without impairing vision. Most working channels of this design offer a working channel ranging between 3 and 6 Fr. Currently, ureteroscopes with two separate working channels are also available.

Most semi-rigid ureteroscopes have a tapered oval or circular tip. Some manufacturers have started producing ureteroscopes with a smooth triangular beveled tip to reduce trauma to the ureteral orifice while introducing the instrument.

Rigid or semi-rigid ureteroscopes can make use of either a fixed or a pendulum-type camera. With a fixed camera, the image orientation can be lost with rotation, similar to the situation in digital flexible ureteroscopy. If present, luminal air bubbles may help the surgeon regain orientation because they always indicate the 12 o'clock position (Fig. 3.1a and b).

Flexible Ureteroscopes

Flexible ureteroscopes are divided into fiberoptic and digital scopes (Table 3.2). It has been demonstrated that digital flexible ureteroscopes result in decreased

Table 3.1 Currently available semi-rigid ureteroscope models and specifications

Model	Brand	Proximal diameter (F)	Tip diameter (F)	Working channel size (F)	Number of working channels	Angle of view (degrees)	Working length (cm)
OES Pro	Olympus	7.8	6.4	4.2	1	7	33, 43
OES Pro	Olympus	9.8	8.6	6.4	1	7	43
OES 4000	Olympus	7.5	7.5	3.4 + 2.4	2	7	33, 43
27,000 K/L	Storz	9.9	6.5	4.8	1	6	34, 43
27,001 K/L	Storz	12.0	7	5.0	1	6	34, 43
27,002 K/L	Storz	12.0	8.0	6.0	1	6	34, 43
27,003 L sec. Michel	Storz	12.0	9.0	6	1	6	43
27,010 K/L	Storz	9.9	7.0	3.4	1	6	34, 43
27,013 L sec. Gautier	Storz	13.5	7.0	5.0	1	6	41
Marberger "E-Line"	Wolf	7.5	6	4.8	1	5	31.5, 43
Marberger "E-Line"	Wolf	9.8	8	6	1	12	31.5, 43
Marberger "E-Line"	Wolf	11.5	8.5	8	1	12	31.5, 43
Bichler "E-Line"	Wolf	7.5	6	4.8	1	5	31.5, 43
Bichler "E-Line"	Wolf	9.8	8	6	1	12	31.5, 43
Bichler "E-Line"	Wolf	6.5	4.5	3.3	1	5	31.5, 43

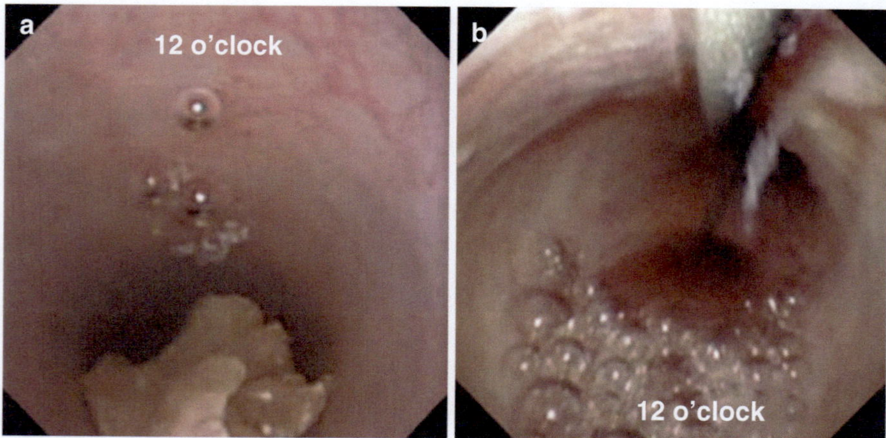

Fig. 3.1 Orientation can be lost during rotation with semi-rigid ureteroscopy using a fixed camera. Air bubbles always indicate 12 o'clock or anterior position (**a**) semi-rigid ureteroscope at neutral position, (**b**) semi-rigid ureteroscope rotated 180 degrees

Table 3.2 Currently available flexible ureteroscopes and specifications

Name	Brand	Type	Imaging	Camera sensor type	Shaft diameter (F)	Distal end outer diameter (F)	Working channel size (F)	Deflection (up/down) (degrees)	Working length (cm)
URF-P5	Olympus	Reusable	Fiberoptic	–	5.4	8.4	3.6	180/275	70
URF-P6	Olympus	Reusable	Fiberoptic	–	7.95	4.9	3.6	275/275	67
URF-P7	Olympus	Reusable	Fiberoptic	–	7.95	4.9	3.6	275/275	67
URF-V	Olympus	Reusable	Digital	CCD	9.9	8.5	3.6	180/275	67
URF-V2	Olympus	Reusable	Digital	CCD	8.4	8.5	3.6	275/275	67
URF-V3	Olympus	Reusable	Digital	CCD	8.4	8.5	3.6	275/275	67
Flex-X2	Storz	Reusable	Fiberoptic	–	8.5	7.5	3.6	270/270	67.5
Flex-XC	Storz	Reusable	Digital	CMOS	8.5	8.5	3.6	270/270	70
Cobra	Wolf	Reusable	Fiberoptic	–	9.9	6.0	3.3	270/270	68
Viper	Wolf	Reusable	Fiberoptic	–	8.8	6.0	3.6	270/270	68
Cobra vision	Wolf	Reusable	Digital	CMOS	–	5.2	3.6 + 2.4	270/270	68
Boa	Wolf	Reusable	Digital	CMOS	–	6.6	3.6	270/270	68
LithoVue	Boston Scientific	Single use	Digital	CMOS	9.5	7.7	3.6	270/270	68
Uscope	Pusen	Single use	Digital	CMOS	9.5	9.0	3.6	270/270	65
Neoflex	Neoscope	Single use	Digital	CMOS	9.0	9.0	3.6	270/270	63
ShaoGang	YouCare	Single use	Digital	CMOS	9	8	4.2	270/270	63
Axis	Dornier	Single use	Digital	NA	9	8.5	3.6	275/275	NA
WiScope	BD/Bard	Single use	Digital	CMOS	8.6	7.4	3.6	275/275	67

NA not available

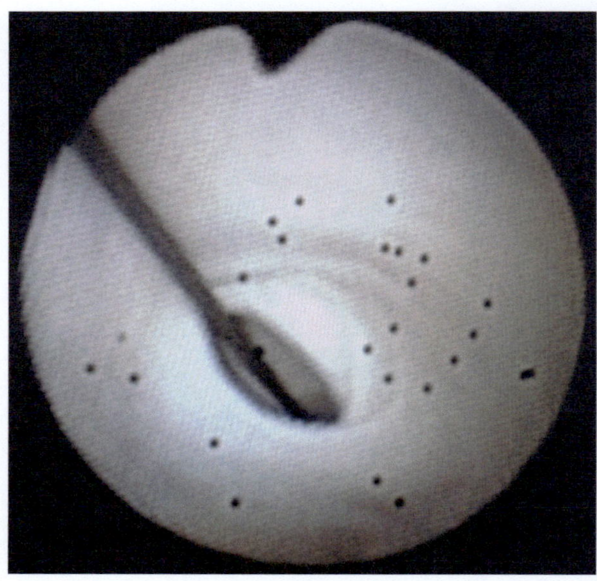

Fig. 3.2 Fiberoptic vision with broken fibers

operative times and improved visibility with similar stone-free rates compared to fiberoptic scopes [8]. As a matter of fact, the quality of vision of fiberoptic flexible ureteroscopes is very variable between designers and depends on the number and quality of the fiberoptic bundles used for illumination and image transmission. Depending on the number of fiberoptic bundles used, a honeycomb effect on the screen could be seen. Currently, the manufacturers have increased the number of bundles in the instruments, decreasing the honeycomb effect, but these smaller fiberoptic bundles may be more prone to breakage, which can lead to loss of image quality (Fig. 3.2). Broken fibers not only limit the visibility but also result in costly repairs [9].

With the advent of digital technology, the quality of vision of digital flexible ureteroscopes has improved dramatically compared with the fiberoptic counterparts. Two different imaging chips are used for digital ureteroscopy: charge-coupled devices (CCD) and complementary metal oxide semiconductors (CMOS). CCD and CMOS image sensors both convert light into electronic signals. The biggest difference is that CCD sensors create high-quality images with low noise. CMOS imagers tend to be higher in noise, require less energy, process images faster, and are less expensive compared to CCD sensors.

The "chip on the tip" carries the digital signal to the image processor via a single wire, where further processing and transmission take place for real-time image viewing, eliminating the need of the bulky camera head placed at the eyepiece of fiberoptic ureteroscopes. Moreover, most digital ureteroscopes do not need an external light source, thanks to the LED (light-emitting diode) light source at their tip, just adjacent to the distal lens, minimizing shadowing and giving the sensation of depth of field. These characteristics result in one combined cable instead of two cables (camera and light cord). This leads to significant reduction in weight [10] and has ergonomic advantages, which are important during longer procedures where minimizing upper limb fatigue becomes fundamental [11]. Importantly, the combined cord of the digital ureteroscope permits only exclusive use of the respective manufacturer's tower, which may be considered a limitation of digital ureteroscopes.

The use of a digital chip at the tip of the instrument makes digital ureteroscopes have larger distal tips compared to the fiberoptic counterparts. Moreover, the chip on the tip makes digital flexible ureteroscopes less effective in accessing a sharp-angled calyx, and they have lesser end-tip deflection compared with the fiberoptic scopes [12]. When approaching a difficult lower calyx, it might be better to use a fiberoptic flexible ureteroscope and consequently to have it as a part of the endourological armamentarium in the operating room (Fig. 3.3).

Even though all the flexible ureteroscopes are indeed flexible, the newer generation has a shaft more rigid than the previous ones and consequently tends to be "semi-flexible" in order to negotiate and navigate the upper urinary tract easily and more precisely.

Image flickering, due to the effect of acoustic waves produced during laser lithotripsy on the digital chip, was reduced by amortizing the digital imager with the application of shock waves absorbers. This effect can still occur with modern digital flexible ureteroscopes when the holmium:YAG laser and the new thulium fiber laser are activated near the tip of the instrument.

Considering that all the flexible ureteroscopes have a 0-degree optic, the so-called safety distance in order to avoid the burn back effect of the holmium laser on the tip of the instrument is to place the laser fiber 3 mm outside the ureteroscope. From a practical point of view, that equates to ¼ of the diameter of the screen (Fig. 3.4). In this way, the bubble generated when the holmium laser is activated never rebounds on the camera of the ureteroscope, protecting it from laser damages [13].

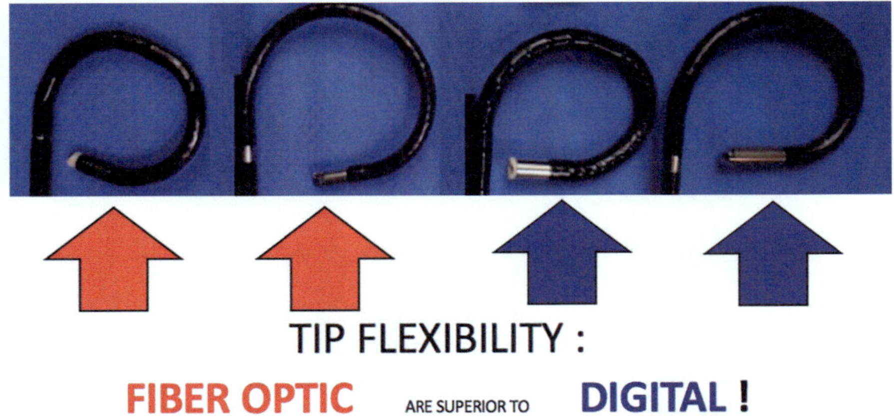

Fig. 3.3 End-tip deflection of fiberoptic and digital ureteroscopes

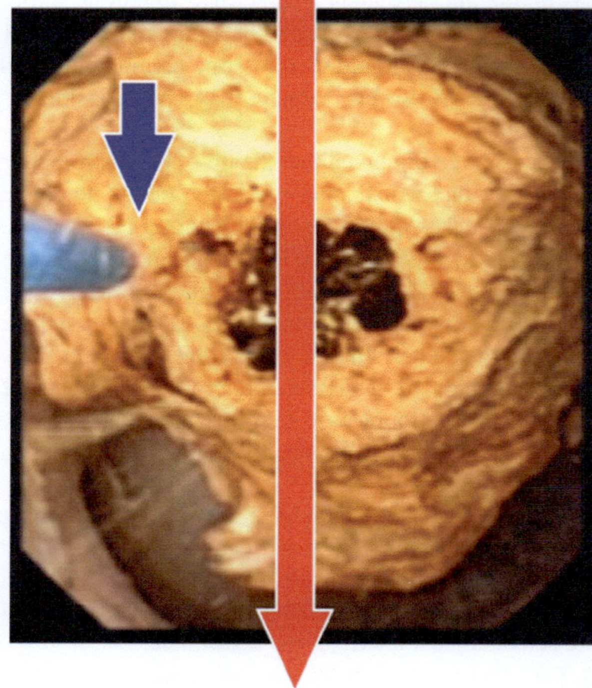

Fig. 3.4 Laser fiber "safety distance" means ¼ of the diameter of the screen

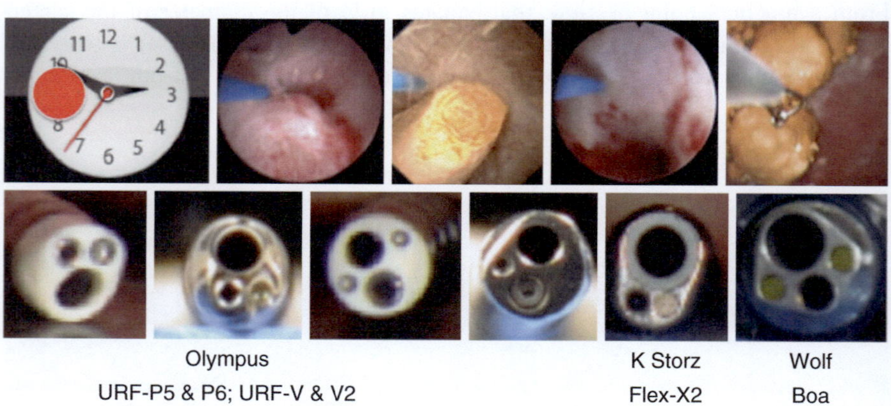

Fig. 3.5 Flexible ureteroscopes with working channel at 9 o'clock

All flexible ureteroscopes have one working channel, 3.6 Fr in diameter, except the Cobra and the Cobra Vision by Wolf Company that have two working channels. The orientation of the working channel is different among the several flexible ureteroscopes available on the market (Fig. 3.5). Some of them have the working channel at 3 o'clock, some at 9 o'clock, and others at 6 o'clock (Figs. 3.5, 3.6, and 3.7).

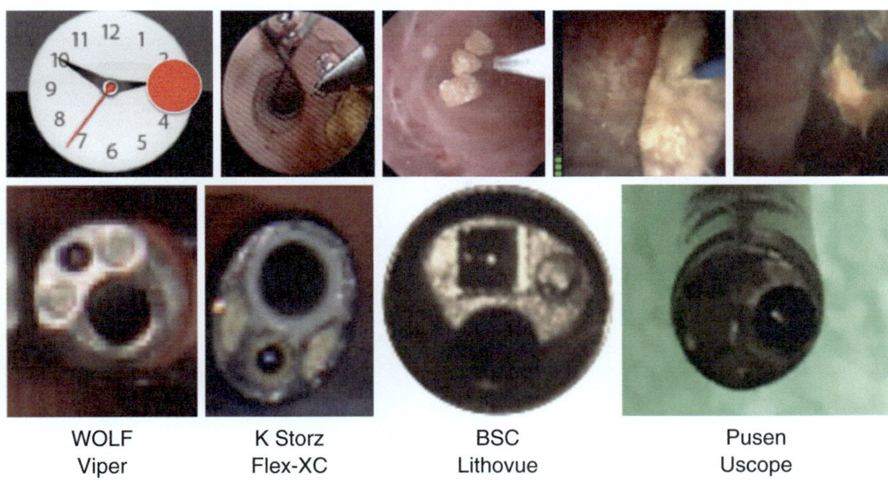

Fig. 3.6 Flexible ureteroscopes with working channel at 3 o'clock

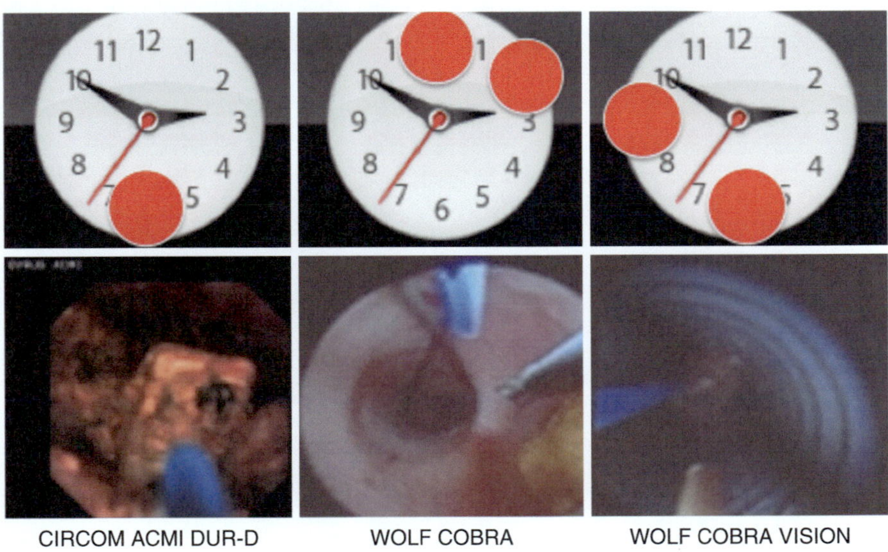

Fig. 3.7 Flexible ureteroscopes with working channel at 6, 12–2, 6–9 o'clock

The reason for this variation in orientation of the working channel among the different manufacturers is unknown. Considering that in the right kidney the calices are located at 9 o'clock and the gravity is at 3 o'clock, it is better to use the flexible ureteroscopes with the working channel at 3 o'clock; for the left kidney, the flexible ureteroscopes to choose are those with the working channel at 9 o'clock (Figs. 3.8 and 3.9).

Fig. 3.8 Position of
calices in the right kidney

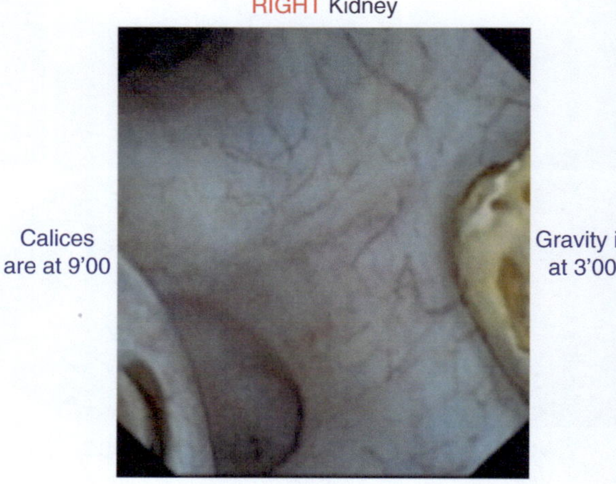

Fig. 3.9 Position of
calices in the left kidney

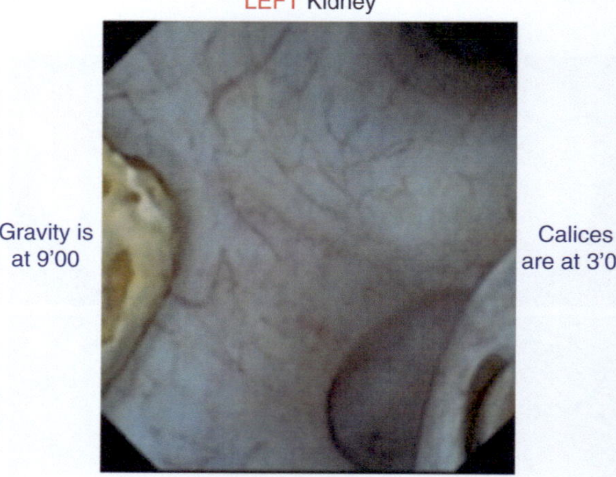

Single-Use Ureteroscopes

As the technology of ureteroscopes advances, durability remains a major concern
[14]. Due to the high cost and limited durability, the cost-benefit of reusable flexible
ureteroscopes continues to be the most important factor for initiating and maintaining endourological surgery programs worldwide.

Several authors have studied the durability of different instruments reporting a
wide range in the number of procedures performed before there was a need for
repair, varying from 5 to 113 [15–17]. Regardless of the manufacturer, the durability of the ureteroscope depends on the overall time of usage, location, size of the
stone or tumor, use of other devices (ureteral access sheath, laser fiber, basket),
surgeons' experience, and the sterilization method used. Furthermore, it has been
demonstrated that brand-new flexible ureteroscopes are more resistant to damage

than devices refurbished by original manufacturer and by outsourced vendors (mean of 44 usages vs. 11.1 vs. 6.9, respectively) [18]. Therefore, the cost of maintaining an older ureteroscope should be considered in addition to the overall cost of the equipment maintenance.

Therefore, to overcome these concerns, single-use ureteroscopes have been introduced. Some fiberoptic semi-disposable flexible ureteroscopes have been already present on the market since 2010 [19], but the real breakthrough in terms of single-use ureteroscopes has started with the introduction of LithoVue by Boston Scientific (Marlborough, MA). It is the first commercially available digital, single-use, flexible ureteroscope on the market. LithoVue is comparable to other conventional ureteroscopes in terms of maneuverability [20, 21], but in terms of quality of vision, it still seems to be slightly less than digital reusable flexible ureteroscopes, probably due to problems related to over-illumination and dark areas in the field and much more impaired visibility in case of bleeding compared with the reusable counterparts.

Recently, several digital single-use flexible ureteroscopes have been launched on the market, but so far, limited data comparing these instruments in terms of quality of vision and maneuverability are available [22] (Fig. 3.10). It has been

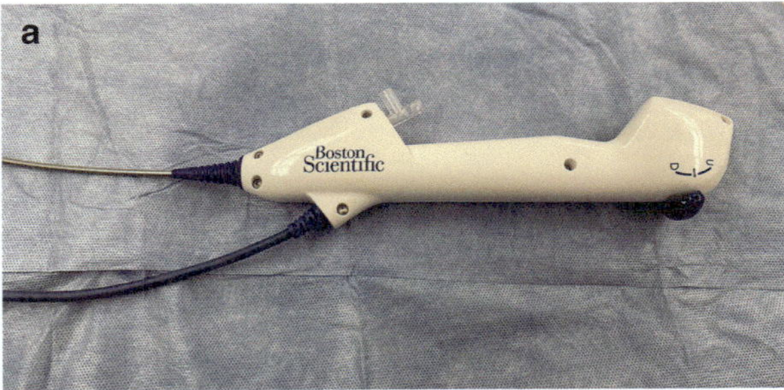

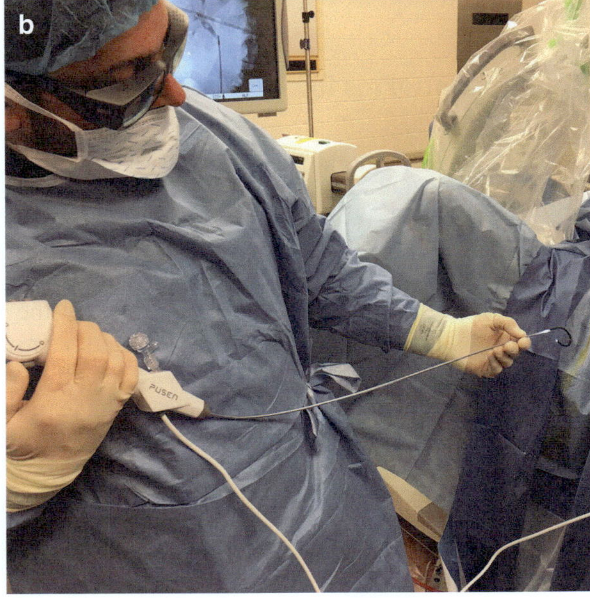

Fig. 3.10 Examples of single-use digital flexible ureteroscopes. (**a**) LithoVue (Boston Scientific, Marlborough, MA). (**b**) Uscope (Zhuhai Pusen Medical Technology Co. Ltd. Zhuhai, Guangdong Province, China)

demonstrated that the use of single-use ureteroscopes may be cost beneficial at centers with lower case volume per year, whereas high-volume centers may find reusable ureteroscopes cost-beneficial [23].

Regardless the cost per endoscope, selective utilization of single-use ureteroscopes in difficult cases, for teaching purposes, and particular situations becomes cost-effective because it allows for preservation of costly reusable endoscopes. The single-use ureteroscopes completely bypass the process of sterilization, thereby saving on cost, time, and labor and moreover avoiding the risk of cross-contamination of the instruments. Current recommendations for single-use flexible ureteroscopes at our institutions include any case in which damage to a reusable instrument is anticipated. Cases such as these include those with large stone burdens (>15 mm, greatest dimension) requiring extended lasering times, dependent lower pole stone position, need for bilateral upper tract access in a single procedure, antegrade ureteroscopic access, retrograde ureteroscopy through a urinary diversion, or any other situation in which significant torque will be applied to the ureteroscope shaft. Not surprisingly, it has been anecdotally observed that selective use of single-use ureteroscopes can significantly decrease repair costs of reusable flexible ureteroscopes.

Conclusion

A wide variety of flexible and semi-rigid ureteroscopes are available. Performance characteristics as well as cost will dictate ureteroscope selection. Single-use flexible digital ureteroscopes are currently available and may offer cost savings if used selectively.

Robotic Platforms for Ureteroscopy

Salvatore Buttice, Vincent De Coninck, and Olivier Traxer

Introduction

In recent years, urology has been revolutionized by the introduction of robotics, and endourology has been no exception. Flexible ureteroscopy (f-URS) has been the rising star for endourologists thanks to safe and efficient outcomes and its ability to adapt to technological advancements. Due to endourologists' passion for new technology and innovations, development of robotic platforms has been inevitable.

Two devices have been reported for flexible ureteroscopic stone surgery. The first device was developed in 2008; the Sensei Magellan robotic catheter system (Hansen Medical, Mountain View, USA), which was originally designed for intracardiac applications by Fred Moll, the inventor of the da Vinci system. In 2012, ELMED (Ankara, Turkey) started working on a robot specifically designed for flexible ureteroscopy, called the Avicenna Roboflex. This became the second robotic flexible ureteroscopy platform on the market.

The Sensei Magellan Robotic Catheter System

The Sensei Magellan system consists of the surgeon console, flexible catheter system, remote manipulation system, and the electronic rack that contains the computer hardware and power supplies. The robotic flexible catheter system has an outer catheter sheath of 12/14 F and an inner guide of 10/12 F. The fiberoptic flexible ureteroscope that has a diameter of 7.5 F is inserted through the inner catheter guide, and the tip of the ureteroscope, which is glued to the inner guide, can be remotely manipulated. The outer sheath tip is stabilized at the ureteropelvic junction. The guide catheter and the ureteroscope can be deflected up to 270 degrees in all directions without compromise by using accessories in the working channel [24].

The first robotic f-URS series was reported in 18 patients by Desai et al. after performing appropriate software modifications [25]. Although the results of this study were encouraging due to successfully accessing 98% of possible calices in a porcine model, the fact that the system is not perfectly compatible with f-URS and that the ureteroscope is only passively manipulated, the Sensei Magellan flexible ureteroscopy project was discontinued.

The Avicenna Roboflex

The concept of the Avicenna Roboflex hasn't changed significantly from the prototype to the latest version, which is operated by a surgeon's console and a manipulation arm for the flexible ureteroscope (Fig. 3.11). In the first version, the console consisted of an adjustable seat where the urologist could utilize two different joysticks to control the endoscope. The right joystick permitted tip deflection as in a standard f-URS, while the left joystick allowed rotation, advancement, and retraction of the endoscope. The direction of deflection (upward, downward) was adjustable between the United States (steering lever toward the surgeon results in downward deflection of the tip) and the European version (steering lever toward the surgeon results in upward deflection of the tip). The controls allowed four functions: adaptation to the US or European mode, change of the speed of rotation and advancement, advancement and retraction of the laser fiber, and adjustment of the irrigation flow rate. The pedals controlled the fluoroscopy and the laser generator. The insertion of the endoscope needed a ureteral access sheath to be in place. Small motors moved the tip of the endoscope and allowed it to perform basic movements inside the ureteral access sheath. The height of the manipulation arm was also

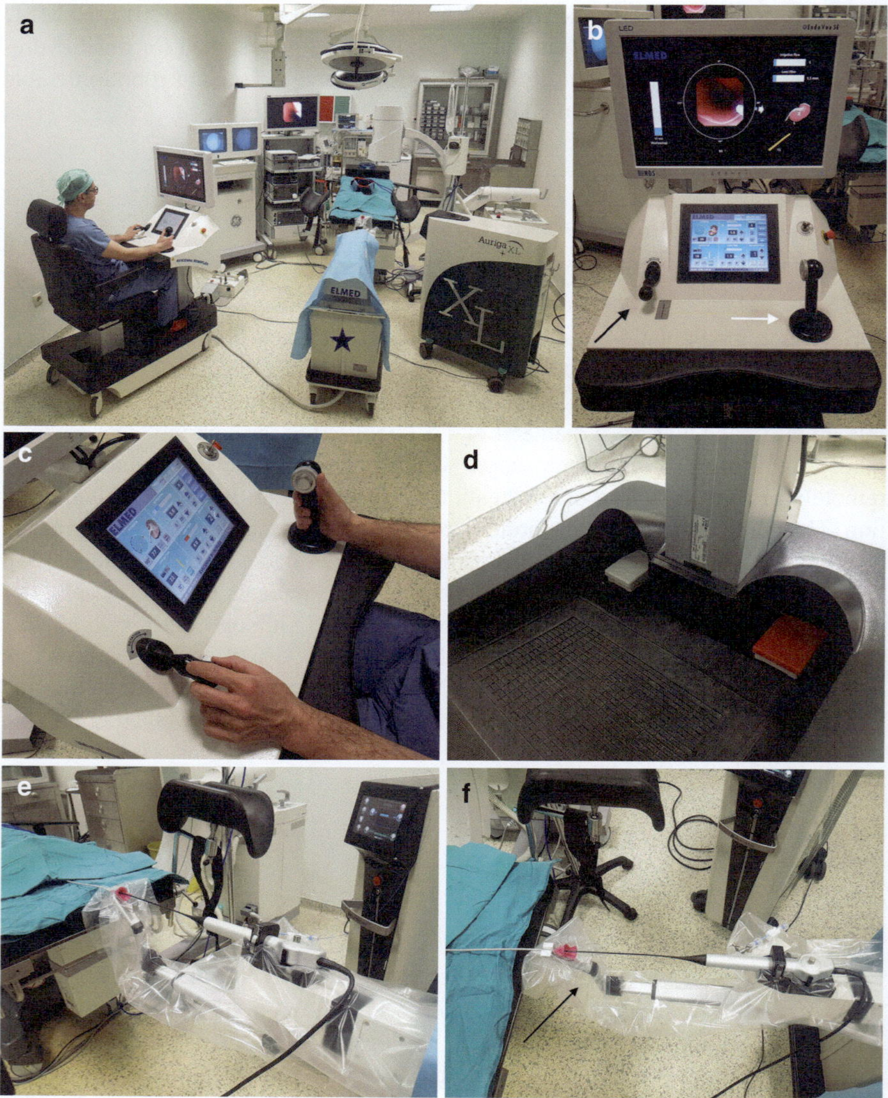

Fig. 3.11 (**a**) Avicenna Roboflex Platform (ELMED, Ankara, Turkey). Room set-up demonstrates surgeon's console (far left) with manipulation arm (black star). (**b**) Surgeon's console includes left joystick (black arrow), which allows for rotation as well as advancement and retraction, while the right joystick (white arrow) allows for bilateral tip deflection of the flexible ureteroscope. (**c**) Console also controls advancement of laser fiber and control of irrigation flow. (**d**) Foot pedal controls allow for activation of the laser and fluoroscopy. (**e**) The robotic manipulation arm is designed to hold any model of flexible ureteroscope since interchangeable endoscope holders are available. The most distal portion of the arm is designed to stabilize a ureteral access sheath. (**f**) The height of the manipulation arm is adjustable (black arrow) to accommodate unique patient anatomy

adjustable according to the patient's anatomy. The endoscope was attached to the arm and further stabilized by two brackets, while the distal stabilizer fixed the ureteral access sheath. The arm permitted the use of any type of flexible ureteroscope, and the robotic arm could be rotated $210°$ in each direction to allow overlap. Small rotators moved the steering lever for deflection and enabled precise movements of the string-based tip of the endoscope. The applied forces were limited to 1 N/mm^2 to minimize the risk of injury to the collecting system as well as to the endoscope. Additionally, the arm provided a system for advancement of the laser fiber, which was connected to the working channel of the flexible ureteroscope.

Comparatively, the latest version of the Avicenna Roboflex has a new interchangeable endoscope holder system so that it is compatible with the different brands and models of flexible ureteroscopes on the market. There is a new deflection right handle with a thumb wheel, which can also be adjusted from the console as well as a new right handle to control the rotation and two-stage speed control for forward/backward movements. Precision or scale of the rotation is selectable from the touch screen as well. Additionally, the model has a new foot pedal unit to control any type of laser or fluoroscopy foot pedals and allows visual guidance on the screen of the video monitor to realize the position of the flexible ureteroscope (horizontal distance, rotation angle, and deflection part 3D simulation and angle).

The irrigation system has also changed throughout the various versions [26]. In the first one, it was operated by a 25-speed mechanical pump, whereas in the latest version (the fourth), the irrigation system is controlled by a 12-speed mechanical pump and can be attached to a regular rod for gravitational irrigation. This pump is powered electronically and has two small rotors in the front connected to an infusion tube that is compatible with others on the market or with the included piece itself. The system is connected to a console with four buttons: one to start and stop, one to increase, another to decrease the flow, and another to flush. The "flush" allows a rapid increase in flow for about 1 second and is different from other mechanical systems that permit a saline adjustment. The flush can be operated approximately every 2 seconds after it has been activated; a refractory time that varies from 1.5 to 2 seconds by switching from low to high speed.

There is limited published experience on the Avicenna Roboflex available in the literature. The first study by Saglam et al. demonstrated complete stone disintegration in 79 out of 81 patients with mean stone volume of 1296 mm^3 [27]. According to a validated questionnaire rating 12 different domains of ergonomics, all seven participating surgeons reported a significant ergonomic advantage ($p < 0.01$) with the robotic platform. The second study was performed by Geavlete et al. on 132 randomized patients who underwent conventional f-URS (66 cases) versus robotic f-URS (another 66 cases) [28]. They showed that treatment time was relatively similar between the two types of procedures, while fragmentation time of the stone was somewhat better for robotic f-URS. The stone-free rate after 3 months was 89.4% for conventional f-URS and 92.4% for robotic f-URS – a slight improvement. The acquisition of basic skills with the robot was also compared by Proietti et al. in another study, which tested how subjects with no prior surgical training were able to acquire basic ureteroscopic skills with and without robotic f-URS in the K-box simulator [29]. The study divided medical students into two groups: Group 1 was trained with Avicenna Roboflex, and Group 2 was trained with conventional flexible ureteroscopy. Participants were then rated by a third party on their ability to perform (or not) two exercises in light of the time for each procedure. Participants were also evaluated on the quality of their performance along the following parameters: respect of the surrounding environment, flow of the operation, orientation, vision centering, and stability. The first exercise was completed by only three out of five students in Group 1 and by four out of five students in Group 2. Stability with the scope was significantly more accurate in the first group compared to that of the second ($P = 0.02$), but there were no differences in timing, flow, or orientation between the two groups. Although not significant, a tendency to respect the surrounding tissue and maintain centered vision was perceived more frequently in the first group. As for the second exercise, there were no differences between groups in orientation, flow, respect for the surrounding tissue, stability, or the ability to maintain centered vision. The second group tended to perform the exercise faster, albeit not to a significant extent. Concerning X-ray exposure to the operator, there are no studies showing any benefits of the Avicenna Roboflex, but it is unquestionable that the surgeon sits on the console far away from the fluoroscopy unit, reducing the risk of radiation exposure. Finally, the latest study published on robotic-assisted f-URS with Avicenna Roboflex illustrates the most robust experience of its clinical use. In a consecutive series of 240 patients with renal stones with an average stone load of 1798 mm^3, Klein et al. demonstrated non-inferiority compared to published conventional series of f-URS in terms of OR time, stone-free rate, re-treatment rate, and complications [30]. There was a 1% technical failure rate of the robotic system, which was circumvented with conventional f-URS when needed. The study concluded that the robotic system may help further push the limit of flexible ureteroscopy in terms of treating medium to large stone burdens, mostly due to alleviating unfavorable ergonomics for the treating surgeon.

There remain some limitations on the use of Avicenna Roboflex. The first is not having tactile feedback for the surgeon while handling the ureteroscope. Another issue is the cost of the system. It is logical that the use of this device is much more expensive than a standard flexible ureteroscope. Even the operating room must be suitable in terms of size to accommodate the robot, and a dedicated technician or another urologist is required to cooperate in assembling the device.

Technology has always been exciting for urologists and has a prominent place at the heart of urological practice. From the studies and results we have seen so far, it appears that the Avicenna Roboflex is a promising platform for f-URS. Currently available reports seem encouraging and demonstrate a potential improvement for the surgeon in terms of ergonomics and less exposure to radiation. For patients, stone disintegration and the stone-free rate also saw some minor improvements.

Conclusions

Robotic-assisted flexible ureteroscopy has been available for almost 10 years, and limited published experience is available. The current platforms seem most beneficial in making the ergonomic situation better for the treating surgeon and can potentially reduce radiation exposure as well. Patient outcomes seem to be equivalent to that of conventional flexible ureteroscopy for medium to large stone volumes. Robotic platforms can help push the limit of conventional flexible ureteroscopy in terms of comfortably treating larger stone burdens, but currently cost is a barrier to widespread acceptance. Future robotic designs will attempt to enhance access within the luminal collecting system beyond what current flexible ureteroscopic technology offers.

Guidewires

Jan Brachlow, Etienne Xavier Keller, and Olivier Traxer

Introduction

Guidewires were initially developed for the percutaneous placement of central venous catheters over 60 years ago [31]. Since the development of Seldinger technique, guidewires have undergone significant improvements with stiffer shafts [32] and flexible hydrophilic tips and have been used in endourological applications since the 1970s [33, 34]. Since then, the placement of a guidewire is an essential step in endourological procedures involving the upper urinary tract. The wire maintains the access to the upper tract during the procedure and facilitates immediate drain placement in case of ureteric or collecting system injury, such as ureteral perforation or excessive bleeding. In this chapter we will describe the existing types of guidewires and the materials of which they are composed and discuss their advantages and possible disadvantages.

Size and Tip Design

There are different types of guidewires with various tip shapes and materials. The specific design for each wire is made for different clinical scenarios. Clayman et al. compared structural properties of various guidewires on the market and showed that those wires with soft, hydrophilic tips are least likely to perforate the ureter and most likely to bend around a point of obstruction. Meanwhile, super-stiff wires are least likely to slip out of the ureter and allow for most reliable placement of access sheaths, since they are least likely to buckle [35].

The standard wire length for endourological application is 150 cm, but versions up to 180 cm long are available. If the wire is shorter than 150 cm, the potential for inability to pass a flexible ureteroscope becomes higher, and one can lose access to the upper urinary tract. The standard guidewire diameters are 0.035 and 0.038 inch (2.7 F and 2.9 F; 0.89 mm and 0.97 mm). Thinner diameter versions exist at 0.025 inch (1.9 F; 0.64 mm). The design of the tip exists in three different shapes: straight, angled, and J-type.

In daily endourological practice, the straight tip is used most frequently. For special situations like difficult access to the ureteral orifice, the angled tip can be used. Both angled tips and J-type tips are useful to bypass impacted ureteral calculi or a tortuous ureter [36]. The distal tip of all types should be soft and flexible so as to minimize ureteral perforations or abrasions. The wire tips are often soft on only one end and frequently quite stiff on the opposite end. As the responsible surgeon, it is always wise to check the character of the tip of the wire prior to insertion into the ureter or ureteroscope (Fig. 3.12). Inserting the stiff end of a guidewire can easily result in ureteral perforation or damage to the working channel of a flexible ureteroscope, leading to failure of leak testing and costly endoscope repairs, which would otherwise be avoidable. Wires with double floppy-tip designs are ideal for placing flexible ureteroscopes when advancement up the ureter is challenging given ureteral narrowing or tortuosity. The double floppy-tip design helps protect against working channel perforations.

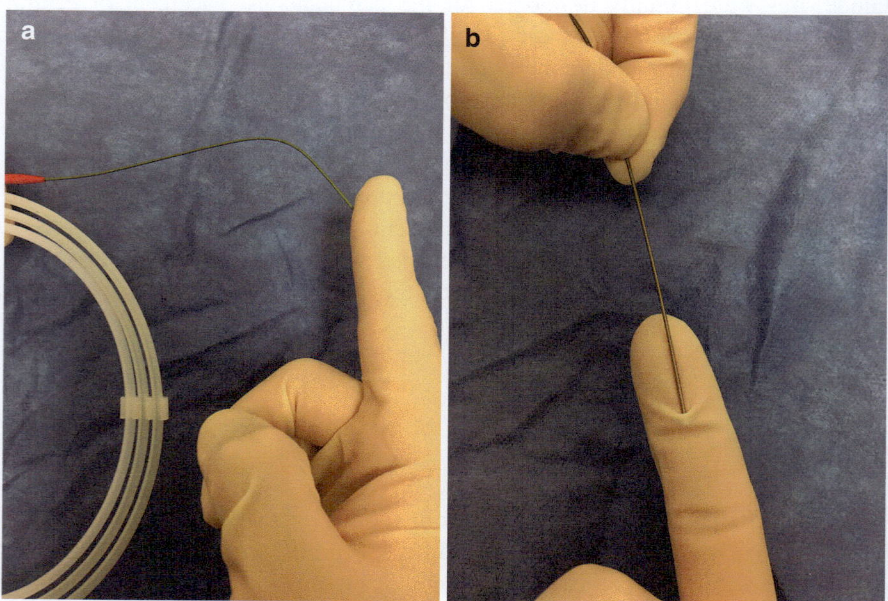

Fig. 3.12 (**a**) Note the soft flexible tip of this 0.038-inch PTFE wire against the surgeon's finger. (**b**) The opposite tip of the same wire is very stiff and would easily perforate the ureteral wall or ureteroscope working channel

Material

Guidewires have two components: an inner core, which is responsible for the inner stiffness, and an outer coating, which is responsible for the interface lubricity. Both of these factors need to be considered when placing drains or endoscopes over a guidewire. The inner core can be made out of stainless steel or of nitinol (a metal alloy of nickel and titanium). The newest product for inner cores is Triton alloy, which is a "next-generation" form of nitinol with a higher bending modulus. A stiffer shaft is very useful for straightening a kinked ureter (Fig. 3.13) or when passing retrograde ureteral drains in a patient with a tortuous urinary diversion such as an ileal conduit.

As for coating materials, there are three different substances: PTFE (polytetrafluorethylene or Teflon), hydrophilic polymer, and slip coat. Their main goal is to decrease the friction between the wire and the instrument or the tissue. All hydrophilic guidewires have to be lubricated with sterile water or saline during the intervention (Fig. 3.14). In order to minimize friction or "drag," a hydrophilic wire is necessary when placing a silicon stent. Despite this advantage, a potential downside to hydrophilic wires is a tendency for them to slip out of the ureter. Therefore some surgeons prefer not to use them as safety wires. Hybrid wires have been developed to address this issue. Hybrid wires combine the advantageous properties of individual wires into one wire that has a hydrophilic flexible tip to enhance access and a stiffer PTFE-coated shaft over a nitinol core to reduce wire slippage (Fig. 3.15). Many have suggested that a hybrid wire is the best first choice guidewire to access the ureter from below, as it minimizes the need to open a second wire given its beneficial structural properties. Furthermore, hybrid wires have been purported to simplify equipment choice for operating room staff and urologist alike, thus decreasing the need to maintain a large inventory of wires [37]. Given the relatively greater expense compared to some other wires, exclusive use of hybrid wires for every case may not be a cost-effective option.

Should Safety Wires Still Be Used?

In recent years there has been an on-going debate whether a safety guidewire (SG) should routinely be used in endourological procedures or not [38–41]. SG is recommended in the AUA and EAU guidelines [42, 43] based on experience and expert opinions rather than level 1 evidence. The clear advantage of a SG during retrograde ureteroscopy is that it enables immediate drain placement if any worrisome violation of the ureteral mucosa or muscular wall is encountered or if significant bleeding is present and prevents completion of the operative case. In most of these situations, stent placement allows for safe termination of the case and allows for adequate drainage and avoidance of serious infection. Eventual return for a potential second-stage procedure is then possible.

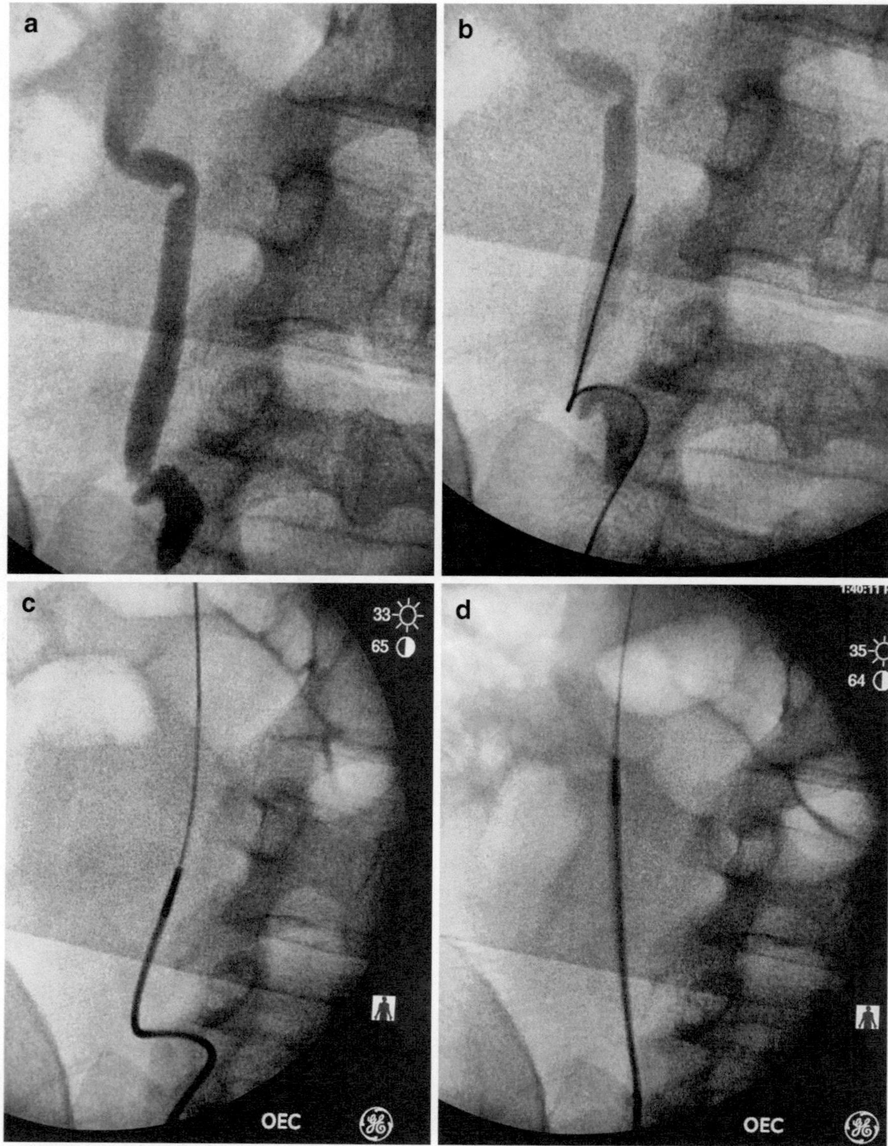

Fig. 3.13 (**a**) Retrograde pyelogram shows a chronically dilated ureter with multiple tortuosities. (**b**) A super-stiff glidewire is hydrophilic at the tip and along the shaft, allowing for negotiation of ureteral tortuosities. (**c**) Retrograde ureteral catheter aids in stabilization. (**d**) Further advancement of the super-stiff wire shaft straightens the ureter

Fig. 3.14 Hydrophilic
wires require adequate
application of sterile saline
or water to maximize
lubricity

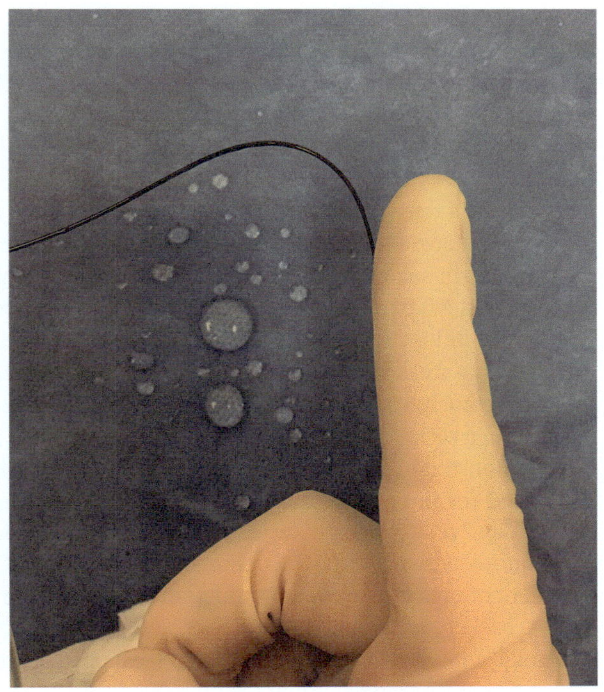

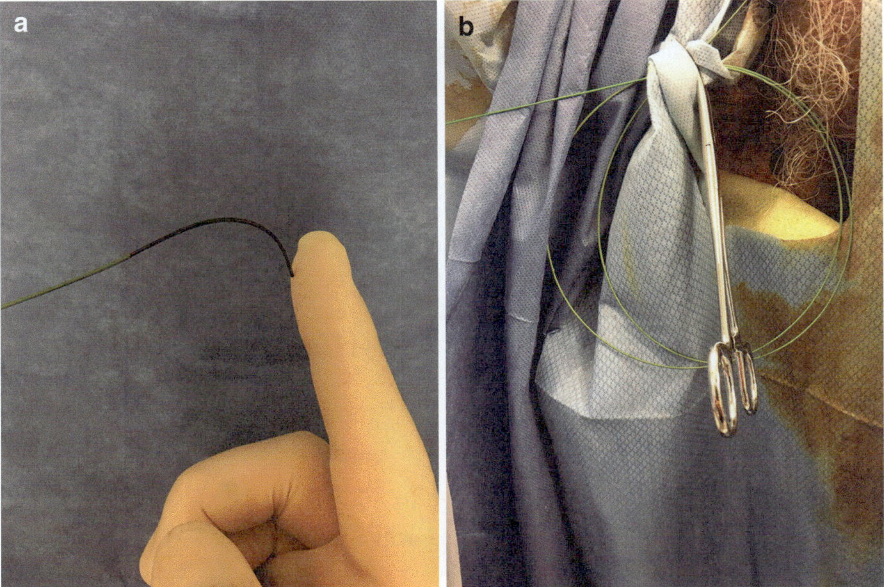

Fig. 3.15 (**a**) Hybrid wire with flexible hydrophilic tip to enhance access around upper urinary tract obstructions, while (**b**) PTFE-coated shaft reduces slippage of safety wire

With experience however, some groups have pointed out potential disadvantages of the routine use of a SG. Eandi et al. demonstrated in a porcine model that there was an increased amount of force required to place either a semi-rigid or flexible ureteroscope alongside an existing guidewire [44]. In a separate study, Ulvik et al. showed a statistically significant increase of 52%–113% for advancement and retraction forces during endoscopic treatment with a SG [45]. Clearly, situations exist in which retrograde access to the kidney is limited or not possible when trying to pass a ureteroscope alongside a safety wire, validating the observations of these two studies. In such cases, the surgeon may consider the slimmest available safety wire, such as a 0.025-inch wire. Alternatively, the ureteroscope can be passed to the level of the kidney without a SG. In the absence of active ureteral pathology, when the goal is to treat stone or tumor in the kidney, it is reasonable to forego a SG in order to obtain retrograde access. In this manner, the ureteroscope acts as the "safety device." In a series of 268 retrograde ureteroscopies for renal stone treatment, Patel et al. demonstrated safe procedure performance without the use of a SG. Guidewires were used for initial access only. For larger stones, ureteral access sheathes were utilized, and relatively smaller stones were refined to dust. There were no ureteral perforations or avulsions. The authors conceded that SGs should be utilized in the treatment of ureteral stones, any situation in which stone fragments will be removed with a basket, incisional procedures such as endopyelotomies, in patients with abnormal anatomy, and any situation in which the ureter requires dilation [46]. Dickstein et al. reported similar results in a consecutive series of 305 patients treated with retrograde ureteroscopy for stones and also had success without the use of a routine SG. In addition to criteria listed by Patel et al., they added situations in which SG placement is prudent including cases with encrusted ureteral stents and those patients with urinary diversions [39].

Therefore, experience has shown that safety wires can be omitted in some carefully selected cases, particularly in the treatment of relatively low stone burdens confined to the kidney, when there is no intention to extract fragments with a basket. However, in the opinion of the authors, safety wire use in retrograde ureteroscopy should always be considered as the "default mode," especially if the wire does not limit initial access to the kidney or impair visualization. Safety wire utilization is very much like a seat belt: it may be useful only once in your lifetime, and at that time, you will never regret to always have used it [47].

Conclusion

Guidewires are essential tools in the armamentarium of the advanced ureteroscopist. They provide access to the upper urinary tract and allow for expeditious drain placement when necessary. Guidewires vary in the shape and composition of their tips as well as shafts. Knowledge of specific nuances will empower the surgeon to make optimal choices to maximize case safety and success. The use of safety wires should always be encouraged although it is not unreasonable to omit them in very carefully selected cases.

Ureteral Access Sheaths

Vincent De Coninck, Etienne Xavier Keller, and Olivier Traxer

Introduction

Retrograde intrarenal surgery has undergone many technological advances during the past three decades. The development of flexible ureteroscopes, laser lithotripters, and instruments like ureteral access sheaths (UASs) has expanded our ability to treat pathologies of the upper urinary tract. The UAS was developed in 1974 by Hisao Takayasu and Yoshio Aso to facilitate the insertion of their completely passive flexible ureteroscope in the ureter [48]. Afterward, UASs were developed with a kink-resistant and streamlined design. Currently, they consist of an inner dilator that is fixed to an outer sheath with a locking hub. It allows a fluent introduction of the UAS over a guidewire in the ureter under fluoroscopic control and to perform a retrograde ureteropyelography through the dilator after introduction.

Characteristics/Specifications

UASs are produced with multiple specifications. They differ in diameter, length, material, stiffness, radiopaque marker, and dilator design (straight or articulated, single or dual lumen, axial or radial dilating system). To minimize friction with tissue during insertion, they all have a hydrophilic coating of the outer surface [49]. Some UASs are produced with a slit and a notch in the exposed part of the dilator, allowing the use of a single working wire as a safety guidewire [50, 51]. This may save material costs and operative time [52].

Of the above specifications, choosing UAS length and diameter will influence the success of the case, if the goals are to save time and maximize the stone-free rate. Ideal UAS length is long enough to allow for the sheath to traverse the majority of the ureter in order to facilitate reinsertions and withdrawals, but not too long as to limit maneuverability (Fig. 3.16). Selection of UAS diameter will depend on the exact model of flexible ureteroscope being used. A useful generalization is that the cross-sectional size of a sheath will require about 2F for the wall and an additional 1–3F for the ureteroscope to be able to clear the inner sheath diameter [53]. A sheath that measures 12F inner diameter and 14F outer diameter (12/14F) will accommodate almost any contemporary flexible ureteroscope [54]. Smaller diameter sheaths can be utilized with slimmer flexible ureteroscopes, but it is essential for the

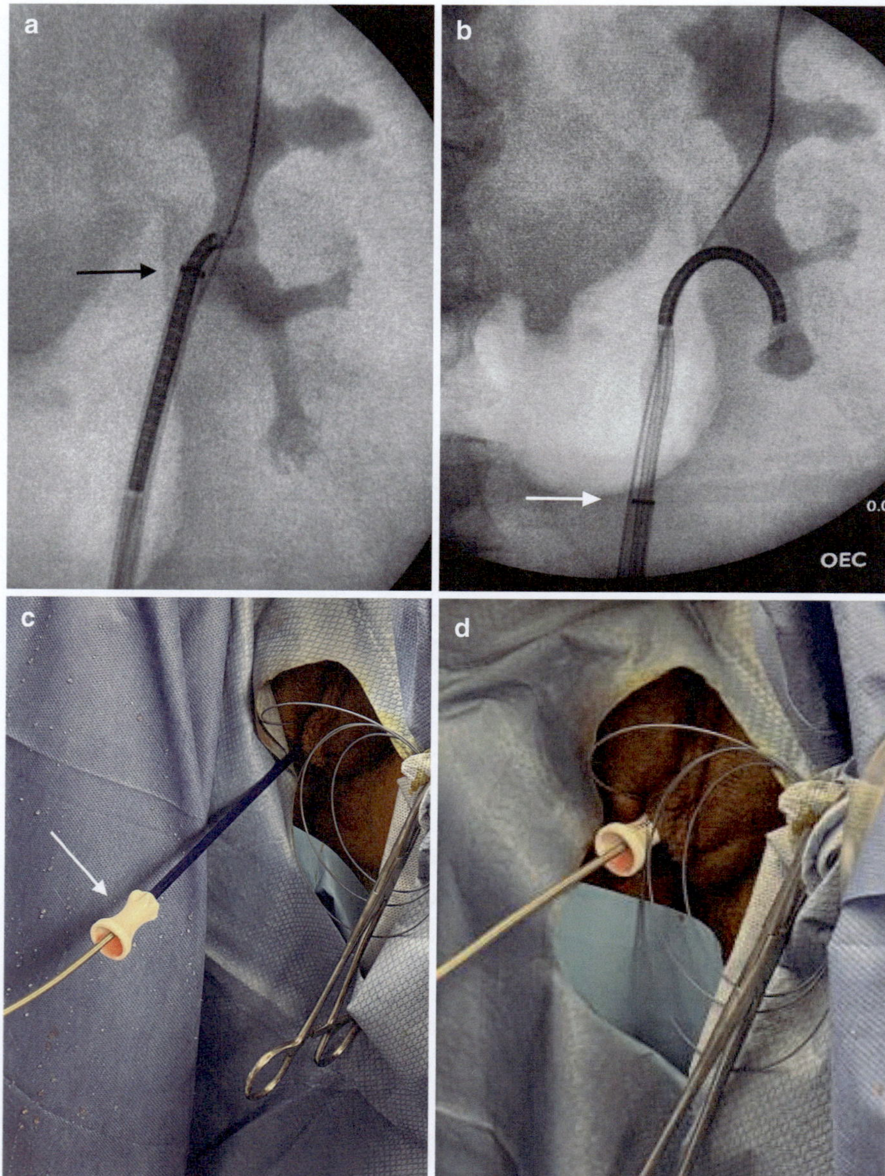

Fig. 3.16 (**a**) Black arrow points to the radio-opaque marker on the proximal end of the ureteral access sheath, just above the ureteropelvic junction. Mobility of the flexible ureteroscope is compromised with over-advancement of the sheath, in this particular collecting system morphology. (**b**) White arrow shows the radio-opaque marker of the access sheath has been moved more distally into the proximal ureter which now allows full deflection into the dependent lower pole calyx. (**c**) Excess ureteral access sheath length can result in placement of the sheath introducer (white arrow) relatively farther away from the patient's urethra, therefore compromising maneuverability of the flexible ureteroscope. (**d**) When appropriate ureteral access sheath length is selected, the introducer is in very close proximity to the patient's urethral meatus, which maximizes the surgeon's ability to maneuver the flexible ureteroscope and is ergonomically favorable

advanced ureteroscopist to appreciate the specifications of both in order to maximize successful outcomes.

Impact on Multiple Instrument Reinsertions and Withdrawals

It is commonly cited that a UAS facilitates multiple withdrawals and reinsertions of a ureteroscope into the upper urinary tract. However, a ureteroscope can also be backloaded over a working guidewire under fluoroscopic control or alongside a safety guidewire. It remains controversial if using a UAS for this reason is cost- and time-efficient [55, 56], although for larger stone volumes requiring multiple passes, UAS use is likely to be beneficial.

Impact on Irrigation and Intrarenal Pressure

Using a UAS increases irrigation flow by 35% to 80% compared to an unsheathed ureteroscope [57]. Outflow increases with wider UAS diameters in case of an empty ureteroscope working channel. However, this is not the case when the working channel is occupied [58, 59].

Ideally, intrarenal pressure should be kept below 40 cm H_2O (or 30 mmHg) during ureteroscopy to prevent complications like bleeding, hematoma, urinoma, sepsis, and post-operative pain. This can be achieved by using a UAS that lowers irrigation pressure to the renal pelvis and parenchyma by increasing outflow [60]. Using a 10/12 Fr or 12/14 Fr UAS will keep intrapelvic pressures below 30 and 20 cmH_2O (or 22 and 15 mmHg), respectively, even when applying forced irrigation pressures of 200 cm H_2O (or 147 mmHg) [57]. Since intrarenal pressure depends on inflow and outflow, the lowest intrarenal pressures are acquired using a small-sized flexible ureteroscope [58] (Fig. 3.17).

When the tip of the ureteroscope and UAS are close to each other, the lowest pressure and highest inflow and outflow are observed. Because of this, UAS's length should be chosen based on the ureteral length and location of the pathology [57].

Impact on Stone-Free Rate

It is unclear if using a UAS or not influences stone-free rates. Some authors found increased stone-free rates, and others did not [55, 56, 61, 62]. A limitation of these studies is that stone-free rates were not determined by a computerized tomography in most patients.

UAS's Insertion Success Rate

Primary insertion of a UAS is not always possible since its outer diameter varies between 11.5 and 18 Fr, whereas the diameter of a native ureter is approximately 6 to 9 Fr [63]. Pre-stenting will facilitate UAS insertion and reduce ureteral injuries [64]. Failure from UAS insertion decreases from 16–42% to 0–12% in pre-stented patients [65–67]. Alternatively, the ureter can be dilated actively by using the inner UAS dilator, a semi-rigid ureteroscope, serial coaxial tapered dilators, or a balloon dilator [61, 65, 67–69]. Currently, the risk of long-term ureteral damage between active and passive dilation remains unclear.

The Impact on Ureteroscope Durability

Some authors mention that using a UAS protects and reduces the strain on flexible ureteroscopes. Others report that it may damage the ureteroscope at the interface between the deflecting tip and the extremity of the UAS. Currently, it is unclear if using a UAS influences ureteroscope durability or not [15, 70, 71].

Coagulopathy

It is unclear if UAS should be recommended in patients under continuous anticoagulation/antiplatelet therapy or with uncorrected bleeding diatheses. Some prefer not using a UAS since damaging the ureteral wall during insertion may provoke bleeding, and spontaneous hemorrhage of the urothelium is rare when working at intrapelvic pressures below 40 cm H_2O. Others prefer to use one, based on one study in which no more hemorrhagic complications were encountered using a UAS

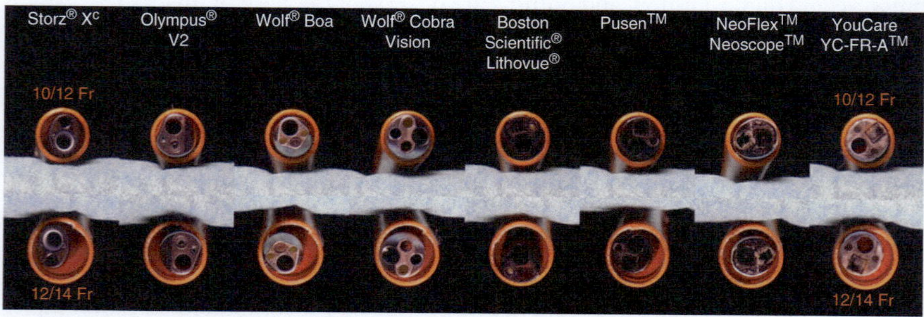

Fig. 3.17 Digital flexible ureteroscopes inside UASs of 10/12 Fr and 12/14 Fr. Larger sheath diameter allows better irrigation movement along the ureteroscope and the ability to remove larger resultant fragments

in patients taking anticoagulants [72]. However, safety and complications were not a primary endpoint in this study.

Children

It is unclear if using a UAS should be recommended during retrograde intrarenal surgery in children or not. Some authors noticed increased complications (ureteral perforation, stent migration), and others did not [73, 74]. An argument for not using a UAS may be the significant levels of ionizing radiation required during sheath insertion [75].

Complications

The influence of using a UAS on ureteral damage is generally underreported. UASs provoke ureteral wall injuries visualized during ureteroscopy in up to half of patients. The risk decreases when using smaller diameter UASs or in pre-stented patients [64, 76, 77]. In one study, there was no long-term correlation between using a UAS and ureteral stricture formation [78].

In a prospective study over a 1-year period, Traxer et al. found a decrease of infectious complications (fever, urinary tract infection, sepsis) when a UAS was used. The decreased intrapelvic pressure may explain this when a UAS is applied [56]. The effect a UAS has on diminishing post-operative pain remains controversial [55, 79].

Guideline Recommendations

The guidelines of the American Urological Association recommend using a UAS for lengthy procedures with prolonged high intrarenal pressures since this increases the risk of hemorrhage and infections. The guidelines of the European Association of Urology (EAU), Société Internationale d'Urologie, and International Consultation on Urology Disease state that its use should depend on surgeon's preference.

Conclusions

Using a UAS increases irrigation outflow during retrograde intrarenal surgery and decreases intrapelvic pressure and infectious complications. Data are controversial about its cost-effectiveness, impact on stone-free rates, ureteroscope durability, post-operative pain, and ureteral strictures. Therefore, inserting a UAS should not be an automatic step when performing flexible ureteroscopy but should be considered on a case-specific basis.

Stone Retrieval Devices

Kymora B. Scotland, Bree'ava Limbrick, and Demetrius H. Bagley

Introduction

Evolution in the endoscopic treatment and management of urinary lithiasis has been aided by the development of stone extraction devices. Ureteroscopes alone without a working channel or working instruments can function only as a visual diagnostic instrument. The addition of a channel that can accept instruments, such as endoscopic lithotriptors, laser fibers, electrodes, and stone or tissue retrieval devices, offers therapeutic options. The sizes of the channel and the working instruments must be compatible. The combination of endoscope and working instrument forms a useful diagnostic and therapeutic device.

Many of the devices presently available have been downsized from those used cystoscopically. Since they must pass through the generally standard channel of 3.6 F, they must be 3 F or less to leave room for irrigant. Some are available in designs as small as 1.3 F. Additionally, there are many specifically designed for the size and purpose of ureteroscopic use.

The vast majority of ureteroscopic retrieval devices consist of an inner movable component composed of metal and an outer flexible plastic sheath, which contains the expandable components. The metal, which has long been the standard for the inner component, is stainless steel. It is strong, flexible, and relatively inexpensive, but it can kink.

Nitinol is an alloy of nickel and titanium, characterized by shape memory and super-elasticity. It can be deformed, even repetitively, and return to its original shape. In this way it does not kink, but it is more expensive than stainless steel. These characteristics have explosively expanded the designs and applications for endoscopic working instruments.

The wires composing the internal metal components are generally round in cross section. Other cross-sectional designs include flat or rectangular, triangular, D-shaped, and concave. These confer specific attributes related to function and size.

The sheath of the instrument contains the moving core components and compresses the expansive portions. It requires strength, both radial and compressive; flexibility; and low friction with the metal components and the working channel of the endoscope. The two main sheathing materials are polytetrafluoroethylene (PTFE) or Teflon and polyimide. PTFE is very slippery and flexible but not as strong, thus requiring a larger diameter for similar central components. Polyimide is stronger and therefore can be smaller. It has a higher coefficient of friction and may require coating to function smoothly. It is also relatively more expensive.

Some devices, so-called non-retracting instruments, have a double-layered or coaxial sheath, the inner of which retracts to open the contained metal component. The grasper or basket itself does not move during opening or closing and requires compensatory movement for initial positioning. In a few specific instruments, a wrapped wire sheath has been employed. It is less flexible but considerably stronger than the plastic materials.

Baskets

Stone basket technology has evolved to improve the efficacy in the approaches for renal and ureteral stone retrieval. Contemporary stone basket designs range from simple to complex wire compositions allowing for different grasping strategies. With the many options available, urologists can tailor their choice of basket based on the specific size, number, and location of stones within the urinary system.

Historical Development

Stone retrieval baskets were originally designed for use through a cystoscope to reach and engage stones blindly within the ureter. Early devices include the council extractor, first described in 1926, as well as the Johnson extractor [80, 81]. These were both multiple-wire configurations mounted on a shaft, which was inserted into the ureter. It was claimed that the basket could both dilate the ureter and entrap the stone. X-ray guidance was useful to enable the localization, positioning of the basket, and extraction of the ureteral calculus. Because of the large size of the device, it was often necessary to dilate the ureter prior to placement. Additionally, because there were no devices available at the time for stone fragmentation, it was often not possible to remove larger renal and ureteral calculi, and there was a real risk of ureteral injury or of having to convert to open ureterolithotomy or to use a weight on the basket to extract over several hours [82].

These problems persisted with the introduction of the Dormia basket described in 1958 [83]. This was the first extractor device composed of four wires with a helical configuration contained in a flexible hollow stem for insertion. The tip could be short or with a longer filiform to maintain its position above the stone. The inner, basket portion was advanced beyond the sheath to allow the basket to open, both to dilate the ureter and engage the stone. It could be opened above or adjacent to the stone and rotated for engagement. In 1973 Pfister and Schwartz described a basket with six helical wires composed of a cobalt-nickel-chromium alloy contained in a 3.6 F Teflon sheath [84]. Both of these devices were best used with radiologic guidance, but still the disproportion between the size of the stone and the ureter could not be determined accurately. One of the major disastrous complications was ureteral avulsion [85, 86] (see Chap. 10). Although the recognized complications stimulated attempts to design safer baskets, the Dormia helical model with round wires formed a structural foundation that is still commonly used today.

In 1976, a percutaneous approach to renal calculi was described [87]. The Segura stainless steel basket (Boston Scientific Corporation, MA), the first flat wire design, was developed in the 1980s, specifically to engage renal pelvic and calyceal stones in a percutaneous fashion. It was constructed with four flat wires, which could be expanded to grasp a stone. It offered a larger unobstructed area between the wires than the helical models (Fig. 3.18). These baskets have also been used to biopsy urothelial tumors, providing a better sample than forceps or other devices with round wires (see Chap. 6: "Diagnosis of Upper Tract Urothelial Carcinoma"). The basket has a tip preventing safe use in the renal calyx because of the risk of trauma to the papilla. Since it is composed of stainless steel, it can kink, thus trapping the stone although this has been lessened with changing to a wire with a D-shaped cross section.

It was the advent of ureteroscopes with their ability to visualize ureteral or renal calculi within the urinary tract that necessitated and facilitated the development of contemporary stone retrieval devices. These endoscopes also required even smaller devices to fit through the working channels. The introduction and application of flexible ureteroscopes required smaller, longer, and more flexible retrieval devices with other specific features.

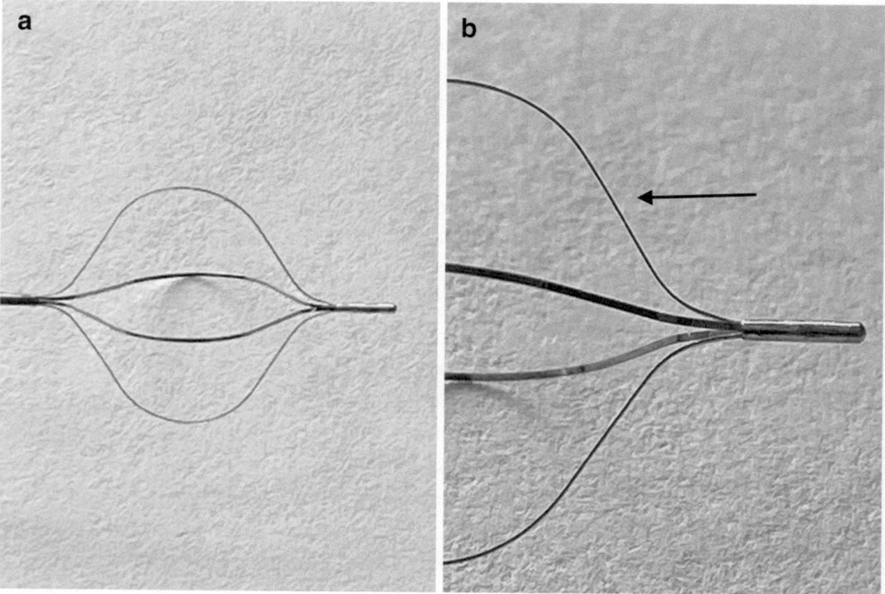

Fig. 3.18 (**a**) Stainless steel flat wire basket. (**b**) Close-up view shows the flat, ribbon-like shape of the basket wire, ideal for biopsy of luminal neoplasms

The introduction of nitinol into the medical device inventory has been one of the most important advances in technology. As noted above, nitinol is an alloy of nickel and titanium possessing the properties of flexibility and shape memory, which have been carried into medical devices.

D'A. Honey described a four-wire basket, which truly had no tip [88]. The two loops forming the wire were joined at the tip by tying a knot, a design only possible with nitinol (Fig. 3.19). This basket, initially available as 3 F, exhibits the characteristics of nitinol wires. In addition to being tipless, it is flexible, non-kinking, durable, and capable of releasing stones. Similar concepts have extended this basket to as small as 1.3 F.

Numerous studies have demonstrated the functional superiority of baskets of this design using in vitro studies throughout the urinary tract. These studies have countered many of the earlier beliefs regarding essential design features of baskets. The soft flexible wires of the basket have been very effective in manipulating around even impacted ureteral stones and have demonstrated that dilating force is not an essential feature. Under direct vision, a filiform tip is not essential and in fact is even detrimental for placement of a basket. The smooth and flexible form of the four-wire basket fits well into the calyx without perforating the mucosa [89, 90].

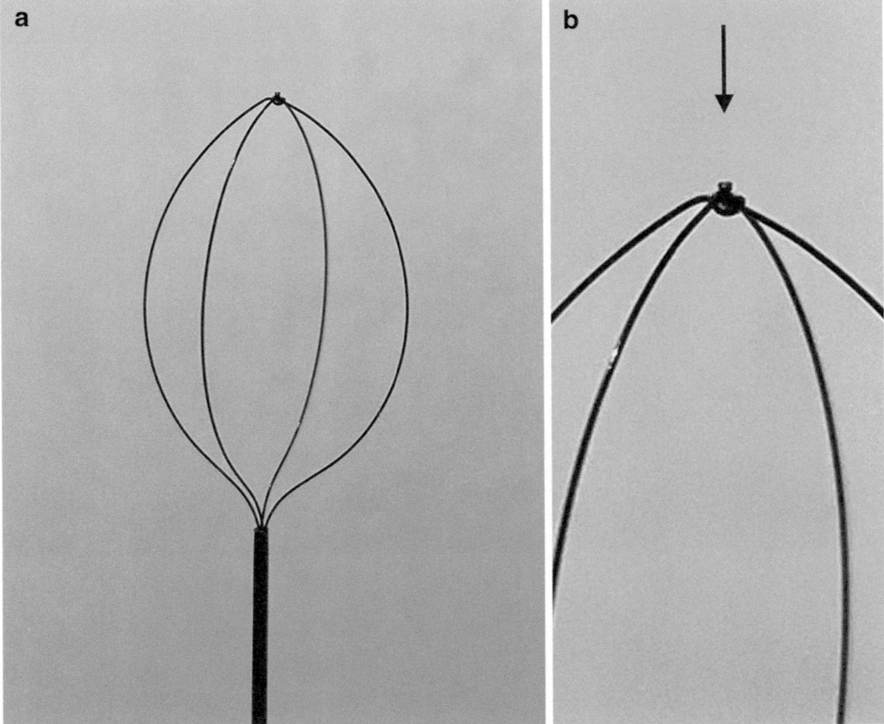

Fig. 3.19 (**a**) Tipless nitinol basket design. (**b**) Close-up view shows the "nitinol knot" allowing for the "tipless" design

One of the greatest benefits of the nitinol's four-wire basket is the ability to disengage a stone. The basket can usually be advanced away from the ureteroscope to remove the wires from a stone by folding them away from the surface. This is not possible with a stainless steel basket since the wires tend to kink if they are sharply angled. It is also not possible with the helical design of a Dormia basket in which the wires cross the stone at an angle [91]. This technique of engaging and disengaging a stone was enhanced with the dimension basket (CR Bard, USA), which has a mechanism to deflect the wires of the basket in opposite directions in the same plane to effectively widen the space between the wires on one side [92] (Fig. 3.20).

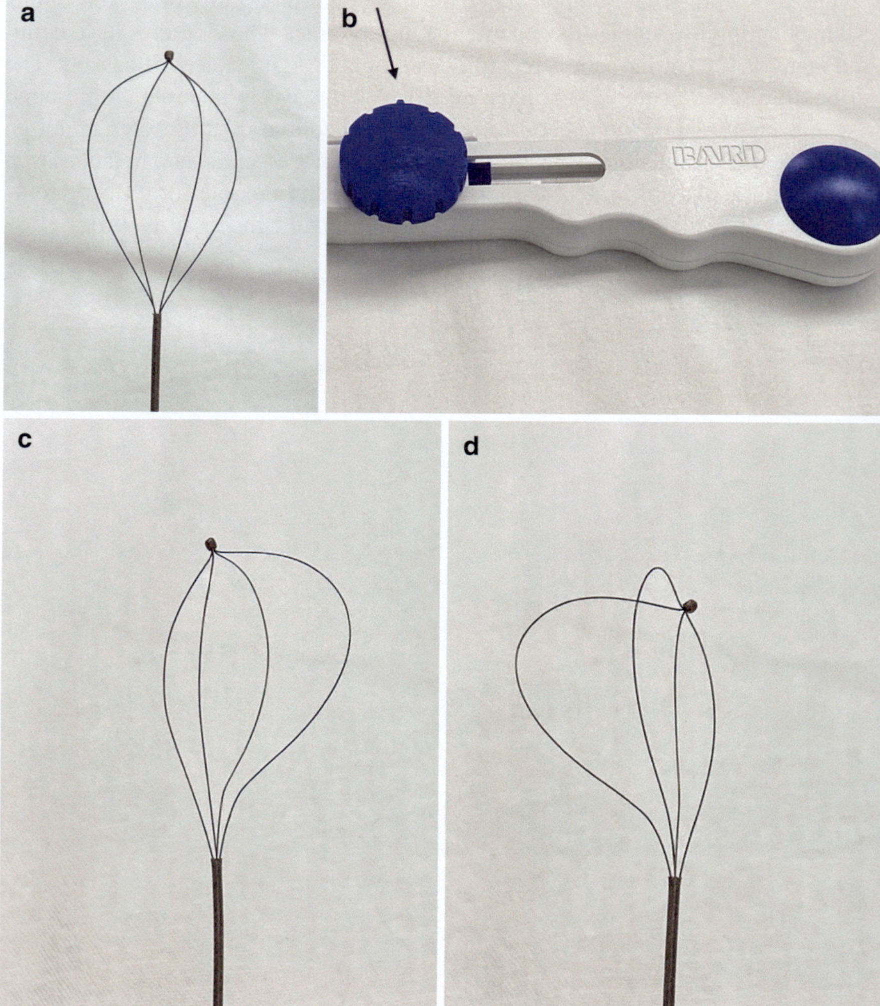

Fig. 3.20 (**a**) Articulating tipless nitinol basket. Dimension basket (BD, Franklin Lakes, NJ). (**b**) The dial on the basket handle (black arrow) allows for articulation of the basket opening. (**c** and **d**) The wires of the basket can be articulated to the left or right in order to provide an exaggerated opening for stone retrieval or release

Numerous baskets have been designed with multiple wires. Some have multiple wires in the distal portion and a single strand on each side more proximally, similar to fingers attached to a wrist and distal arm. These baskets can trap smaller fragments but with the risk of reforming a large stone when multiple fragments are grasped. They have also been shown to be slower to retrieve a stone compared to other simpler designs [93].

Forward Grasping Devices

Often the target to be removed is located directly in front of the endoscope. Examples include a stone fragment in a calyx, a foreign body such as a proximally located ureteral stent, or piece of a stent, basket, or laser fiber. These may be difficult to engage with the more standard baskets and call for other specific retrieval devices.

Standard helical or flat wire baskets made of stainless steel can be difficult or even dangerous for grasping within a calyx. The widest opening between the wires is located significantly proximally from the tip. They are also stiffer and tend to perforate the mucosa. The nitinol baskets have minimized these problems since the wires are flexible enough to bend against the mucosa, but they can be difficult to position accurately. By deflecting, the dimension basket moves the opening and the curvature of the wires forming the basket for better positioning. Other devices have been designed specifically for forward grasping.

The simplest and earliest forward grasping devices are the wire-pronged graspers. These are designed with multiple fingers or prongs forming the active tip. They are compressed as they withdraw into the sheath and separate more widely as they are advanced from the tip (Fig. 3.21). Similar but larger models have been used in the bladder and for industrial applications. Again to fit within a ureteroscope, a much smaller design is needed. Although multiple different numbers of wire prongs have been used, the three-pronged design is most common. It was found that it is difficult to firmly grasp an object with a two-pronged grasper and the four-pronged design is unwieldy with frequent perforation of the ureteral mucosa. Sizes range from 1.9 to 3F for ureteroscopic application.

Forceps have also been employed for a forward grasp. Because of the mechanism involved, it is difficult to miniaturize these below 3F. They have been used most commonly through rigid ureteroscopes.

More recent additions have been the forward grasping NGage (Cook Urology, Indiana) and Dakota (Boston Scientific, Mass) stone retrieval devices. These have a relatively complex appearing design of curved wires with the largest opening at the most distal aspect (Fig. 3.22). They function somewhat as a basket but with a forward grasping capability. A direct in vitro comparison of the two devices showed similar durability but some variation in both grasping and releasing characteristics [94]. These differences have not been confirmed clinically.

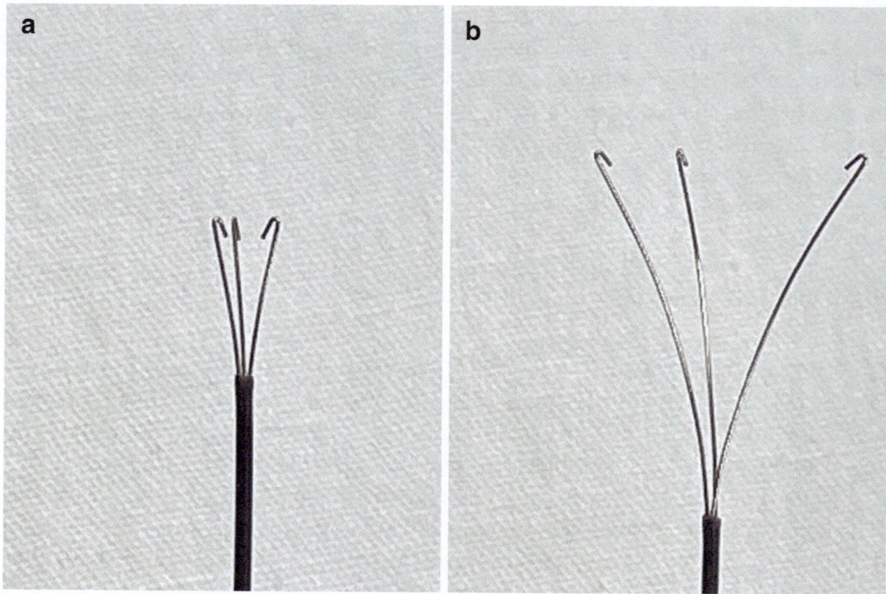

Fig. 3.21 (**a**) Three-pronged grasper in near-closed position. (**b**) Three-pronged grasper fully opened. Note the hook-shaped ends of the grasper wires, which enhance grasp but can snag surface mucosa of the urinary tract

Fig. 3.22 Nitinol hybrid basket/grasper with forward grasping capability ideal for calyceal stones. Dakota (Boston Scientific, Marlborough, MA) and NGage (Cook Medical, Bloomington IN)

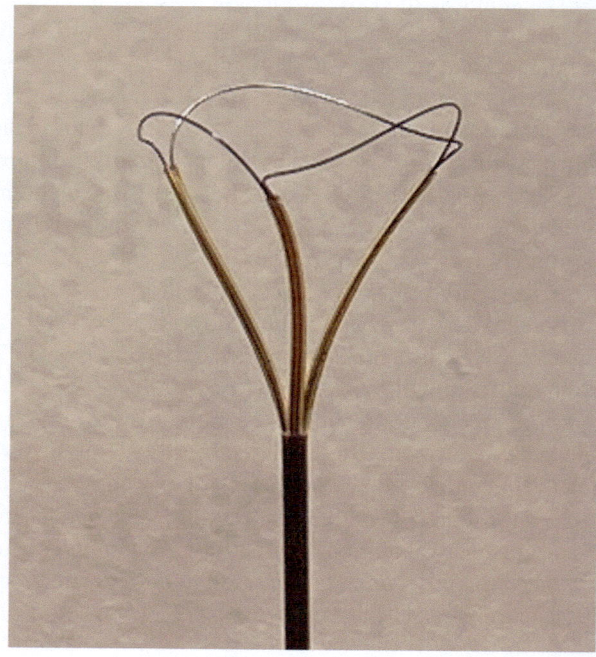

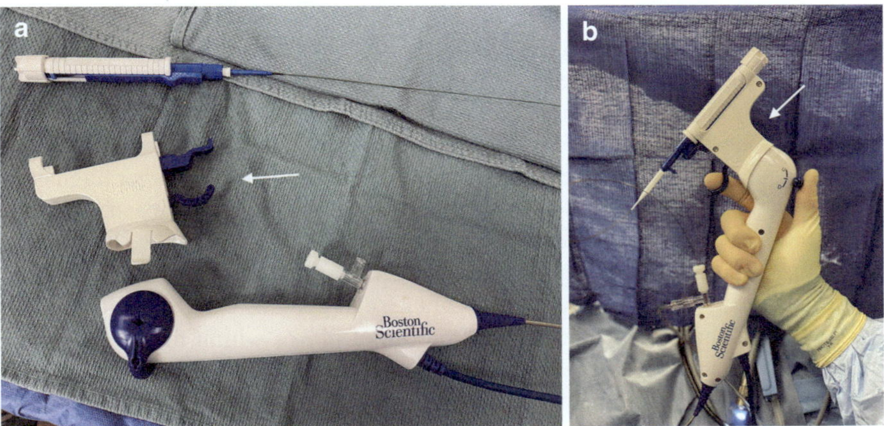

Fig. 3.23 (**a**) LithoVue Empower retrieval deployment device (Boston Scientific, Marlborough, MA) (white arrow). (**b**) The Empower (white arrow) couples the flexible ureteroscope to the handle of a basket or grasper. The surgeon's index finger controls basket/grasper opening and closing while the thumb can deflect the ureteroscope simultaneously as needed

Retrieval Deployment Device

The LithoVue Empower (Boston Scientific, Marlborough, MA) is a novel stone retrieval device, which allows the surgeon to actively open and close a basket or grasper without the aid of an assistant (Fig. 3.23). This allows for a near autonomous process of flexible ureteroscopic maneuvering and stone removal. It is ideal for manual removal of large quantities of resultant fragments following ureteroscopic lithotripsy. The device has been evaluated and compared to ureteroscopy with both an experienced assistant or a naïve, inexperienced assistant, whose task was to open and close the grasper. The Empower had performance characteristics similar to working with an experienced assistant and not surprisingly performed better than working with an inexperienced assistant [95]. It may prove beneficial for treating relatively large stone burdens with ureteroscopic laser lithotripsy when large quantities of resultant fragments need to be manually extracted, especially in the absence of an experienced assistant.

Antiretropulsion Devices

One of the risks of early rigid ureteroscopy for calculi was the proximal movement of the targeted stone. Without effective flexible ureteroscopes or endoscopic lithotrites, the movement of a stone into the lateral or inferior portions of the intrarenal collecting system resulted in failure of the procedure. It was attractive to consider a device to prevent the retrograde movement of calculi during attempted treatment. These remain valuable in situations when flexible endoscopes or other therapeutic options are not available.

Placement of a balloon catheter within the ureter with inflation of the balloon proximal to the stone theoretically could be effective. However the flexibility and elasticity of the balloon allowed surprisingly large stones to migrate beyond the balloon. The only appropriately sized balloons available were the Fogarty embolectomy design, which was then prohibitively expensive. Positioning of a stone basket proximal to the target stone could be effective in preventing migration of larger fragments. However both of these devices occupied precious space within the lumen of the ureter.

The Stone Cone was the first device designed specifically to prevent proximal migration of ureteral stones and fragments during ureteroscopic manipulation and lithotripsy [96]. This device has the appearance of a guidewire but is composed of a wire within a sheath. The central wire of nitinol moves within the sheath and is manipulated to cause the coiled segment to form within the ureter. It can be withdrawn into the stiffer portion of the sheath to remove the coil. The coil (7 or 10 mm diameter) acts as a barrier to prevent proximal migration of a stone or fragments. The device can also be withdrawn with a coil formed to sweep fragments distally within the ureter and into the bladder.

The NTrap is a complex nitinol-woven basket, which can be placed above a ureteral stone to catch mobile fragments and prevent retrograde migration. It also functions as a basket to collect fragments and retrieve them through the ureter. It has been successful in preventing the retrograde movement of stone fragments [97].

Another retropulsion prevention device is the accordion, which like the others is placed through the ureter and positioned proximal to the ureteral calculus. It is composed of a band of plastic film mounted along the distal portion of a shaft. It can be placed through the ureter and beyond the stone as the film collapses during placement. The inner wire of the device is withdrawn into the sheathing portion resulting in grouping of the film to form a mass structure, not unlike the folds of an accordion. It also can function as a sweeping device to remove small fragments as it is withdrawn.

Each of these three devices has been shown to be effective to prevent proximal migration of stones during endoscopic lithotripsy and to improve stone-free rates [96–98]. Results have varied regarding time savings, the need for a stent, and postoperative symptoms. One study suggested net cost saving with the use of a device under certain circumstances [99].

Another technique used to obstruct the ureter and prevent stone migration has been to inject a semi-solid gel into the ureter proximal to the stone. Water-soluble materials, which persist long enough for the lithotripsy, are used. Both lidocaine gel and specific thermosensitive gel have been used with reported success [100]. Both of these discolor with bleeding and become more difficult to use.

Basketing Techniques

There are several steps to consider in using a basket within the ureter. The first is to decide which stone to remove by basketing. Stones to avoid include those too large to move easily within the ureter, others that are impacted within the ureter, or those that must be moved through an infundibulum or a ureter that is too narrow. Stones in these cases must be fragmented before attempts at removal. In contrast, the ideal stone to be removed is the one that is small enough to pass through the ureter but possibly too large to pass spontaneously. Thus many decisions made involve stones measuring 3–4 mm.

Another important choice is which basket to use. In general, stainless steel baskets should be avoided for use in the ureter or intrarenal collecting system. Similarly helical baskets should be avoided above the distal ureter. No basket should be used blindly in the ureter from the level of the bladder. The procedure should always be performed through a ureteroscope under direct vision. Therefore only baskets of 3F or less can be considered. Narrow-shaft diameter baskets, such as those at 1.9F or less, are advantageous for many reasons. Given the slimmer profile, they take up less room in the ureteroscopic working channel. This not only allows for better irritation and visualization but also allows for the simultaneous placement of a 200-µ laser fiber, if needed, to treat an entrapped stone. Finally, they limit deflection of the flexible ureteroscope and may offer an advantage in difficult-to-reach calyces, such as those in very dependent lower pole positions. The disadvantages of slimmer baskets are (1) being relatively more expensive and (2) may be less durable compared to wider counterparts. Therefore, they should be used selectively. In general, the first choice basket in almost any situation is a 3F or less, four-wire nitinol basket. It is useful and safe in nearly every application.

The wires of the basket are compressed into the sheath by withdrawing the central wire portion with the handle, operated by one hand. The tip of the basket is advanced through the channel of the ureteroscope until it enters the field of view. The endoscope and device are then positioned to see the stone and so that the largest opening of the wires will be adjacent to the stone. It is then manipulated by opening and closing or deflecting with the tip of the ureteroscope to encourage the wires to pass around the stone. The basket is then closed as it is advanced to maintain the position of the stone within the wires. If it is just rapidly closed, then the wires may move away from the stone and release it. To extract the stone from the patient, the entire unit of stone, basket, and ureteroscope is withdrawn from the urinary tract. This movement must be monitored visually through the ureteroscope to be certain that the stone and basket are moving within the lumen and not pulling mucosa with it. This is the essential step for safely retrieving stones.

The same type of nitinol basket is the first choice for use within the intrarenal collecting system including the calyces. The atraumatic design and the flexible wires do not damage the mucosa, and the form of the basket fits into the calyx. Again, the widest part should be placed near the stone, and the basket closed to maintain the stone within the confines of the wires. If the stone is not located directly in front of the channel of the endoscope or within the range of deflection of the flexible ureteroscope, the basket can be pressed against the wall of the calyx to direct it toward the stone. The similar basket with a deflecting mechanism (dimension) can do these maneuvers in a similar pattern or has the additional capability of active deflection of the basket itself for positioning onto the stone.

It may be necessary or desirable to release a calculus from the grasping device. Release is performed when repositioning the stone within the kidney is the goal or when it is found that the stone is too large to be removed from the ureter. In either case, the nitinol basket has properties advantageous for releasing. Within the ureter, the basket is opened fully, and the shaft and sheath advanced into the lumen to remove the wires from the stone. Within a calyx, the basket is also opened fully, and the shaft advanced to roll the wires off the stone. This is usually technically straightforward but may be very difficult if the stone is too large, relative to the maximal size of the basket opening. For example, do not try to reposition a 9–10-mm stone within the kidney with a 10-mm basket. It may be engaged but be very difficult to release. It is preferable to use a larger diameter basket, such as 16-mm, which can open widely to disengage from the stone.

Some stones, by which their location directly in front of the ureteroscope cannot be engaged by a basket, call for other devices as noted above. It is also advantageous to use a device, which can easily release a stone. The three-pronged grasper is an excellent choice to be used as a retrieval device through a flexible ureteroscope throughout the upper urinary tract. It does not hold a stone or other objects as firmly as a basket, but that is its major advantage. It is extraordinarily unlikely that it will become entrapped.

Some urologists have noted difficulty using this grasper. As it is opened, the wires move forward and must be carefully positioned to avoid moving the stone. When the three wires are positioned around the stone, the device is closed. Here there is a risk of losing the position as the wires withdraw into the sheath. The operator must compensate by advancing the sheath to keep the wires on the stone. If the wires catch in the mucosa, they are difficult to remove without causing bleeding.

Another category of forward opening retrieval devices includes the NGage and the Dakota baskets. These are circumferentially engaging but open at the end rather than the side as conventional baskets. They are constructed of smooth flexible nitinol wires, which do not harm the intrarenal mucosa (Fig. 3.22). They hold stones more firmly than wire-pronged graspers but may not release them as easily. The Dakota has what has been termed the OpenSure Handle which allows increased opening specifically for otherwise entrapped stones.

Entrapped Basket

A basket containing a stone may become entrapped in the ureter during withdrawal. The first choice in treatment would be to attempt to release the stone from the basket. With the simple nitinol wire designs, the shaft/sheath of the basket is advanced in an attempt to pass the stone and unroll the wires. If this fails, the basket and stone are entrapped and require additional maneuvers. The next step is to try to move the stone proximally to a more dilated part of the ureter. The stone should then be released and fragmented further.

One step, which should be avoided entirely, is to pull harder on the basket. Avulsion of the ureter is a disastrous complication, which has occurred with blind basketing from the level of the bladder. It should never occur with visual ureteroscopic stone retrieval since there are many other options for release of the stone-containing basket.

Further fragmentation in situ can be attempted with the optimal instrumentation. If the basket within the channel has an outer dimension of less than 2F, a small diameter laser fiber may fit through the channel alongside the basket sheath. It should be positioned carefully on the stone and activated to remove the volume of stone to free the basket. The holmium laser can easily cut the wire of the basket. With a nitinol basket, this will usually free the basket for removal. If cutting the wire is done specifically, then it should be cut in the more distal portion to leave less wire distally. Nitinol is sufficiently flexible that it should not engage the mucosa. Stainless steel can form a fishhook configuration, which may become trapped in the ureteral wall.

Another option is to remove the ureteroscope leaving the basket and stone in place. The handle of the basket must be removed to allow the endoscope to be withdrawn, leaving the sheath and basket. On some retrieval devices, the handle can be released with a screw or nut mechanism. If this is not available, the handle can be freed by cutting the sheath and internal wire mechanism above the handle with scissors. The ureteroscope is then withdrawn very carefully from the patient, purposefully leaving the basket in place. The ureteroscope is replaced into the ureter and advanced under vision to laser the stone or to cut the basket. When it is impossible to see or to advance the ureteroscope, it may be necessary to place another wire into the ureter to support passage of the flexible instrument. When the stone is lodged in the mid to distal ureter, a rigid/semi-rigid ureteroscope can give better control.

Another option for release is to dilate the obstructing segment of the ureter. That area may be a short band or a longer narrow segment of the ureter. Either can be dilated to some degree to permit passage of the stone within the basket. A guidewire must be in place to allow passage of any dilator, either a graduated taper or a balloon catheter. If there was already a safety wire in place, the ureteroscope can be withdrawn over the basket shaft leaving the basket and stone in place. The dilator can then be advanced over the safety wire only to the level of the stone. The tapered portion of the balloon can be inflated adjacent to the stone, but the cylindrical portion should definitely not be. Similarly, the graduated dilator should pass only to the stone with no attempt to go beyond it. Dilating at the location of the trapped stone risks forcing it into and through the wall of the ureter. In general, tapered dilators can be used in the mid to distal ureter and a balloon catheter from the mid-ureter proximally.

If there is no safety wire, then the steps above to remove the ureteroscope are followed. A double-lumen catheter is then placed over the shaft of the basket to introduce the second wire into the ureter for dilator placement.

If these steps fail, then an antegrade approach may be best. All steps should be taken to avoid avulsion of the ureter and to avoid an open procedure if possible.

Conclusion

There is a wide range of ureteroscopic retrieval devices including baskets, graspers, and hybrid designs. The introduction of nitinol with its unique properties has made complex designs possible. These have rendered earlier rules of design and technique obsolete. Baskets do not need great opening strength to function, and releasing capability is as important as the engaging ability. Stone and basket entrapment occurs and is best prevented by judicious application of basketing. We can expect more developments in the field of stone retrieval devices.

Intracorporeal Lithotripters for Ureteroscopy

Scott G. Hubosky and Thomas J. Hardacker

Introduction

Ureteroscopy has evolved from once a diagnostic procedure to a therapeutic one for various upper urinary tract pathologies. In order to reliably treat ureteral and renal stones, intracorporeal lithotripters must be utilized together with either semi-rigid or flexible ureteroscopes. Various forms of intracorporeal lithotrites exist, but not all are broadly applicable to ureteroscopy, given the generally small working channel size and need to limit reduction in deflection of flexible instruments. Lasers, by far, are the most common intracorporeal lithotrites used today, with holmium:yttrium aluminum garnet (Ho:YAG) being the most popular, known for its reliable safety profile and practical versatility. Other available intracorporeal lithotrites include electrohydraulic lithotripsy (EHL), ultrasonic lithotripter, and pneumatic/ballistic lithotripter.

Laser Lithotrites

Holmium Laser

The most commonly used laser for the purpose of lithotripsy today is the holmium:yttrium aluminum garnet (Ho:YAG) laser. This is a solid-state pulsed laser in which holmium ions are concentrated on a YAG crystal. When excited from white light generated by a flashlamp in a laser cavity, holmium atoms emit photons at a wavelength of 2140 nm. This laser energy can be transmitted to a stone target by way of a flexible silica laser fiber, ranging in diameter from 200 to 365 microns, which fits through the standard working channel of a flexible or semi-rigid ureteroscope. Due to its emitted wavelength, holmium is significantly absorbed by water and has a shallow depth of tissue penetration at 0.4 mm, although an ex vivo study has shown longer incisional depths, which vary with higher energy and frequency settings [101]. Nevertheless, holmium is still considered one of the safest and most versatile lasers used in urology and has stood the test of time, since its clinical introduction in the early 1990s [102, 103]. In terms of lithotrite performance, holmium is effective on all types of urinary tract stones, is independent of density, and produces the smallest resultant fragments for a given stone composition, when compared to EHL, pulsed dye laser, and pneumatic lithotripters [104]. Although disadvantageous from a cost standpoint, holmium is often considered worth the investment since higher-power systems are versatile enough to support not only lithotripsy cases in the upper and lower urinary tract but also laser incision of ureteral strictures, ablation of upper tract urothelial carcinoma [105], and ablative/enucleation procedures for benign prostatic hyperplasia [106].

The ablative effect of the holmium laser is due to a photothermal mechanism, which chemically decomposes the calculus by way of direct absorbance of radiation by the stone [107, 108]. Stone fragmentation depends on the total power delivered to the target stone, which in turn is determined by the energy applied (measured in joules) and the frequency (Hz). The latest holmium laser platforms are multicavity laser systems, which provide power of up to 120 watts. In general, when choosing holmium laser settings (laser dosimetry), there are three variables, which potentially can be manipulated: the pulse energy (joules), the number of pulses produced by the laser per second or frequency (Hz), and the pulse width (μs). Increasing pulse energy will increase ablative capacity (more volume of stone ablated with less time) but also results in production of relatively larger resultant fragments [109], leads to laser fiber-tip degradation, and target stone retropulsion [110]. Keeping pulse energy relatively low, such as 0.2 joules, will produce the smallest resultant fragments [109] but will also decrease ablative volume, which is why high frequencies are often employed in this situation (dusting settings). Higher-frequency settings will increase the fragmentation rate for a given pulse energy but can cause retropulsion, especially at higher pulse energies. Increasing pulse width has been shown to reduce retropulsion [111], which is useful when treating stones in a dilated ureter or collecting system. Fragmentation rate can also vary with laser fiber size but seems mostly to apply to larger diameter fibers when using pulse energies >1.0 joule [112].

Moses Platform

Pulse modulation with the holmium laser is a process currently being explored and essentially changes how energy is delivered to a calculus. The 120-watt holmium laser generator with "Moses technology" (Lumenis Ltd., Yokneam, Israel) serves to improve efficiency during stone fragmentation by dividing laser energy into two distinct pulses. The initial pulse separates fluid between the fiber and the stone, while the second pulse delivers energy directly to the target calculus. Overall, this results in more efficient energy delivery from the fiber to the stone. In vivo and in vitro studies have demonstrated decreased retropulsion and increased stone ablation with Moses technology, particularly in softer stones [113, 114]. A recent prospective, double-blinded study involving 72 consecutive patients with renal stone burden between 1.4 and 1.7 cm, demonstrated that the use of the Moses mode compared to conventional holmium laser mode resulted in significantly decreased overall procedure time and fragmentation/pulverization time, saving almost 10 minutes and 7 minutes, respectively [115]. Interestingly, between the two groups, there was essentially equal lasing time and laser energy applied. The conclusions were that Moses mode saved time due to less stone retropulsion compared to conventional mode, requiring fewer pauses during laser fragmentation to adjust the laser fiber. An important study limitation was that Moses mode was compared to conventional mode with short pulse width and not long pulse width, which potentially could have altered the results.

Thulium Fiber Laser

While thulium:YAG has been utilized for several decades in benign prostate surgery, thulium fiber laser (TFL) energy is an emerging modality for lithotripsy with a wavelength of 1940 nm, compared to 2140 nm for the holmium laser. This modality confers several benefits over traditional holmium energy, including lower amperage requirements, frequency settings in excess of 600 Hz, decreased stone retropulsion, and laser fibers between 50 and 150 μm that allow for improved irrigation and deflection [116]. TFL results in higher ablation energy at lower pulse width compared to holmium, in part owing to its higher absorption peak in water, which has been hypothesized to correlate with improved fragmentation [117]. TFL produces a smaller vaporization bubble compared to holmium, resulting in decreased retropulsion and more efficient energy delivery to the stone [116, 117].

TFL has been demonstrated in vitro by Blackmon and colleagues to result in two to four times higher fragmentation rates for uric acid and calcium oxalate monohydrate stones when compared to standard holmium [118]. In one of the initial clinical analyses of TFL during stone surgery, Enikeev and colleagues demonstrated that this modality is both safe and effective during PCNL, with limited retropulsion [119]. In addition, efficiency of the thulium laser was independent of stone density, as well. Overall, TFL has properties that in theory yield benefits of increased deflection, increased fragmentation, and decreased retropulsion compared to traditional laser energy sources.

Electrohydraulic Lithotripsy (EHL)

Electrohydraulic lithotripsy (EHL) has been utilized for the treatment of calculi within the genitourinary tract since the 1950s, where it was initially employed in the treatment of bladder stones [120]. EHL employs two electrodes that produce a spark when activated, causing transition of irrigant fluid to gaseous state, resulting in a

360-degree plasma shockwave. Resulting collapse of the shockwave creates a cavitation bubble, causing high-pressure microjets and secondary shockwave to induce stone fragmentation [121].

EHL was initially employed for treatment of upper tract calculi prior to the availability of endoscopic visualization. Significant collateral damage, particularly within the ureter, was noted even after small-caliber ureteroscopes were developed. As a result, EHL was utilized for lower pole renal stones that were inaccessible secondary to reduced deflection with laser fibers in the working channel. EHL probes – available in sizes from 1.9 to 3.3 French – result in improved deflection and increased access in these scenarios, even compared to smaller caliber laser fibers. Importantly, EHL is contraindicated for treatment of ureteral stones, owing to the significant rates of ureteral perforation, which can range from 8.5 to 17.6% [121–123]. Owing to larger working area, EHL can safely be used within the confines of the kidney, though perforation rates remain higher than with other modalities. EHL has been described in combination with holmium laser energy during ureteroscopy for treatment of renal stones greater than 4 cm with reasonable results [124] although this is not a first-line recommendation. Despite its potential for urothelial surface insult, secondary to its mechanism of action, EHL still maintains a select utility for renal stones that are challenging to access with standard laser fibers or when a laser is not available. Additionally, EHL is quite efficacious for removing encrustation from stent curls with less risk of fracturing the stent, relative to the holmium laser. Again, EHL should be avoided in the ureter.

Pneumatic/Ballistic Lithotripsy

Ballistic lithotripsy relies on a projectile physically making contact with a stone and mechanically fragmenting it, similar to a jackhammer. Most ballistic lithotripters used compressed air to propel the projectile. Although more commonly used during PCNL, pneumatic/ballistic lithotripters can be used during semi-rigid URS. Models are available which are light and portable and make use of a detachable cartridge of high-pressure CO_2 [125]. Advantages also include relatively low cost, but the main challenges include retropulsion of the target stone and generation of relatively larger resultant fragments, especially compared to those produced by Ho:YAG lasers [104]. Flexible pneumatic/ballistic probes exist for flexible ureteroscopy, but their impact momentum significantly decreases even with a small amount of deflection [126], essentially making them inferior to other available modalities.

Conclusion

Many intracorporeal lithotripters are available for use during ureteroscopy. Ho:YAG laser is the most widely utilized and the most versatile since it can be used to treat numerous other urologic pathologies. The thulium fiber laser is relatively new, but preliminary studies suggest it may offer additional benefit due to less retropulsion, and its smaller fiber diameter offers better deflection and visualization. Cost is the primary disadvantage of laser lithotripsy. EHL serves a limited role in the kidney, especially when laser fibers limit deflectability or are unavailable. Pneumatic/ballistic lithotripsy is an affordable alternative during semi-rigid URS, but disadvantages include relatively larger resultant fragments and retropulsion.

Disclosures Financial Disclosure: Prof. Olivier Traxer is a consultant for Coloplast, Rocamed, Olympus, EMS, and Boston Scientific.

Financial Disclosure: Prof. Demetrius Bagley receives royalties from Olympus/ACMI and BD/Bard.

Financial Disclosure: Prof. Scott Hubosky is a consultant for Boston Scientific and BD/Bard.

Funding Support: Dr. Vincent De Coninck is supported by a EUSP scholarship from the European Association of Urology and by a grant from the Belgische Vereniging voor Urologie (BVU).

Funding Support: Dr. Etienne Xavier Keller is supported by a travel grant from the University Hospital Zurich and by a grant from the Kurt and Senta Herrmann Foundation.

Dr. Etienne Xavier Keller is supported by a travel grant from the University Hospital Zurich and by a grant from the Kurt and Senta Herrmann Foundation.

References

Ureteroscope Specifications: Flexible, Semi-rigid, and Single Use

1. Young HH, McKay RW. Congenital valvular obstruction of the prostatic urethra. Surg Gynecol Obstet. 1929;48:509.
2. Wickham JEA, Miller RA. Endoscopic instruments and their accessories. In: Wickham JEA, Miller RA, editors. Percutaneous renal surgery. New York: Churchill Livingstone; 1983. p. 45–74.
3. Lyon E, Kyker JS, Schoenberg HW. Transurethral ureteroscopy in women: a ready addition to the urological armamentarium. J Urol. 1978;119:35–6.
4. Pérez-Castro EE, Martinez-Piniero JA. Transurethral ureteroscopy: a current urological procedure. Arch Esp Urol. 1980;33:445–60.
5. Marshall V. Fiber optics in urology. J Urol. 1964;64:1033–8.
6. Takagi T, Go T, Takayasu H, Aso Y. Fiberoptic pyeloureteroscopy. Surgery. 1971;70:661.
7. Dretler SP, Cho G. Semirigid ureteroscopy: a new genre. J Urol. 1989;141:1314–6.
8. Somani BK, Al-Qahtani SM, de Medina SD, Traxer O. Outcomes of flexible ureterorenoscopy and laser fragmentation for renal stones: comparison between digital and conventional ureteroscope. Urology. 2013;82:1017–9.
9. Tosoian JJ, Ludwig W, Sopko N, Mullins JK, Matlaga BR. The effect of repair costs on the profitability of a ureteroscopy program. J Endourol. 2015;29:406–9.
10. Proietti S, Somani B, Sofer M, Pietropaolo A, Rosso M, Saitta G, et al. The "body mass index" of flexible ureteroscopes. J Endourol. 2017;31:1090–5.
11. Ludwig WW, Lee G, Ziemba JB, Ko JS, Matlaga BR. Evaluating the ergonomics of flexible ureteroscopy. J Endourol. 2017;31:1062–6.
12. Dragos L, Somani BK, Sener ET, Butticè S, Proietti S, Ploumidis A, et al. Which flexible ureteroscopes (digital vs. fiber-optic) can easily reach the difficult lower pole calices and

have better end-tip deflection: in vitro study on k-box. A PETRA evaluation. J Endourol. 2017;31:630–7.

13. Talso M, Emiliani E, Haddad M, Berthe L, Baghdadi M, Montanari E, et al. Laser fiber and flexible ureteroscopy: the safety distance concept. J Endourol. 2016;30:1269–74.

14. Monga M, Best S, Venkatesh R, Ames C, Lee C, Kuskowski M, et al. Durability of flexible ureteroscopes: a randomized prospective study. J Urol. 2006;176:137–41.

15. Traxer O, Dubosq F, Jamali K, Gattegno B, Thibault P. New-generation flexible ureterorenoscopes are more durable than previous ones. Urology. 2006;68:276–9; discussion 280–1.

16. Defidio L, De Dominicis M, Di Gianfrancesco L, Fuchs G, Patel A. Improving flexible ureteroscope durability up to 100 procedures. J Endourol. 2012;26:1329–34.

17. Knudsen B, Miyaoka R, Shah K, Holden T, Turk T, Pedro RN, et al. Durability of the next-generation flexible fiberoptic ureteroscopes: a randomized prospective multi-institutional clinical trial. Urology. 2010;75:534–8.

18. Carey RI, Martin CJ, Knego JR. Prospective evaluation of refurbished flexible ureteroscope durability seen in a large public tertiary care center with multiple surgeons. Urology. 2014;84:42–5.

19. Bader MJ, Gratzke C, Walther S, Schlenker B, Tilki D, Hocaoglu Y, et al. The Polyscope. A modular design, semidisposable flexible ureterorenoscope system. J Endourol. 2010;24:1061–6.

20. Proietti S, Dragos L, Molina W, Doizi S, Giusti G, Traxer O. Comparison of new single-use digital flexible ureteroscope versus nondisposable fiber optic and digital ureteroscope in a cadaveric model. J Endourol. 2016;30:655–9.

21. Doizi S, Kamphuis G, Giusti G, Andreassen KH, Knoll T, Osther PJ, et al. First clinical evaluation of a new single-use flexible ureteroscope (LithoVue): a European prospective multicentric feasibility study. World J Urol. 2017;35:809–18.

22. Dragos LB, Somani BK, Keller EX, De Coninck VJM, Rodriguez-Monsalve Herrero M, Kamphuis GM, et al. Characteristics of current digital single-use flexible ureteroscopes versus their reusable counterparts: an *in-vitro* comparative analysis. Transl Androl Urol. 2019 Sep;8(Suppl 4):S359–70.

23. Martin JC, McAdams SB, Abdul-Muhsin H, Lim VM, Nunez-Nateras R, Tyson MD, et al. The economic implications of a reusable flexible digital ureteroscope: a cost-benefit analysis. J Urol. 2017;197:730–5.

Robotic Platforms for Ureteroscopy

24. Rassweiler J, Fielder M, Charalampogiannis N, Kabakci AS, Saglam R, Klein JT. Robot-assisted flexible ureteroscopy: an update. Urolithiasis. 2018;46:69–77.

25. Desai MM, Aron M, Gill IS, Haber GP, Ukimura O, Kaouk JH, et al. Flexible robotic retrograde renoscopy: description of novel robotic device and preliminary laboratory experience. Urology. 2008;72:42–6.

26. Buttice S, Proietti S, Dragos L, Traxer O. Are you familiar with the flow of the Roboflex Avicenna pump? Allow me to explain. J Endourol. 2017;31:418–9.

27. Saglam R, Muslumanoglu AY, Tokatli Z, Caskurlu T, Sarica K, Tasci A, et al. A new robot for flexible ureteroscopy: development and early clinical results (IDEAL stage 1-2b). Eur Urol. 2014;66:1092–100.

28. Geavlete P, Saglam R, Georgescu D, Multescu R, Iordache V, Kabakci AS, et al. Robotic flexible ureteroscopy versus classic flexible ureteroscopy in renal stones: the initial Romanian experience. Chirurgia. 2016;111:326–9.

29. Proietti S, Dragos L, Emiliani E, Buttice S, Talso M, Baghdadi M, et al. Ureteroscopic skills with and without Roboflex Avicenna in the K-box((R)) simulator. Cent Eur J Urol. 2017;70:76–80.

30. Klein J, Charalampogiannis N, Fiedler M, Wakileh G, Gozen A, Rassweiler J. Analysis of performance factors in 240 consecutive cases of robot-assited flexible ureteroscopic stone treatment. J Robotic Surg. 2021;15:265–74.

Guidewires

31. Seldinger SI. Catheter replacement of the needle in percutaneous arteriography; a new technique. Acta Radiol. 1953;39:368–76.
32. Schroder J. The mechanical properties of guidewires. Part 1: stiffness and torsional strength. Cardiovasc Intervent Radiol. 1993;16:43–6.
33. Smith AD, Lange PH, Miller RP, Reinke DB. Introduction of the Gibbons ureteral stent facilitated by antecedent percutaneous nephrostomy. J Urol. 1978;120:543–4.
34. Fritzsche P, Moorhead JD, Axford PD, Torrey RR. Urologic applications of angiographic guidewire and catheter techniques. J Urol. 1981;125:774–80.
35. Clayman M, Uribe CA, Eichel L, Gordon Z, McDougall EM, Clayman RV. Comparison of guide wires in urology. Which, when and why? J Urol. 2004;171:2146–50.
36. Rosenberg BH, Averch TD. Ancillary instrumentation for ureteroscopy. Urol Clin North Am. 2004;31:49–59.
37. Holden T, Pedro RN, Hendlin K, Durfee W, Monga M. Evidence-based instrumentation for flexible ureteroscopy: a review. J Endourol. 2008;22:1423–6.
38. Warde N. Stones: safety guidewire unnecessary during flexible ureteroscopy for routine cases of nephrolithiasis. Nat Rev Urol. 2010;7:645.
39. Dickstein RJ, Kreshover JE, Babayan RK, Wang DS. Is a safety wire necessary during routine flexible ureteroscopy? J Endourol. 2010;24:1589–92.
40. Liguori G, Antoniolli F, Trombetta C, Biasotto M, Amodeo A, Pomara G, et al. Comparative experimental evaluation of guidewire use in urology. Urology. 2008;72:286–9; discussion 289–90.
41. Dutta R, Vyas A, Landman J, Clayman RV. Death of the safety guidewire. J Endourol. 2016;30:941–4.
42. Assimos D, Krambeck A, Miller NL, Monga M, Murad MH, Nelson CP, et al. Surgical management of stones: American Urological Association/Endourological Society guideline, part 1. J Urol. 2016;196:1153–60.
43. Turk C, Petrik A, Sarica K, Sietz C, Skolarikos A, Straub M, et al. EAU guidelines on interventional treatment for urolithiasis. Eur Urol. 2016;69:475–82.
44. Eandi JA, Hu B, Low RK. Evaluation of the impact and need for use of a safety guidewire during ureteroscopy. J Endourol. 2008;22:1653–8.
45. Ulvik O, Wentzel-Larsen T, Ulvik NM. A safety guidewire influences the pushing and pulling forces needed to move the ureteroscope in the ureter: a clinical randomized, crossover study. J Endourol. 2013;27:850–5.
46. Patel SR, McLaren ID, Nakada SY. The ureteroscope as a safety wire for ureteronephroscopy. J Endourol. 2012;26:351–4.
47. Doizi S, Herrmann T, Traxer O. Death of the safety guidewire. J Endourol. 2017;31:619–20.

Ureteral Access Sheaths

48. Takayasu H, Aso Y. Recent development for pyeloureteroscopy: guide tube method for its introduction into the ureter. J Urol. 1974;112:176–8.
49. Pedro RN, Weiland D, Reardon S, Monga M. Ureteral access sheath insertion forces: implications for design and training. Urol Res. 2007;35:107–9.

50. Doizi S, Knoll T, Scoffone CM, Breda A, Brehmer M, Liatsikos E, et al. First clinical evaluation of a new innovative ureteral access sheath (Re-Trace (TM)): a European study. World J Urol. 2014;32:143–7.
51. Breda A, Emiliani E, Millan F, Scoffone CN, Knoll T, Osther PJS, et al. The new concept of ureteral access sheath with guidewire disengagement: one wire does it all. World J Urol. 2016;34:603–6.
52. Delto JC, Wayne G, Sidhu A, Yanes R, Bhandari A, Nieder AM. The single wire ureteral access sheath, both safe and economical. Adv Urol. 2016;2016:6267953. https://doi.org/10.1155/2016/6267953.
53. Hubosky SG, Healy KA, Grasso M, Bagley DH. Assessing the difficult ureter and the importance of ureteroscope miniaturization: history is repeating itself. Urology. 2014;84:740–2.
54. Al-Qahtani SM, Letendre J, Thomas A, Natalin R, Saussez T, Traxer O. Which ureteral access sheath is compatible with your flexible ureteroscope? J Endourol. 2014;28:286–90.
55. Kourambas J, Byrne RR, Preminger GM. Does a ureteral access sheath facilitate ureteroscopy? J Urol. 2001;165:789–93.
56. Traxer O, Wendt-Nordahl G, Sodha H, Rassweiler J, Meretyk S, Tefekli A, et al. Differences in renal stone treatment and outcomes for patients treated either with or without the support of a ureteral access sheath: the Clinical Research Office of the Endourological Society Ureteroscopy Global Study. World J Urol. 2015;33:2137–44.
57. Rehman J, Monga M, Landman J, Lee DI, Felfela T, Conradie MC, et al. Characterization of intrapelvic pressure during ureteropyeloscopy with ureteral access sheaths. Urology. 2003;61:713–8.
58. Sener TE, Cloutier J, Villa L, Marson F, Buttice S, Doizi S, et al. Can we provide low intrarenal pressures with good irrigation flow by decreasing the size of ureteral access sheaths? J Endourol. 2016;30:49–55.
59. Ng YH, Somani BK, Dennison A, Kata SG, Nabi G, Brown S. Irrigant flow and intrarenal pressure during flexible ureteroscopy: the effect of different access sheaths, working channel instruments, and hydrostatic pressure. J Endourol. 2010;24:1915–20.
60. Auge BK, Pietrow PK, Lallas CD, Raj GV, Santa-Cruz RW, Preminger GM. Ureteral access sheath provides protection against elevated renal pressures during routine flexible ureteroscopic stone manipulation. J Endourol. 2004;18:33–6.
61. L'Esperance JO, Ekeruo WO, Scales CD, Marguet CG, Springhart WP, Maloney ME, et al. Effect of ureteral access sheath on stone-free rates in patients undergoing ureteroscopic management of renal calculi. Urology. 2005;66:252–5.
62. Berquet G, Prunel P, Verhoest G, Mathieu R, Bensalah K. The use of a ureteral access sheath does not improve stone-free rate after ureteroscopy for upper urinary tract stones. World J Urol. 2014;32:229–32.
63. Zelenko N, Coll D, Rosenfeld AT, Smith RC. Normal ureter size on unenhanced helical CT. AJR Am J Roentgenol. 2004;182:1039–41.
64. Traxer O, Thomas A. Prospective evaluation and classification of ureteral wall injuries resulting from insertion of a ureteral access sheath during retrograde intrarenal surgery. J Urol. 2013;189:580–4.
65. Mogilevkin Y, Sofer M, Margel D, Greenstein A, Lifshitz D. Predicting an effective ureteral access sheath insertion: a bicenter prospective study. J Endourol. 2014;28:1414–7.
66. Kawahara T, Ito H, Terao H, Ishigaki H, Ogawa T, Uemura H, et al. Preoperative stenting for ureteroscopic lithotripsy for a large renal stone. Int J Urol. 2012;19:881–5.
67. Viers BR, Viers LD, Hull NC, Hanson TJ, Mehta RA, Bergstralh EJ, et al. The difficult ureter: clinical and radiographic characteristics associated with upper urinary tract access at the time of ureteroscopic stone treatment. Urology. 2015;86:878–84.
68. Kuntz NJ, Neisius A, Tsivian M, Ghaffar M, Patel N, Ferrandino MN, et al. Balloon dilation of the ureter: a contemporary review of outcomes and complications. J Urol. 2015;194:413–7.
69. Mahajan PM, Padhye AS, Bhave AA, Sovani YB, Kshirsagar YB, Bapat SS. Is stenting required before retrograde intrarenal surgery with access sheath. Indian J Urol. 2009;25:326–8.

70. Multescu R, Geavlete B, Georgescu D, Geavlete P. Improved durability of flex-xc digital flexible ureteroscope: how long can you expect it to last? Urology. 2014;84:32–5.
71. Pietrow PK, Auge BK, Delvecchio FC, Silverstein AD, Weizer AZ, Albala DM, et al. Techniques to maximize flexible ureteroscope longevity. Urology. 2002;60:784–8.
72. Turna B, Stein RJ, Smaldone MC, Santos BR, Kefer JC, Jackman SV, et al. Safety and efficacy of flexible ureterorenoscopy and holmium: YAG lithotripsy for intrarenal stones in anticoagulated cases. J Urol. 2008;179:1415–9.
73. Singh A, Shah G, Young J, Sheridan M, Haas G, Upadhyay J. Ureteral access sheath for the management of pediatric renal and ureteral stones: a single center experience. J Urol. 2006;175:1080–2.
74. Wang HH, Huang L, Routh JC, Kokorowski P, Cilento BG, Nelson CP. Use of the ureteral access sheath during ureteroscopy in children. J Urol. 2011;186(4 SUPPL):1728–33.
75. Kokorowski PJ, Chow JS, Strauss K, Pennison M, Routh JC, Nelson CP. Prospective measurement of patient exposure to radiation during pediatric ureteroscopy. J Urol. 2012;187:1408–14.
76. Miernik A, Wilhelm K, Ardelt PU, Adams F, Kuehhas FE, Schoenthaler M. Standardized flexible ureteroscopic technique to improve stone-free rates. Urology. 2012;80:1198–202.
77. Guzelburc V, Guven S, Boz MY, Erkurt B, Soytas M, Altay B, et al. Intraoperative evaluation of ureteral access sheath-related injuries using post-ureteroscopic lesion scale. J. Laparoendosc. Adv. Surg. Tech. 2016;26:23–6.
78. Delvecchio FC, Auge BK, Brizuela RM, Weizer AZ, Silverstein AD, Lallas CD, et al. Assessment of stricture formation with the ureteral access sheath. Urology. 2003;61:518–22; discussion 522.
79. Oguz U, Sahin T, Senocak C, Ozyuvali E, Bozkurt OF, Resorlu B, et al. Factors associated with postoperative pain after retrograde intrarenal surgery for kidney stones. Turkish J Urol. 2017;43:303–8.

Stone Retrieval Devices

80. Council WA. A new ureteral stone extractor and dilator. JAMA. 1926;86:1907–8.
81. Johnson FP. A new method of removing ureteral calculi. J Urol. 1937;37:84–9.
82. Rusche CF, Bacon SK. Injury to the ureter due to cystoscopic intraureteral instrumentation: report of sixteen cases. J Urol. 1940;44:777–93.
83. Dormia E. Due nuovi apparecchi per la rimozione dei calculi dall' uretere. Urologia. 1958;25:225–33.
84. Pfister RR, Schwartz R. Development of ureteral stone basket. Urology. 1975;3:337–8.
85. Hart JB. Avulsion of distal ureter with Dormia basket. J Urol. 1967;97:62–3.
86. Hodge J. Avulsion of long segment of ureter with Dormia basket. Br J Urol. 1973;45:328.
87. Fernstrom I, Johansson B. Percutaneous pyelolithotomy. A new extraction technique. Scan J Urol Nephrol. 1976;10:257–9.
88. Honey RJ. Assessment of a new tipless nitinol stone basket and comparison with an existing flat-wire basket. J Endourol. 1998;12:529–31.
89. el-Gabry EA, Bagley DH. Retrieval capabilities of different stone basket designs in vitro. J Endourol. 1999;13:305–7.
90. Lukasewycz S, Skenazy J, Hoffman N, Kuskowski M, Hendlin K, Monga M. Comparison of nitinol tipless stone baskets in an in vitro caliceal model. J Urol. 2004;172:562–4.
91. Chenven ES, Bagley DH. Retrieval and releasing capabilities of stone-basket designs in vitro. J Endourol. 2005;19:204–9.
92. Zeltser IS, Bagley DH. Basket design as a factor in retention and release of calculi in vitro. J Endourol. 2007;21:337–42.

93. Ptashnyk T, Cueva-Martinez A, Michel MS, Alken P, Köhrmann KU. Comparative investigations on the retrieval capabilities of various baskets and graspers in four ex vivo models. Eur Urol. 2002;41:406–10.

94. Bechis SK, Abbott JE, Sur RL. *In vitro* head-to-head comparison of the durability, versatility and efficacy of the NGage and novel Dakota stone retrieval baskets. Transl Androl Urol. 2017;6:1144–9.

95. Matlaga B, Healy KA, Kaplan A, Leavitt D. MP 27-9 moving from four hands to two during flexible ureteroscopy with stone manipulation. J Endourol. 2018;32:A273–4.

96. Eisner BH, Dretler SP. Use of the stone cone for prevention of calculus retropulsion during holmium:YAG laser lithotripsy: case series and review of the literature. Urol Int. 2009;82:356–60.

97. Jiang K, Male M, Yu X, Chen Z, Sun F, Yuan H. Efficacy and safety of NTrap® stone entrapment and extraction device for ureteroscopic lithotripsy. Urol J. 2020; https://doi.org/10.22037/uj.v0i0.5584. Epub ahead of print.

98. Pagnani CJ, El Akkad M, Bagley DH. Prevention of stone migration with the accordion during endoscopic ureteral lithotripsy. J Endourol. 2012;26:484–8.

99. Ursiny M, Eisner BH. Cost-effectiveness of anti-retropulsion devices for ureteroscopic lithotripsy. J Urol. 2013;189:1762–6.

100. Elashry OM, Tawfik AM. Preventing stone retropulsion during intracorporeal lithotripsy. Nat Rev Urol. 2012;9:691–8.

Intracorporeal Lithotripters for Ureteroscopy

101. Emiliani E, Talso M, Haddad M, Pouliquen C, Derman J, Côté JF, et al. The true ablation effect of Holmium YAG laser on soft tissue. J Endourol. 2018;32:230–5.

102. Johnson DE, Cromeens DM, Price RE. Use of the holmium:YAG laser in urology. Lasers Surg Med. 1992;12:353–63.

103. Wolf JS. Editorial: laughing all the way…Ho, Ho, Holmium. J Urol. 1998;159:695.

104. Teichman JM, Vassar GJ, Bishoff JT, Bellman GC. Holmium: YAG lithotripsy yields smaller fragments than Lithoclast, pulsed dye laser or electrohydraulic lithotripsy. J Urol. 1998;159:17–23.

105. Erhard MJ, Bagley DH. Urologic applications of the Holmium laser: preliminary experience. J Endourol. 1995;9:383–6.

106. Gilling PJ, Cass CB, Cresswell MD, Fraundorfer MR. Holmium laser resection of the prostate: preliminary results of a new method for the treatment of benign prostatic hyperplasia. Urology. 1996;47:48–51.

107. Chan KF, Vassar GJ, Pfefer TJ, Teichman JM, Glickman RD, Weintraub ST, et al. Holmium:YAG laser lithotripsy: a dominant photothermal ablative mechanism with chemical decomposition of urinary calculi. Lasers Surg Med. 1999;25:22–37.

108. Vassar GJ, Chan KF, Teichman JM, Glickman RD, Weintraub ST, Pfefer TJ. Holmium:YAG lithotripsy: photothermal mechanism. J Endourol. 1999;13:181–90.

109. Sea J, Jonat LM, Chew BH, Qiu J, Wang B, Hoopman J, et al. Optimal power settings for Holmium:YAG lithotripsy. J Urol. 2012;187:914–9.

110. Lee H, Ryan RT, Teichman JM, Kim J, Choi B, Arakeri NV, et al. Stone retropulsion during holmium:YAG lithotripsy. J Urol. 2003;169:881–5.

111. Kang HW, Lee H, Teichman JM, Oh J, Kim J, Welch AJ. Dependence of calculus retropulsion on pulse duration during Ho:YAG laser lithotripsy. Lasers Surg Med. 2006;38:762–72.

112. Kuo RL, Aslan P, Zhong P, Preminger GM. Impact of holmium laser settings and fiber diameter on stone fragmentation and endoscope deflection. J Endourol. 1998;12:523–7.

113. Elhilali M, Badaan S, Ibrahim A, Andonian S. Use of Moses Technology to improve holmium laser lithotripsy outcomes. J Endourol. 2017;31:598–604.

114. Winship B, Wollin D, Carlos E, Li J, Peters C, Simmons WN, et al. Dusting efficiency of the Moses holmium laser: an automated in vitro assessment. J Endourol. 2018;32:1131–5.
115. Ibrahim A, Elhilali M, Fahmy N, Carrier S, Andonian S. Double-blinded prospective randomized clinical trial comparing regular and Moses modes of holmium laser lithotripsy. J Endourol. 2020;34:624–8.
116. Traxer O, Keller EX. Thulium fiber laser: the new player for kidney stone treatment? A comparison with Holmium: YAG laser. World J Urol. 2020;38:1883–94.
117. Aldoukhi AH, Black KM, Ghani KR. Emerging laser techniques for the management of stones. Urol Clin N Am. 2019;46:193–205.
118. Blackmon RL, Irby PB, Fried NM. Holmium:YAG (lambda = 2,120 nm) versus thulium fiber (lambda = 1,908 nm) laser lithotripsy. Lasers Surg Med. 2010;42:232–6.
119. Enikeev D, Taratkin M, Klimov R, Alyaev Y, Rapoport L, Gazimiev M, et al. Thulium-fiber laser for lithotripsy: first clinical experience in percutaneous nephrolithotomy. World J Urol. 2020;38:3069–74.
120. Grocela JA, Dretler SP. Intracorporeal lithotripsy. Instrumentation and development. Urol Clin North Am. 1997;24:13–23.
121. Vorreuther R, Corleis R, Klotz T, Bernards P, Engelmann U. Impact of shock wave pattern and cavitation bubble size on tissue damage during ureteroscopic electrohydraulic lithotripsy. J Urol. 1995;153:849–53.
122. Hofbauer J, Höbarth K, Marberger M. Electrohydraulic versus pneumatic disintegration in the treatment of ureteral stones: a randomized, prospective trial. J Urol. 1995;153:623–5.
123. Assimos D, Krambeck A, Miller NL, Monga M, Murad MH, Nelson CP, et al. Surgical Management of Stones: American Urological Association/Endourological Society guideline, part I. J Urol. 2016;196:1153–60.
124. Mariani A. Combined electrohydraulic and holmium:YAG laser ureteroscopic nephrolithotripsy of larger (greater than 4 cm) renal calculi. J Urol. 2007;177:168–73.
125. Nerli RB, Koura AC, Prabha V, Kamat G, Alur SB. Use of LMA stonebreaker as an intracorporeal lithotrite in the management of ureteral calculi. J Endourol. 2008;22:641–3.
126. Zhu S, Kourambas J, Munver R, Preminger GM, Zhong P. Quantification of the tip movement of lithotripsy flexible pneumatic probes. J Urol. 2000;164:1735–9.

Chapter 4
Basic Techniques

Steeve Doizi, Etienne Xavier Keller, Scott G. Hubosky, Olivier Traxer, Nitin Sharma, Michael Grasso III, and Edward J. Kloniecke

Fundamental Maneuvering During Ureteroscopy

Steeve Doizi, Etienna Xavier Keller, Olivier Traxer, and Scott G. Hubosky

Introduction

During the last four decades, patients with upper urinary tract stones have benefited from many technological advances including the development of ureteroscopy (URS), in both semi-rigid and flexible forms. In turn, there has been a widening of ureteroscopic indications including both the diagnostic and therapeutic management of upper urinary tract pathologies such as urolithiasis and urothelial tumors. Certain fundamental principles are necessary to employ in order to ensure safe and effective outcomes during ureteroscopy.

S. Doizi · E. X. Keller · O. Traxer
Sorbonne Université, GRC n°20, Groupe de Recherche Clinique sur la Lithiase Urinaire, Hôpital Tenon, Paris, France
e-mail: steeve.doizi@aphp.fr; olivier.traxer@aphp.fr

S. G. Hubosky (✉) · E. J. Kloniecke
Department of Urology, Sidney Kimmel Medical College at Thomas Jefferson University Hospital, Philadelphia, PA, USA
e-mail: scott.hubosky@jefferson.edu; Edward.Kloniecke@jefferson.edu

N. Sharma
Phelps Memorial Hospital, Sleepy Hollow, NY, USA

M. Grasso III
Department of Urology, New York Medical College, Valhalla, NY, USA

© Springer Nature Switzerland AG 2022
S. G. Hubosky et al. (eds.), *Advanced Ureteroscopy*,
https://doi.org/10.1007/978-3-030-82351-1_4

General Considerations

Whether it is semi-rigid or flexible ureteroscopy (fURS), the procedure begins with cystoscopy to rule out any significant pathology in the bladder and to identify the location and configuration of the ureteric orifices. At this point, performance of a baseline retrograde pyelogram (RGP) is considered, especially if any ureteral pathology is anticipated. A cone-tipped catheter or similar device can provide a high-quality RGP without cannulating the ureteral orifice with a wire (Fig. 4.1). At this point, a guidewire can be placed with fluoroscopic guidance to function as either a working wire or a safety wire, depending on the situation. A dual-lumen catheter can be placed to allow for both a working and a safety wire, if desired. Both the European Association of Urology and American Urological Association guidelines generally recommend the use of a safety wire [1, 2] but acknowledge that groups have published on safe performance of ureteroscopy without it [3–8]. In general, a safety wire is particularly useful anytime the ureter is considered at risk, especially if ureteral pathology is present or manual ureteroscopic removal of stone fragments is planned without the use of a ureteral access sheath. Moreover, the use of a safety guidewire ensures access to the collecting system and facilitates the insertion of a stent in case of ureteric or collecting system injury such as ureteral perforation or excessive bleeding. Although considered a routine step, safety wire insertion should not be treated as an insignificant, rote, or mundane maneuver.

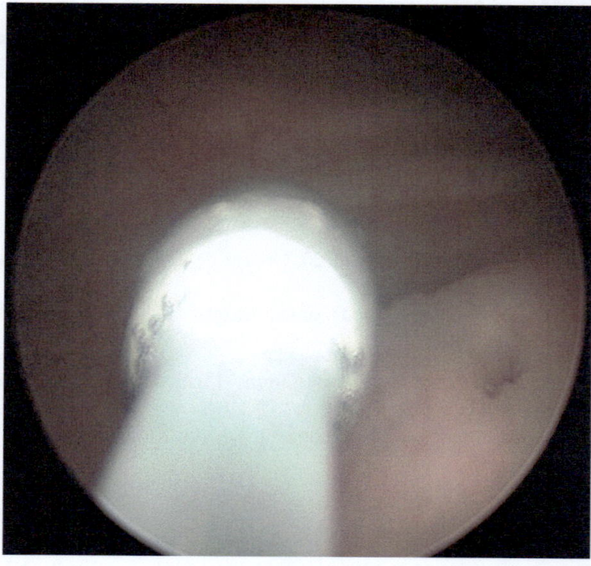

Fig. 4.1 Cone-tipped catheters provide a seal at the ureteral orifice to allow for retrograde pyelogram

Advancement of too great a length of wire can cause surface abrasions and lead to collecting system bleeding with resultant impaired visualization of the intrarenal luminal compartment, making simple cases unnecessarily difficult (Fig. 4.2). After the guidewire is placed, the bladder should be emptied to avoid compression of the intramural ureter, which will facilitate ureteroscope passage.

Semi-rigid Ureteroscope Insertion

Semi-rigid ureteroscopy is preferred for pathology that affects the distal ureter, since flexible ureteroscopes traditionally tend to buckle in this area, although newer flexible models with improved durometer are less likely to do so [3]. After confirming the presence, condition, and general location of the ureteral orifice with cystoscopy, a semi-rigid ureteroscope can be inserted. With a guidewire in place, the ureteric orifice is readily identified, thereby facilitating ureteroscope introduction. It is important for urology residents/trainees to appreciate that small movements of the semi-rigid ureteroscope lead to large movements on the video screen due to the magnification provided by these devices, which ranges from 30 to 50 times, depending on the model [9]. In case of difficult insertion at the level of the ureteral orifice, there are two options to facilitate scope introduction. Either placing a second

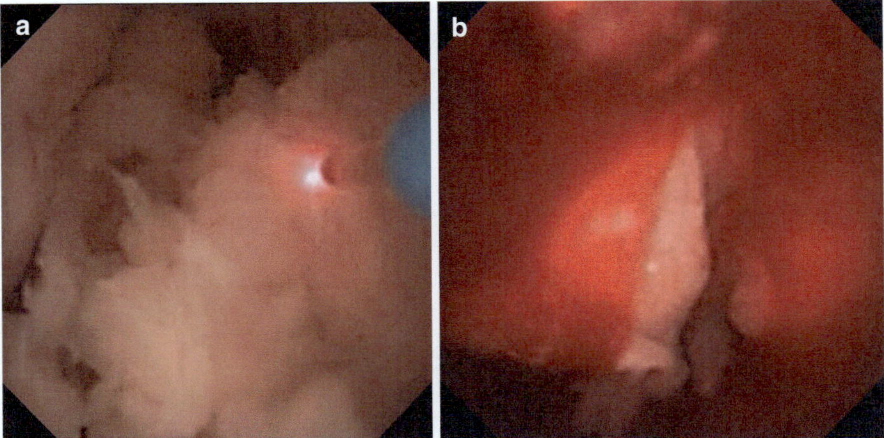

Fig. 4.2 (**a**) Ureteroscopic visualization of upper tract urothelial carcinoma. (**b**) The same tumor with obscured ureteroscopic visualization due to surface bleeding from excessively advanced safety wire placement

guidewire to widen access for the scope (scope passing between the two wires) or the URS can be gently guided over a second wire under direct vision [10, 11].

When performing a semi-rigid URS, it is important to note that the ureter is not a straight tube but rather has an S-shaped course in both lateral to medial and posterior to anterior directions [12]. Thus, advancement of the semi-rigid URS is often limited to the lower and mid-ureter below the pelvic brim. It is imperative not to force the endoscope if trying to advance above the pelvic brim, which can cause severe bending and resultant damage to the semi-rigid ureteroscope (Fig. 4.3). Also, if the ureter is tight and endoscope advancement difficult, it is important not to force the instrument, as there is a risk of ureteric perforation. When any resistance is felt and advancement of the URS compromised, it is safer to place a ureteral stent for passive ureteral dilation, making a secondary procedure much easier to perform at a later date.

Flexible Ureteroscopy

Currently, we can distinguish two types of flexible ureteroscopes (fURS): fiberoptic and digital. The difference between them is the image relay and light transmission. In both fiberoptic and digital fURS, most manufacturers have models with a 3.6 Fr working channel (for irrigation and use of accessory instruments) and usually bilateral 270° active deflection of the tip.

Once the guidewire is in place, the procedure may begin with a semi-rigid ureteroscopy, which has the advantage of passively dilating the distal ureter and may help the surgeon choose the most appropriate ureteral access sheath (UAS) size, if one is to be used [13, 14]. Whether a semi-rigid ureteroscopy has been performed or not initially, different options are feasible for fURS insertion into the urinary tract.

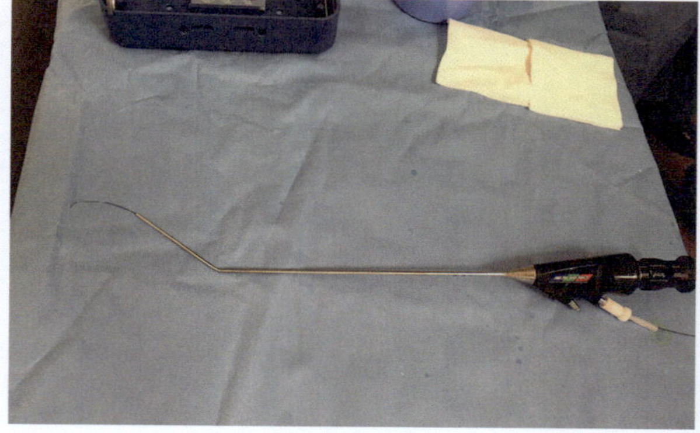

Fig. 4.3 Semi-rigid ureteroscope shaft damage secondary to excessive torque encountered during ureteroscope advancement

First, the fURS may be passed up to the kidney alongside the guidewire. Another possibility is to introduce the fURS over a second guidewire, or "working wire," placed through a dual-lumen catheter under fluoroscopic guidance. Another option is to place a UAS under fluoroscopic guidance and insert the fURS through the UAS. In case of upper urinary tract tumor management, the "no-touch" technique can be performed. In this technique, the fURS is directly introduced into the urinary tract without previous guidewire insertion to avoid any trauma [3]. The choice among these different options for fURS insertion depends on the surgical indication, stone burden (if applicable), upper urinary tract anatomy, and surgeon's preference.

When placing a UAS, the goals are to facilitate multiple passes for stone fragment removal and most importantly providing irrigation with better fluid outflow, thereby decreasing intrarenal pressure [15–18]. The choice of the UAS, including size and diameter, depends on the patient's anatomy, ureteroscope utilized, and surgeon's preference [19, 20]. Instead of placing two guidewires for UAS insertion, some newly designed UAS use only one guidewire, where the working guidewire turns into safety guidewire [21, 22] (Fig. 4.4). Attention has to be paid to the force applied during UAS placement because ureteral abrasions or perforations may be the consequence of forced maneuvers. The best position of the UAS is with its tip in the proximal ureter or just below the ureteropelvic junction but not through it since this is the portion of the ureter at greatest risk for avulsion because of the least muscular tissue support. Taking these data into consideration, the use of the smallest UAS as possible, in accordance with the fURS shaft size, is suggested.

Once the fURS has been placed into the kidney, the collecting system is explored starting with the upper calices followed by the middle and lower calices. Virtually any position in the potential luminal space of the upper urinary tract can be reached with flexible ureteroscopy using the correct combination of three-dimensional movements: (1) advancement/retreat, (2) ureteroscope deflection, and (3) ureteroscope rotation. It is essential for the surgeon to recall the normal rotational axes of the kidneys in order to anticipate the location of calyces when performing flexible

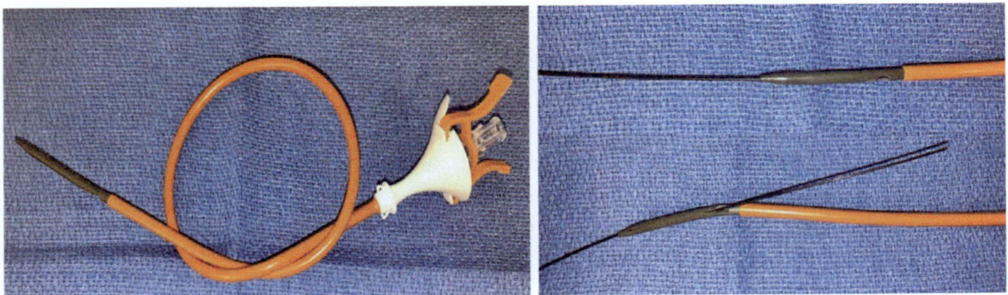

Fig. 4.4 Ureteral access sheath. The removal of the inner tip automatically converts the working guidewire as a safety guidewire laterally to the sheath

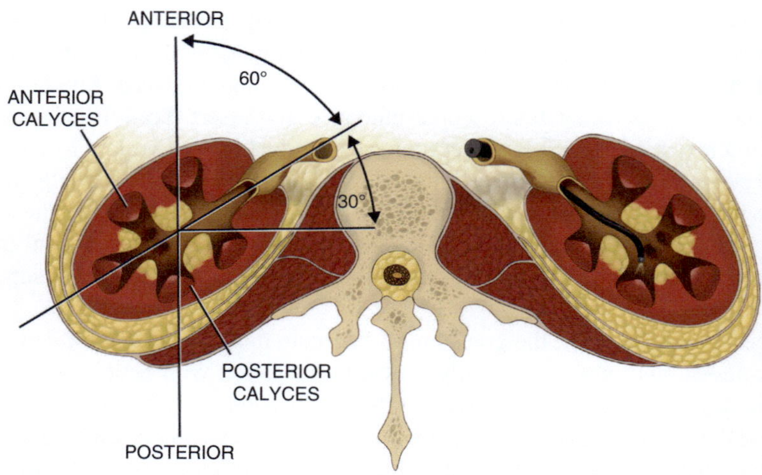

Fig. 4.5 Transverse view of the kidneys demonstrating anterior rotation of the renal hilum by 30°. Note posterior calyces are directed downward, while anterior calyces are directed laterally

nephroscopy. In the transverse plane, the renal hilum is rotated approximately 30° anteriorly, which means that posterior calyces of both the right and the left kidneys are directed towards the floor when the patient is in the dorsal lithotomy position. Anterior calyces are directed laterally (Fig. 4.5). In the right kidney, the calyces are seen on the left of the endoscope screen. Thus, supination is the essential movement to explore the anterior right renal calyces for the endourologist with a right-sided dominant hand. Conversely, the anterior left renal calyces are seen on the right of the endoscope screen, meaning that pronation is essential when exploring the left kidney (Fig. 4.6). Keeping these parameters in mind, the skilled observer can predict the location of the tip of the flexible ureteroscope merely by watching the hands of the operating surgeon, an important principle when training urology residents and fellows.

Another ureteroscopic specification to consider during laser lithotripsy is the position of the working channel as it exits at the tip of the ureteroscope. Most of the fURS have a 3:00 or 9:00 working channel position. When performing laser lithotripsy in the right kidney, a 3:00 position is more favorable to ablate stones because gravity is located at 3:00. However, to better fragment stones located in right anterior calyces, a 9:00 working channel position is advised. Conversely, a 9:00 working channel is advised for left renal stones except for anterior calyces where a 3:00 working channel is preferable (Fig. 4.7). It is fundamental to appreciate that the working channel outlet position can be manipulated simply by rotating the flexible ureteroscope. The surgeon can turn a 3:00 outlet to a 9:00 outlet by rotating the ureteroscope by 180°. When using a fiberoptic fURS with a pendulum camera, the screen view stays the same, as long as the camera stays fixed at the 6:00 position, while the exiting position of the working channel changes (Fig. 4.8). When using a digital flexible ureteroscope, the exiting position will stay constant at the 3:00 position, but the anatomy will rotate by 180°, since the digital camera is at a fixed position on the ureteroscope tip.

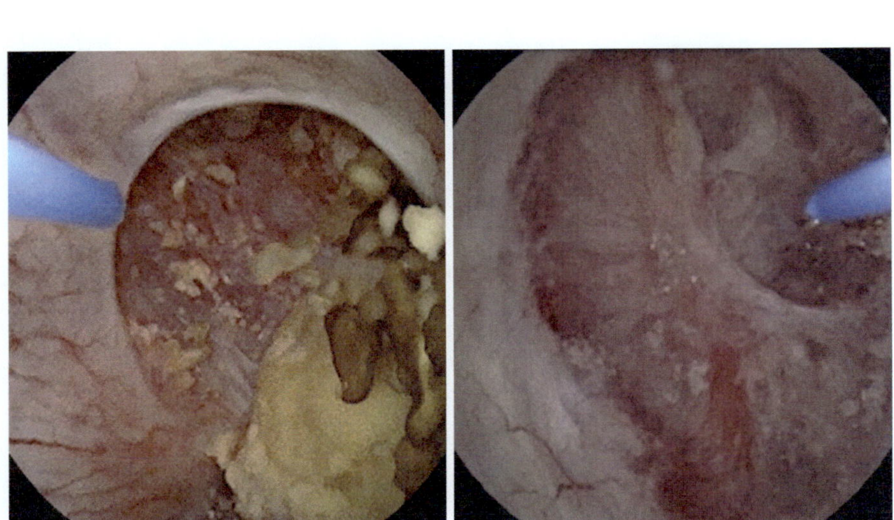

Fig. 4.6 Dominant-hand pronation and supination to change the direction of the distal tip of the flexible ureteroscope (fURS). Supination is essential for the fURS to access the anterior right renal calyces, and pronation is essential when the fURS enters the anterior left renal calyces

Fig. 4.7 Working channel position. (Left) Nine o'clock working channel. (Right) Three o'clock working channel

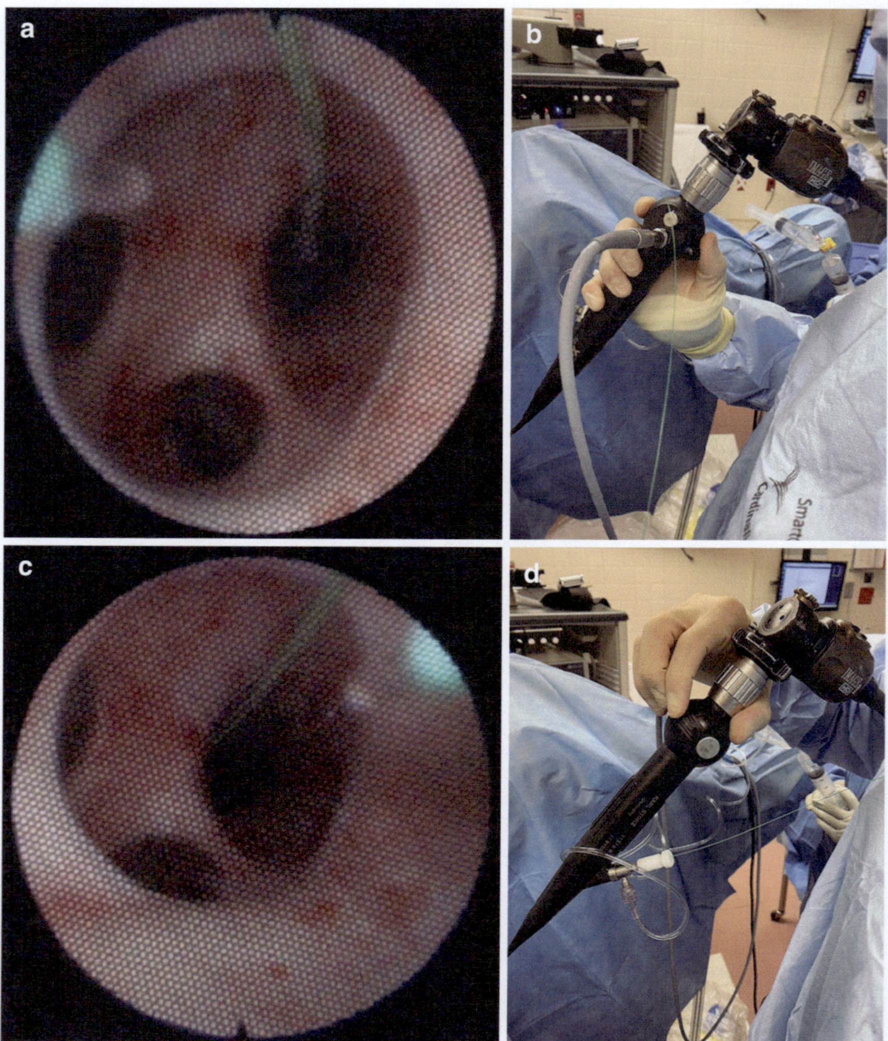

Fig. 4.8 (**a**) View from flexible *fiberoptic* ureteroscope with a *pendulum camera*. Note the reticle at 12:00 with laser fiber exiting at 9:00 position. (**b**) This corresponds to the thumb lever at the 6:00 position in the surgeon's hand. (**c**) Rotation of the flexible ureteroscope by 180° changes the position of the reticle to 6:00 with the laser fiber exiting at the 3:00 position and (**d**) the thumb lever rotated in the surgeon's hand. *Note that the visualized anatomy does not change in its appearance.* (**e**) Same anatomic view with *digital flexible ureteroscope* shows wire at 12:00 and laser fiber exiting at 3:00. (**f**) This corresponds to the surgeon's hand with thumb lever in 6:00 position. (**g**) *With 180° rotation of a digital ureteroscope, the anatomy rotates, but not the exiting position of the laser fiber*, still at 3:00, (**h**) while the thumb lever is at 12:00 in the surgeon's hand

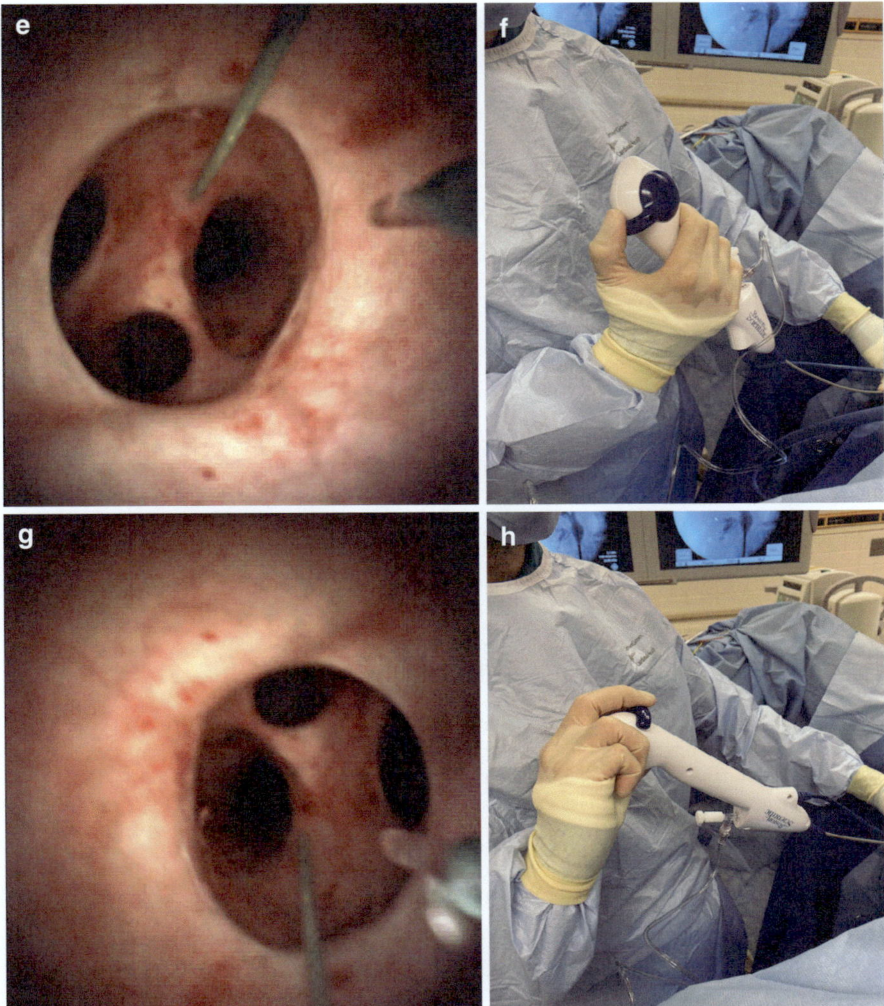

Fig. 4.8 (continued)

A final nuance of flexible ureteroscopic operative technique is the absolute importance of actively using both hands during the procedure. While this may seem obvious during endoscope advancement or retreat, it is not always appreciated in terms of endoscope rotation. When considering a right-handed dominant ureteroscopist, the large-scale rotations are accomplished by the right hand. The left hand, however, is responsible for smaller-scale, more precise rotation, which can be accomplished by rotating the ureteroscope shaft between the left thumb and index finger in close proximity to the urethral meatus. It is mastery of this left-handed maneuvering which makes for the most precise ureteroscopists. Concern for damaging the shaft of flexible ureteroscopes is legitimate with left-handed rotation,

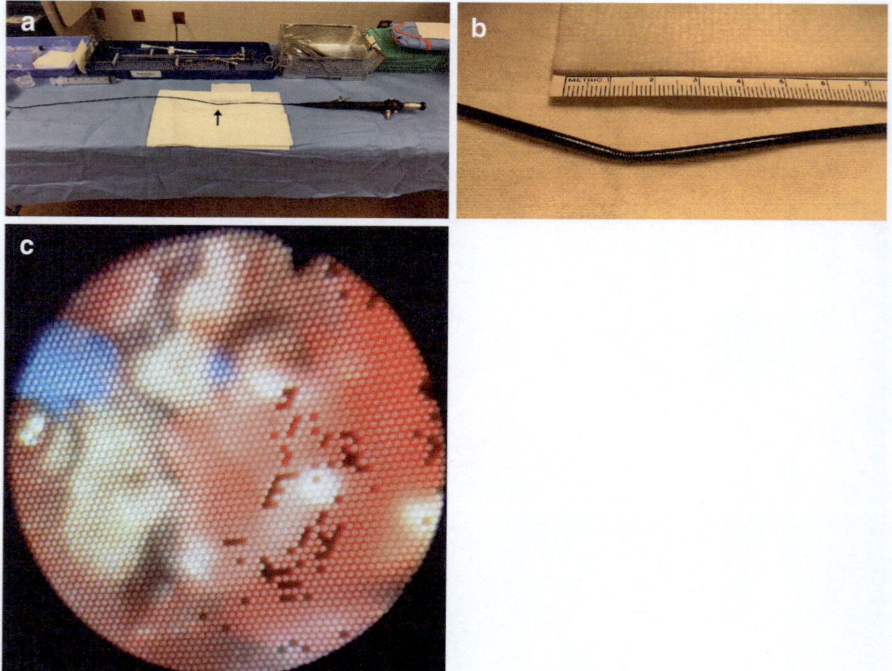

Fig. 4.9 (**a**) Note the crushed proximal shaft of this flexible ureteroscope, marked by the black arrow. (**b**) Close-up view of proximal shaft crush. This problem is seen when the surgeon is torqueing on the proximal shaft with his/her left hand to try and rotate the ureteroscope against a tight ureter with narrow diameter. (**c**) Usually this results in broken fiberoptics

especially when ureteral narrowing exists and causes resistance to shaft rotation. It is in this manner we see breakage of fiberoptic bundles or significant kinking of the ureteroscope shaft (Fig. 4.9). In such situations, it may be best to leave a stent and return when the ureter has been passively dilated or alternatively to use a single-use flexible ureteroscope.

Conclusion

With an appreciation for intrarenal anatomy and ureteroscope design, almost any portion of the upper urinary tract can be accessed with ureteroscopy. Although different in their conception, semi-rigid and flexible ureteroscopes share common steps when a procedure is performed but have inherently unique nuances in terms of maneuvering. This review provided some tips and tricks to facilitate their use in current practice.

Basic Techniques of Ureteroscopy: No-Touch Ureteroscopy

Nitin Sharma and Michael Grasso III

Introduction

No-touch ureteroscopy is also known as "wireless and sheathless" ureteroscopy. The technique, first described for atraumatic diagnostic ureteroscopy, is based on defining the ureteral orifice and under direct vision, intubating and traversing the intramural ureter with an actively deflectable flexible ureteroscope. This maneuver is performed without using a guidewire, ureteral dilator, or ureteral access sheath, which may cause trauma, thus obscuring visualization of any potential urothelial lesions.

Bagley et al. was the first to introduce no-touch endoscopic surveillance in those patients treated ureteroscopically with upper tract urothelial cancers (UTUC) with the aim of avoiding any incidental trauma from a guidewire or dilator (Fig. 4.10) and hence missing small ureteral lesions [23, 24]. In his technique, Bagley described first placing a small diameter semi-rigid ureteroscope to inspect the distal ureter, introducing a guidewire through the rigid endoscope only up to the level of the distal ureter, and finally passing a flexible ureteroscope over that wire to inspect the more proximal collecting system. With broader experience and improved flexible ureteroscopic design, specifically smaller shaft diameter, greater shaft durometer (stiffness), improved two-way tip deflection, and larger deflecting radius, direct intubation of the ureteral orifice without a guidewire or dilation can frequently be

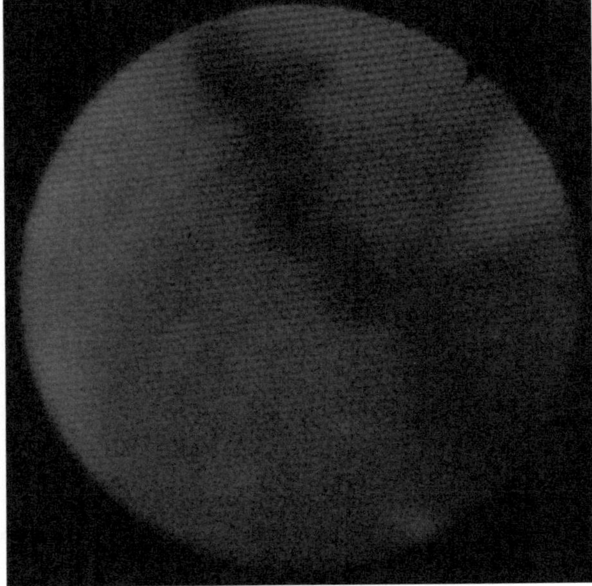

Fig. 4.10 Flexible ureteroscopic view showing linear erythema on the urothelial surface secondary to wire trauma, thus potentially complicating diagnostic ureteroscopy

performed [3, 25]. No-touch ureteroscopy, solely performed with a flexible uretero-scope, was first described by Grasso and Johnson in 2004 [25]. Indications quickly expanded from diagnostic to most therapeutic applications including treatment of UTUC and endoscopic lithotripsy.

Technique and Instrumentation

Instrumentation

A small diameter ≤8 Fr actively deflectable flexible ureteroscope is essential for direct endoscope intubation of the ureteral orifice. Fiberoptic-based flexible uretero-scopes tend to be of smaller caliber as compared to digital instruments and thus are often more successfully placed into the upper urinary tract employing this tech-nique. A standard 3.6 Fr working channel is inherent with most flexible uretero-scopes, allowing for passage of clearing sterile saline irrigant simultaneously with a broad range of endoscopic accessories (e.g., baskets, electrodes, laser fibers, etc.). Primary endoscope tip deflection has evolved with thumb lever control of up to 270° in two directions. US standard is thumb lever down, endoscope tip down, while in Europe this is reversed by convention. Secondary deflection is an inherent weakness in the durometer of the endoscope approximately 4–6 cm from the tip which allows for exaggerated angulation within the intrarenal collecting system for access to the most dependent lower pole calyces. If this secondary deflecting segment is too soft, for example, direct access above the intramural ureter using a no-touch technique may be limited secondary to endoscope buckling. Placing a guidewire through the working channel just to the endoscope tip will increase shaft stiffness and often help in this setting.

Technique

Flexible ureteroscopy, particularly for diagnostic purposes, begins with cystoscopy in the standard dorsal lithotomy position. Anatomic landmarks are defined includ-ing trigonal ridge, and barbotage sample of bladder urine is collected for cytologic evaluation in those with suspicion of a urothelial malignancy. A retrograde uretero-pyelogram is often performed with a 5 Fr open-ended ureteric catheter and dilute radio-opaque contrast material employing real-time fluoroscopy, care being taken not to over-distend the collecting system. The bladder is then completely drained before the flexible ureteroscope is passed to minimize pressure along the intramu-ral ureter.

The actively deflectable flexible ureteroscope is passed directly into the decom-pressed bladder. Sufficient sterile saline irrigant (typically 50–60 cc) is then instilled through the working channel to minimally lift the back wall of the bladder off of the trigone, thus facilitating the identification of the ureteral orifice. Once again, if the bladder is over distended and the intramural tunnel compressed, ureteral cannulation will be that much more challenging. The endoscope is straightened in the midline and then rolled toward the orifice, as if cannulating with a straight angiographic catheter. Trying to maximally deflect toward the orifice will cause shaft buckling during intubation and may prohibit passage through a tortuous or J-hooked intramural segment. The ureteral orifice is gently cannulated with the flexible ureteroscope under direct vision and then directed proximally, often by deflecting up and medially first to engage and then lateral and down to traverse the intramural ureter. If a ureteral peristaltic wave is encountered, a transient pause until the wave has passed is often all that is required.

Upper urinary tract mapping employing the no-touch technique increases the sensitivity of diagnostic ureteroscopy, minimizing false positives associated with guidewire or dilator trauma. The endoscope is passed directly into the intrarenal collecting system, which is meticulously evaluated and mapped. Lower pole calyces can be more challenging to visualize, particularly if associated with an acute infundibulopelvic angle or long (i.e., >3 cm) infundibula. The combination of maximal active tip deflection and passive proximal shaft buckling (i.e., secondary deflection) will often facilitate endoscope placement in this setting. Small aliquots of sterile saline irrigant can be employed through the working channel of the endoscope to clear the optical field of debris and to distend the collecting system sufficiently for inspection. A simple irrigation system commonly utilized is based on two refillable 60 cc syringes joined to a three-way stopcock attached to the endoscope with standard Luer-lock ended tubing (Fig. 4.11). The assistant instills minimal sufficient irrigant to just clear the optical field, varying the pressure and flow as needed based on the specific clinical presentation.

In a 1994 series of more than 500 diagnostic ureteroscopies, complete inspection of the upper urinary tract collecting system by no-touch technique was achieved in the majority of patients [26].

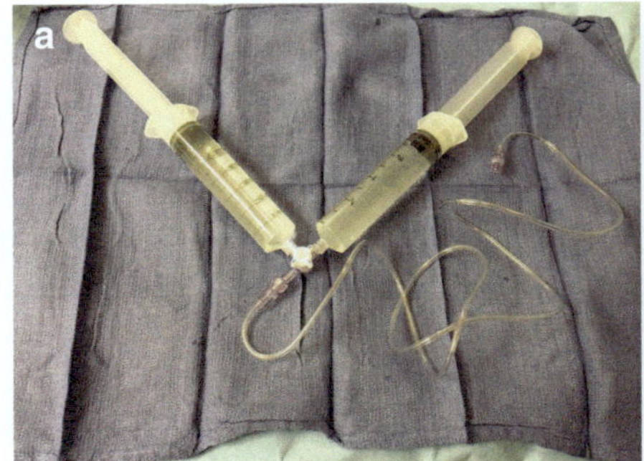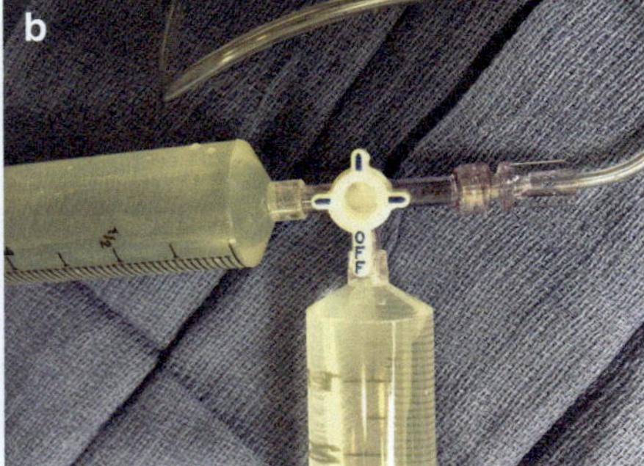

Fig. 4.11 (**a**) Two 60-mL syringes are connected to irrigation tubing by way of a three-way stopcock, which allows for seamless, virtually uninterrupted irrigation with an infinite range of pressure variation. (**b**) Close-up view of a three-way stopcock

Modifications for Difficult Ureteral Access: When to Employ a Guidewire and Dilator

No-touch flexible ureteroscopy should always be earnestly attempted in order to maximize diagnostic sensitivity, but may not always be technically feasible. Many clinical presentations will prohibit direct endoscope intubation. Promptly defining these and employing an access algorithm will increase the efficiency of each procedure. Cystoscopic evaluation is an essential first step. Lower urinary tract findings including pinhole or stenotic ureteral orifice, ureterocele, intrusive median lobe of the prostate, and trabeculated bladder with thickened wall and thus tortuous intramural ureter will often inhibit direct endoscope tip intubation. In these settings more standard access techniques should be used.

If the endoscope can be passed just into the orifice but intramural tortuosity causes buckling, thus prohibiting proximal passage, a guidewire is placed through the working channel to increase the durometer or stiffness of the endoscope shaft and to act as a minimal tip filiform. An angled-tipped Teflon-coated nickel titanium guidewire (i.e., Zebra guidewire, Boston Scientific, Natick, MA) is relatively unkinkable and steerable and has a sufficiently low coefficient of friction to facilitate endoscope passage over it. After traversing the intramural ureter, tortuous segment, or narrow orifice, the guidewire is withdrawn, and endoscopic inspection continues in a no-touch fashion.

If the ureteroscope will not pass through a narrow intramural ureter, then dilation is required. The smallest diameter dilator ($\leq$12 Fr) will cause the least trauma to the urothelium and is thus preferential. Typically, a 6–12 Fr Nottingham graduated dilator passed over a 0.035-inch angled-tipped Zebra guidewire is placed just through the intramural tunnel. Alternatively, a 12-Fr, 4-cm-long dilation balloon can be employed. If these two maneuvers are unsatisfactory, then direct inspection with a small caliber semi-rigid ureteroscope, akin to the technique described historically by Bagley, will allow for distal ureteral inspection, as well as dilation of the intramural segment under direct vision based on the graduated shaft of this instrument.

Need for Staged Procedure

When all else fails, with regard to ureteral access, placement of an internal stent and returning for second stage ureteroscopic inspection is an important strategy to minimize ureteral trauma and associated complications. It has been shown that in the absence of ureteral pathology, the inability to ureteroscopically access the upper urinary tract is 1.4% when using small diameter endoscopes. Active ureteral pathology will increase this rate to about 6.5% in our experience [27]. Certain clinical presentations including prior retroperitoneal surgery, fibrosis from radiotherapy, or adjacent neoplastic or inflammatory processes may inhibit ureteroscope placement in a non-dilated ureter. In such cases, staged procedures with interval ureteral stenting will often facilitate passive dilation and subsequent no-touch diagnostic ureteroscopy.

Procedural Algorithm

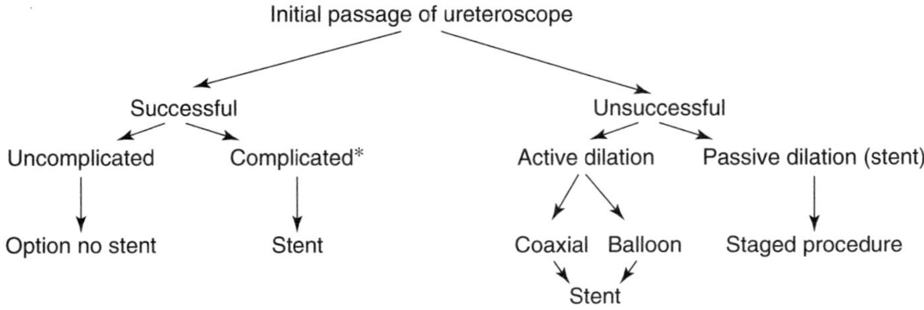

Indications for No-Touch Ureteroscospy

Diagnostic

1. Evaluating abnormal imaging and "filling defects" of the upper urinary tract.
2. Evaluation of lateralized "essential" hematuria: hematuria localized to the upper urinary tract without a discernible lesion or "filling defects" on contrast-based urography with bloody efflux defined cystoscopically from a ureteral orifice. Diagnostic ureteroscopy is the investigation of choice for its evaluation. No-touch technique is of particular importance in this scenario, with the greatest diagnostic sensitivity. Differential diagnosis includes papillary tip hemangioma, treated with electrocautery fulguration.
3. Urothelial malignancy: diagnostic ureteroscopy is employed to assess patients with suspicious lesions or lateralizing cytology to define urothelial neoplasms.
4. Surveillance ureteroscopy after ureteroscopic treatment of UTUC.

Therapeutic

1. Treatment of UTUC
2. Ureteroscopic lithotripsy

Results

In comparison to diagnostic ureteroscopy, therapeutic endeavors commonly begin with no-touch ureteroscopic mapping of the upper urinary tract. From tumor treatment, to endoscopic lithotripsy, therapeutic ureteroscopy is commonly performed without the application of retrograde catheter and guidewire manipulation or an access sheath. For example, a series of ureteroscopic lithotripsy procedures were performed without an access sheath with stone clearance of 95% and without major complications [28].

In 2006, Grasso et al. published results of 460 no-touch ureteroscopies (wireless and sheathless) and also compared it with an established database of 1000 standard flexible ureteroscopy [3]. Of the 460 cases, a stent was in place before hand in 108 [24%] cases. Of the remaining 352 cases, only 11% [54 cases] required guidewire or ureteral dilation to enter the ureter. In that series, success rate of ureteral stones was 99%–100% (proximal stones 99%, mid- and distal ureteral stones 100%), and success rate for renal stones was 91%–99% depending on stone size (<1 cm 99%, 1–2 cm 95%, 2 cm and above 91%). Larger renal stones invariably required more than one stage. No false passages or ureteral perforations were reported in that series. None of the patients had any major complication. Only five patients had postoperative pyelonephritis, requiring antibiotics, and three had hematuria, which resolved spontaneously,

whereas other series describing the use of routine application of a ureteral access sheath have defined a higher rate of complications secondary to ureteral wall trauma [29–31]. Moreover, in year 2000, in our series of 1000 consecutive cases of flexible ureteroscopy routinely employing a no-touch access technique, there were no perforations or avulsions, with a ureteral stricture rate of 0.4% [32].

Conclusions

No-touch technique should be utilized in cases of diagnostic ureteroscopy, whenever possible, in order to maximize visualization and minimize patient morbidity. With smaller diameter flexible ureteroscopes with appropriate durometer, semi-rigid ureteroscopes can often be omitted during diagnostic ureteroscopy. A stepwise approach to retrograde ureteral access should be followed, and patients should be counseled that even with contemporary small-profile endoscopes, second-stage procedures are sometimes necessary due to intrinsic ureteral narrowing.

Safety Considerations During Ureteroscopy

Edward J. Kloniecke and Scott G. Hubosky

Introduction

The use of ureteroscopy in endourology as a diagnostic and therapeutic procedure has increased over the last several years as ureteroscopy has overtaken extracorporeal shockwave lithotripsy (ESWL) for treatment of urolithiasis [33, 34]. It is widely accepted to be a safe procedure with complication rates ranging from 7.4 to 25%, with the majority of complications being minor (Clavien Grade I–II) and related to pain, hematuria, or urinary tract infection [35, 36]. These reported complications result directly from instrumentation and manipulation of the genitourinary tract. Less frequently discussed are the dangers posed by the supplemental technology used during the procedure to both the operating room staff and patient. The ureteroscope itself, radiation, and lasers used to treat malignancy and calculus disease all pose risks to the surgeon, the operating room staff, and the patient. By understanding these risks and developing strategies to mitigate them, the procedure can become even safer for all involved.

For the Surgeon

Radiation

With the increase in ureteroscopic case volume comes an increase in intra-operative fluoroscopy used to guide these procedures. This exposure to ionizing radiation carries with it well-documented risks of DNA and tissue damage leading to an increased risk of malignancy, cataract formation, congenital anomalies, and other issues [37]. Despite these known risks, most urologic training programs do not have formalized curricula in place to ensure an appropriate level of understanding of the risks inherent to the routine use of fluoroscopy and strategies, which can be used to minimize exposure. This is especially concerning since the operating urologist ultimately controls the dose of radiation used during any particular case.

The American Urologic Association (AUA) advocates for minimizing radiation dosing using the principles of "as low as reasonably achievable" or ALARA. This acknowledges that some risk of danger from the use of radiation is expected and necessary in order to perform the task at hand. By adopting these principles, the operator can limit the necessary exposure to the patient and operating room staff.

The first principle for achieving ALARA radiation dose levels is limiting the time that ionizing radiation is used. Pulsed dosing should be used, at as low a rate as possible, with spot fluoroscopic images obtained and held using the last image hold feature, rather than obtaining continuous images. The use of the physician foot pedal at critical portions of the case can allow for a decreased need for repeat images if a radiation technologist was not able to capture the image at the time intended by the physician, although one study suggests there is no difference in overall operative time and fluoroscopic dose based on who is in control of fluoroscopy. Additionally, the use of markings on the floor, standardized handoffs between radiation technologists, or, ideally, avoiding switching staff during a case will decrease the need for additional images and thereby lower time of exposure [38, 39]. Finally, fluoroscopy time should be tracked, and the operating surgeon should be provided feedback on their usage, as this awareness has been shown to decrease fluoroscopy time and dose by up to 24% [39].

The next way to achieve the lowest reasonable radiation dose is to increase distance from the source. The dose of radiation is inversely proportional to the square of the distance from the source. This means that every time distance from the radiation source is doubled, the radiation dose is decreased by 25%. Practically, distance can be increased by stepping back when obtaining fluoroscopic images and ensuring those who are not actively involved in the patient's care are as far from the radiation source as possible [40]. Of note, the use of video cameras and screens rather than direct visualization through lenses has made increasing distance from radiation source much easier as compared to the early years of urologic practice.

Shielding is the final component of achieving ALARA dose levels. This serves as an additional safety mechanism when fluoroscopy time has been minimized and increasing distance is no longer feasible. Shielding includes the traditional lead apron or gown to protect the chest, torso, and pelvis, as well as a thyroid shield, lead gloves, and lead glasses [37]. Chest, abdomen, and pelvic shields protect the gonads and the majority of active bone marrow. Depending on thickness, they can decrease scatter radiation by 90–99.5% [37]. Thyroid shields can reduce the delivered dose of radiation to the thyroid up to 100-fold, reducing the dose of radiation to near background levels and the risk of thyroid cancer to that of the general population [37]. Lead-impregnated gloves can reduce the dose of radiation to the hands by up to 50%, but this does vary with the brand used [41]. For endourologists using a C-arm during ureteroscopy, protective lead aprons can be fitted to the operating room table and are successful in significantly decreasing scatter radiation [42]. Another potential benefit of these table aprons could be to enable the operator to wear less dense, lighter-weight personal protective lead aprons, thereby reducing musculoskeletal strain.

The International Commission on Radiation Protection has provided universally accepted annual occupational dose limits regarding radiation exposure; any one organ or region of the body is limited to a dose of 500 millisieverts (mSv), with sieverts being functionally equivalent to gray, a more familiar unit of measurement to the urologist [43]. Using the above principles, a study estimated that a urologist who performs 50 ureteroscopies per year receives a yearly dose of radiation of 580 *micro*-gray to the lower legs, with a dose of 325, 135, and 95 *micro*-gray reaching the foot, hand, and eye, respectively, making it nearly impossible for even the busiest endourologist to reach their yearly limit [44].

Ergonomics

Work-related musculoskeletal disorders (WRMD) are common throughout the general population and medicine. Procedural specialists are especially at risk due to long hours on their feet, repetitive motions, and the need to be in static, non-neutral positions for prolonged periods. Ergonomists estimate the working environment for a proceduralist to be as harsh as an industrial labor job. Common pathologies include degenerative cervical and lumbar spine disease, rotator cuff injury, carpal tunnel syndrome, tendinitis, neuropathies, and pain syndromes [45].

Endourologists suffer from WRMD at a substantial rate, with 38.1% reporting back problems, 27.6% reporting neck problems, and 17.2–32% reporting hand issues [46, 47]. The lead gown worn as protection from radiation likely contributes to the back issues, as a 15-pound lead gown can exert as much as 300 pounds per square inch of pressure on the intervertebral discs [46]. Consideration should be given to weight when deciding on purchasing lead protective garments for use during ureteroscopy.

The characteristics of the ureteroscope may play a role in the development of hand issues. Current options for ureteroscopes include single-use digital, reusable digital, and reusable fiberoptic instruments. Digital ureteroscopes incorporate the camera and light cable, so are often considerably lighter than fiberoptic ureteroscopes (less than 300 g compared to greater than 1400 g) when considering the additional weight of separate cables [47]. A study compared the electromyography measured muscle activity for completing a number of in vitro tasks using a flexible ureteroscope from each of these categories, and the lighter, digital ureteroscopes consistently required less muscle work per second and cumulative muscle work across all muscle groups than the heavier, fiberoptic counterparts. Additionally, the time it took to complete tasks was shorter using the digital instruments, possibly due to less fatigue [48]. Digital ureteroscopes do have drawbacks and are not necessarily the best option for every case, but their ergonomic advantages should seriously be considered.

Ergonomic issues lead to considerable burden for endourologists. In one study, 84.6% of the endourologists reporting hand problems ultimately required intervention in the form of medication, physical therapy, or surgery [49]. Throughout all specialties, WRMD contribute to the early retirement, practice restriction or modification, or leave of absence for 12% of affected physicians [45].

Eye Safety

Urologist's eyes have long been at risk from a number of potential hazards. Using cameras rather than direct visualization has served to provide additional distance between the eye and the potential danger, but risks still remain. Fortunately, the use of appropriate eyewear can reduce the odds of suffering a significant injury.

Laser Injury

The use of lasers for treating urologic pathologies began in the 1970s. Since that time, many different laser technologies have been used or are being investigated for use, including neodymium-doped yttrium aluminum garnet (Nd:YAG), potassium titanyl phosphate (KTP), holmium:YAG (Ho:YAG), diode, thulium:YAG (Th:YAG), and thulium fiber laser (TFL) [50, 51]. Ho:YAG has become the most commonly used laser in contemporary ureteroscopy. Not only is holmium widely adopted for its versatility and effectiveness but equally essential is its excellent safety profile. A search of two major adverse event databases returned a total of 433 adverse events related to the use of lasers in urology. One hundred sixty-four events were eye injuries, attributed to the use of the Nd:YAG, KTP, or diode lasers; none occurred with the use of the Ho:YAG laser. These eye injuries ranged from minor corneal abrasions to total vision loss, and most were thought to be associated with the improper use of eye protection [50]. The most common injury to the medical operator using the Ho:YAG laser was minor skin burns from firing with a broken fiber (Fig. 4.12).

These injuries are due to the fact that energy from the Nd:YAG, KTP, and diode lasers is absorbed by oxyhemoglobin, whereas the energy from the Ho:YAG laser is absorbed by water [50]. Any stray energy from a broken or unintentionally activated laser fiber is then available to damage to the first structure it encounters containing oxyhemoglobin, which may be the retina or lens of the eye and cause catastrophic injury. For that reason, it is recommended that everyone in the operating room wears wavelength-specific safety goggles with the use of surgical lasers [50, 52, 53].

Multiple guideline statements and manufacturers of Ho:YAG lasers recommend wearing laser protective goggles with the use of this technology, despite limited evidence of possibility of injury. An ex vivo study on porcine eyes showed that Ho:YAG laser could not cause damage to the lens or retina in any scenario, and corneal abrasions were only possible if the laser fiber was very close to the unprotected eye. Eyeglasses alone were sufficient to protect the cornea from damage in this scenario. Based on this, the authors of that study concluded that surgeons should wear goggles, or at least eye glasses, to essentially eliminate any risk posed by the Ho:YAG laser [51].

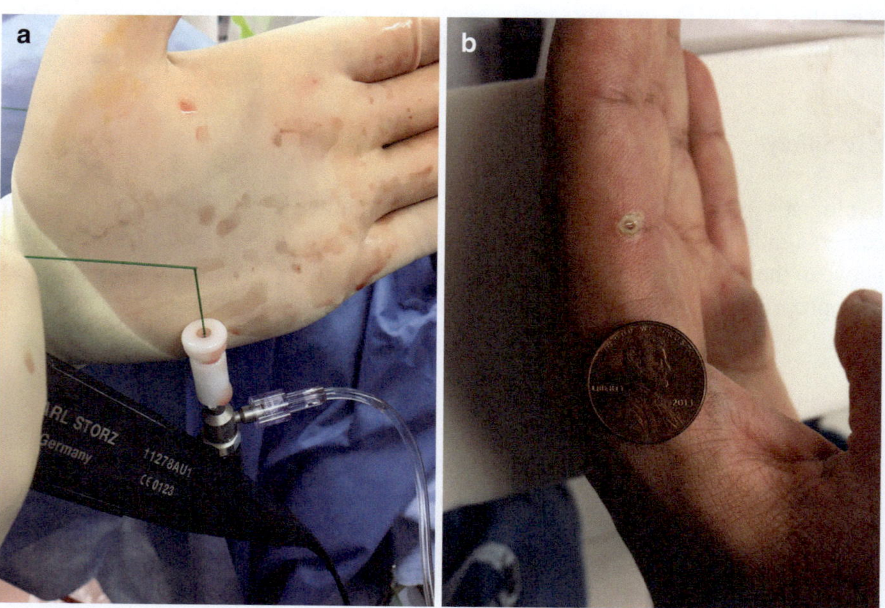

Fig. 4.12 (**a**) Undue strain on laser fibers during ureteroscopic handle manipulation can result in fiber breakage. Particular points of vulnerability are at the insertion of the working channel or areas that are incidentally crushed by hemostats when secured to drapes. (**b**) Minor skin burn encountered by the surgeon when firing through a broken laser fiber while utilizing Ho:YAG

Radiation-Induced Eye Injury

As previously mentioned, the use of ionizing radiation during fluoroscopy can have many deleterious effects. One unique consideration is the risk of cataract formation after repeated exposure. The yearly limit for radiation dose to the lens of the eye is less than 150 mSv per year, and assuming 50 ureteroscopies per year and a distance of 75 cm from the source of the radiation, the eye would receive a dose of 95 *micro-gray*, so well within the yearly limit [44, 54]. This does not account for the cumulative effect of multiple years of practice. Studies have demonstrated that, over a lifetime of exposure, 2000 mSv can cause lens opacification and 2500 mSv can cause cataracts. Based on a study that included stent changes and ureteroscopy, it would take an endourologist who performed 20 cases a week approximately 50 years to accumulate the dose necessary to cause cataracts [54]. It is conceivable that young, very busy endourologists could accumulate this dose. Lead-lined glasses, in line with the ALARA concept of shielding, have been proven to decrease radiation dose by 95% and reduce the risk of cataracts in those with chronic radiation exposure and should be worn, or at least considered by young, busy endourologists and any urologist would not be faulted for their use [44, 52, 54].

Fluid Splash Contamination

Blood-borne pathogens represent an additional hazard for endourologists. Historically, with direct visualization cystoscopy, the risk of contamination with patient's blood or contaminated irrigant fluid was likely higher, but the risk still remains with video-based endoscopic procedures. One study examining blood splash injury in urology specifically found that macroscopic blood was present on 8.3% of masks and face shields after flexible ureteroscopy. Microscopic blood was identified using a chemical reagent and was present on an additional 50% of masks and shields. Macroscopic and microscopic blood was present on the masks and shields 9% and 31.8% of the time, respectively, after semi-rigid ureteroscopy [55].

Urologists have, historically, preferred to forego eye protection as it was felt to negatively impact visualization through the ureteroscope, and the risk of contamination was thought to be low. Additionally, it was believed that glasses worn by physicians provided adequate protection, but this has been proven false, and droplets of blood have been found on the inside of glasses worn during procedures [55]. No pathogen transmission has been recorded from eye splash injury in urology, but the use of goggles can reduce the risk of contamination to zero and eliminate any chance of infection, small as it may be [52, 55].

Prioritizing Eye Protection

Given the many risks to the eye present during ureteroscopy, it may be difficult to choose which eye protection is most appropriate. A very busy endourologist should certainly protect his/her eyes from radiation using lead-lined goggles in any case where fluoroscopy is to be utilized. These goggles are likely sufficient to protect the eye from stray energy from the Ho:YAG laser, so it is recommended that lead-lined glasses be worn if the use of both Ho:YAG laser and fluoroscopy is anticipated. Since significant and sometimes catastrophic injury has been documented with the use of other lasers, specifically the Nd:YAG, KTP, and diode lasers, the surgeon must wear wavelength-specific laser goggles if these lasers are to be utilized. Given the relatively small individual dose of radiation in any single case and the lack of proven efficacy of lead-lined goggles in preventing laser injury, priority must be given to protecting the eye from stray laser energy [52]. Finally, if no fluoroscopy or laser use is anticipated, goggles should be worn to prevent contamination from pathogen-containing fluid [52, 55].

For the OR Staff

The OR staff is at risk for many of the same injuries as the surgeon; although given the nature of ureteroscopy and the limited working space when a patient is in dorsal lithotomy, the OR staff is often further from the potential safety hazard and, therefore, less likely to be harmed. For example, a person who assists in 50 ureteroscopies per year receives an estimated dose of radiation to the lower legs of 40 *micro*-gray, compared to the surgeon's dose of 580 *micro*-gray [44]. Those assisting in procedures where the use of fluoroscopy is intended should observe the same precautions of ALARA, maximizing distance, minimizing time exposed (e.g., the number of people in the room should be limited to those necessary), and wearing all appropriate shielding [37].

Regarding eye protection, the OR staff should wear wavelength-specific goggles if the use of Nd:YAG, KTP, or diode lasers is anticipated. While assistants are more likely to be further from the source of radiation and therefore receive a lower dose of radiation to the lens and be at a lower lifetime risk of cornea opacification and cataract formation, lead-lined goggles can be offered to anyone in the OR [56]. Finally, if no radiation or laser use is anticipated, assisting staff should wear protective goggles as masks and shields of assisting nurses have been found to be contaminated with blood in up to 31.8% of urologic procedures [55].

For the Patient

Patient's undergoing ureteroscopy may have pathology that requires repeat exposure to ionizing radiation to monitor their disease process. In all patients, the surgeon should take care to achieve ALARA radiation doses during surgical procedures. Data from interventional radiology studies suggest that, while not routinely used, lead-lined eye protection and thyroid shields do decrease radiation doses and provide benefit to patients undergoing fluoroscopically guided procedures. One study found the dose of radiation to the thyroid decreased by half with the use of a thyroid shield [57].

Pregnant patients who need procedural intervention can be offered sonographic guidance if institutional structure allows. The American College of Gynecology recognizes that ionizing radiation may be necessary and allows for its use if necessary. If possible, the surgeon should consider shielding the pelvis and developing fetus with a lead apron [38].

The patient's eyes are also at risk of injury from stray laser energy. Perioperative guidelines recommend taping the patient's eyes per normal anesthesia protocol and the use of soft, laser wavelength-specific protective goggles. The use of standard laser goggles is not advised, as these often have too much open space under the lens and could potentially permit laser energy to damage critical tissue [57].

Conclusion

Unique safety risks of ureteroscopy exist beyond those secondary to direct manipulation of the upper urinary tract. Awareness of the principles of "ALARA" can help minimize exposure to ionizing radiation by limiting the amount of time it is used, increasing distance from the radiation source whenever possible and maximizing shielding. Digital flexible ureteroscopes may improve surgeon ergonomics since they are much lighter compared to fiberoptic counterparts with heavier pendulum camera heads. Wavelength-specific safety goggles or glasses should be used during cases employing lasers to maximize eye protection.

Disclosures Financial disclosure: Prof. Olivier Traxer is a consultant for Coloplast, Rocamed, Olympus, EMS, and Boston Scientific. Steeve Doizi is a consultant for Coloplast.

Funding support: Dr. Etienne Xavier Keller is supported by a travel grant from the University Hospital Zurich and by a grant from the Kurt and Senta Herrmann Foundation. Dr. Hubosky is a consultant for Boston Scientific and BD/Bard.

References

Fundamental Maneuvering During Ureteroscopy

1. EAU Guidelines. Edn. Presented at the EAU Annual Congress Amsterdam 2020. ISBN 978-94-92671-07-3. EAU Guidelines Office, Anhem, The Netherlands. http://uroweb.org/guidelines/compilations-of-all-guidelines/.
2. Assimos D, Krambeck A, Miller NL, Monga M, Murad MH, Nelson CP, et al. Surgical management of stones: American Urological Association/Endourological Society guideline, part 1. J Urol. 2016;196:1153–60.
3. Johnson GB, Portela D, Grasso M. Advanced ureteroscopy: wireless and sheathless. J Endourol. 2006;20:552–5.

4. Dickstein RJ, Kreshover JE, Babayan RK, Wang DS. Is a safety wire necessary during routine flexible ureteroscopy? J Endourol. 2010;24:1589–92.
5. Patel SR, McLaren ID, Nakada SY. The ureteroscope as a safety wire for ureteronephroscopy. J Endourol. 2012;26:351–4.
6. Ulvik Ø, Rennesund K, Gjengstø P, Wentzel-Larsen T, Ulvik NM. Ureteroscopy with and without safety guide wire: should the safety wire still be mandatory? J Endourol. 2013;27:1197–202.
7. Dutta R, Vyas A, Landman J, Clayman RV. Death of the safety guidewire. J Endourol. 2016;30:941–4.
8. Doizi S, Herrmann T, Traxer O. Death of the safety guidewire. J Endourol. 2017;31:619–20.
9. Buscarini M, Conlin M. Update on flexible Ureteroscopy. Urol Int. 2008;80:1–7.
10. Rukin NJ, Somani BK, Patterson J, Grey BR, Finch W, McClinton S, et al. Tips and tricks of ureteroscopy: consensus statement part I. Basic ureteroscopy. Cent Eur J Urol. 2015;68:439–46.
11. Whitehurst LA, Somani BK. Semi-rigid ureteroscopy: indications, tips, and tricks. Urolithiasis. 2018;46:39–45.
12. Sampaio FJ. Renal anatomy. Endourologic considerations. Urol Clin North Am. 2000;27:585–607.
13. Giusti G, Proietti S, Villa L, Cloutier J, Rosso M, Gadda GM, et al. Current standard technique for modern flexible ureteroscopy: tips and tricks. Eur Urol. 2016;70:188–94.
14. Doizi S, Traxer O. Flexible ureteroscopy: technique, tips and tricks. Urolithiasis. 2018;46:47–58.
15. Newman RC, Hunter PT, Hawkins IF, Finlayson B. The ureteral access system: a review of the immediate results in 43 cases. J Urol. 1987;137:380–3.
16. Rehman J, Monga M, Landman J, Lee DI, Felfela T, Conradie MC, et al. Characterization of intrapelvic pressure during ureteropyeloscopy with ureteral access sheaths. Urology. 2003;61:713–8.
17. Auge BK, Pietrow PK, Lallas CD, Raj GV, Santa-Cruz RW, Preminger GM. Ureteral access sheath provides protection against elevated renal pressures during routine flexible ureteroscopic stone manipulation. J Endourol. 2004;18:33–6.
18. Kaplan AG, Lipkin ME, Scales CD Jr, Preminger GM. Use of ureteral access sheaths in ureteroscopy. Nat Rev Urol. 2016;13:135–40.
19. Al-Qahtani SM, Letendre J, Thomas A, Natalin R, Saussez T, Traxer O. Which ureteral access sheath is compatible with your flexible ureteroscope? J Endourol. 2014;28:286–90.
20. Emre Sener T, Cloutier J, Villa L, Marson F, Butticè S, Doizi S, et al. Can we provide low intrarenal pressures with good irrigation flow by decreasing the size of ureteral access sheaths? J Endourol. 2016;30:49–55.
21. Doizi S, Knoll T, Scoffone CM, Breda A, Brehmer M, Liatsikos E, et al. First clinical evaluation of a new innovative ureteral access sheath (Re-Trace™): a European study. World J Urol. 2014;32:143–7.
22. Breda A, Emiliani E, Millán F, Scoffone CM, Knoll T, Osther PJ, et al. The new concept of ureteral access sheath with guidewire disengagement: one wire does it all. World J Urol. 2016;34:603–6.

No-Touch Ureteroscopy

23. Keeley FX Jr, Bibbo M, Bagley DH. Ureteroscopic treatment and surveillance of upper urinary tract transitional cell carcinoma. J Urol. 1997;157:1560–5.
24. Bagley DH. Ureteroscopic laser treatment of upper urinary tract tumors. J Clin Laser Med Surg. 1998;16:55–9.
25. Johnson GB, Grasso M. Exaggerated primary endoscope deflection: initial clinical experience with prototype flexible ureteroscopes. BJU Int. 2004;93:109–14.
26. Grasso M, Bagley D. A 7.5/8.2 actively deflectable, flexible ureteroscope: a new device for both diagnostic and therapeutic upper urinary tract endoscopy. Urology. 1994;43:435–41.

27. Hubosky SG, Healy KA, Grasso M, Bagley DH. Accessing the difficult ureter and the importance of ureteroscope miniaturization: history is repeating itself. Urology. 2014;84:740–2.
28. Grasso M, Conlin M, Bagley D. Retrograde uretero- pyeloscopic treatment of 2 cm or greater upper urinary tract and minor staghorn calculi. J Urol. 1998;160:346–51.
29. Breda A, Ogunyemi O, Leppert JT, Lam JS, Schulam PG. Flexible ureteroscopy and laser lithotripsy for single intrarenal stones 2 cm or greater—is this the new frontier? J Urol. 2008;179:981–4.
30. Ricchiuti DJ, Smaldone MC, Jacobs BL, Smaldone AM, Jackman SV, Averch TD. Staged retrograde endoscopic lithotripsy as alternative to PCNL in select patients with large renal calculi. J Endourol. 2007;21:1421–4.
31. Hyams ES, Munver R, Bird VG, Uberoi J, Shah O. Flexible ureterorenoscopy and holmium laser lithotripsy for the management of renal stone burdens that measure 2 to 3 cm: a multi-institutional experience. J Endourol. 2010;24:1583–8.
32. Grasso M. Ureteropyeloscopic treatment of ureteral and intrarenal calculi. Urol Clin North Am. 2000;27:623–31.

Safety Considerations During Ureteroscopy

33. Heers H, Turney BW. Trends in urological stone disease: a 5-year update of hospital episode statistics. BJUI. 2016;118:785–9.
34. Oberlin DT, Flum AS, Bachrach L, Matulewicz RS, Flury SC. Contemporary surgical trends in the management of upper tract calculi. J Urol. 2015;193:880–4.
35. Türk C, Petřík A, Sarica K, Seitz C, Skolarikos A, Straub M, et al. EAU guidelines on interventional treatment for urolithiasis. Eur Urol. 2016;69:475–82.
36. Somani BK, Giusti G, Sun Y, Osther PJ, Frank M, Sio MD, et al. Complications associated with ureterorenoscopy (URS) related to treatment of urolithiasis: the Clinical Research Office of Endourological Society URS global study. World J Urol. 2016;35:675–81.
37. Friedman AA, Ghani KR, Peabody JO, Jackson A, Trinh Q-D, Elder JS. Radiation safety knowledge and practices among urology residents and fellows: results of a nationwide survey. J Surg Ed. 2013;70:224–31.
38. Chrouser K, Foley F, Goldenberg M, Hyder J, Maranchie JK, Moore JM, et al. Optimizing outcomes in urological surgery: intraoperative patient safety and physiological considerations. Urol Practice. 2020;7:309–18.
39. Ngo TC, Macleod LC, Rosenstein DI, Reese JH, Shinghal R. Tracking intraoperative fluoroscopy utilization reduces radiation exposure during ureteroscopy. J Endourol. 2011:763–7.
40. Strom DJ. Ten principles and ten commandments of radiation protection. Health Phys. 1996;70:388–93.
41. Wagner LK, Mulhern OR. Radiation-attenuating surgical gloves: effects of scatter and secondary electron production. Radiology. 1996;200:45–8.
42. Inoue T, Komenmushi A, Murota T, Yoshida T, Taguchi M, Kinoshita H, et al. Effect of protective lead curtains on scattered radiation exposure to the operator during ureteroscopy for stone disease: a controlled trial. Urology. 2017;109:60–6.
43. Andonian S. Radiation safety. AUA University; 2020. https://university.auanet.org/modules/webapps/core/index.cfm#/corecontent/71. Accessed 1 Jun 2020.
44. Hellawell G, Mutch S, Thevendran G, Wells E, Morgan R. Radiation exposure and the urologist: what are the risks? J Urol. 2005;174:948–52.
45. Epstein S, Sparer EH, Tran BN, Ruan QZ, Dennerlein JT, Singhal D, et al. Prevalence of work-related musculoskeletal disorders among surgeons and interventionalists. JAMA Surg. 2018; https://doi.org/10.1001/jamasurg.2017.4947.
46. Elkoushy MA, Andonian S. Prevalence of orthopedic complaints among endourologists and their compliance with radiation safety measures. J Endourol. 2011;25:1609–13.

47. Proietti S, Somani B, Sofer M, Pietropaolo A, Rosso M, Saitta G, et al. The "body mass index" of flexible ureteroscopes. J Endourol. 2017;31:1090–5.
48. Ludwig WW, Lee G, Ziemba JB, Ko JS, Matlaga BR. Evaluating the ergonomics of flexible ureteroscopy. J Endourol. 2017;31:1062–6.
49. Healy KA, Pak RW, Cleary RC, Colon-Herdman A, Bagley DH. Hand problems among endourologists. J Endourol. 2011;25:1915–20.
50. Althunayan AM, Elkoushy MA, Elhilali MM, Andonian S. Adverse events resulting from lasers used in urology. J Endourol. 2014;28:256–60.
51. Kronenberg P, Traxer O. The laser of the future: reality and expectations about the new thulium fiber laser – a systematic review. Trans Andol Urol. 2019;8:S398–417.
52. Doizi S, Audouin M, Villa L, Rodriguez-Monsalve Herrero M, DeConinck V, Keller EX, et al. The eye of the endourologist: what are the risks? A review of the literature. World J Urol. 2019;37:2639–47.
53. Villa L, Cloutier J, Compérat E, Kronemberg P, Charlotte F, Berthe L, et al. Do we really need to wear proper eye protection when using holmium:YAG laser during endourologic procedures? Results from an ex vivo animal model on pig eyes. J Endourol. 2016;30:332–7.
54. Taylor ER, Kramer B, Frye TP, Wang S, Schwartz BF, Köhler TS. Ocular radiation exposure in modern urological practice. J Urol. 2013;190:139–43.
55. Wines MP, Lamb A, Argyropoulos AN, Caviezel A, Gannicliffe C, Tolley D. Blood splash injury: an underestimated risk in endourology. J Endourol. 2008;22:1183–8.
56. Jindal T. The risk of radiation exposure to assisting staff in urological procedures: a literature review. Urol Nur. 2013;33:136–47.
57. Andersen K. Safe use of lasers in the operating room – what perioperative nurses should know. AORN J. 2004;79:171–88.

Chapter 5
Stones

Etienne Xavier Keller, Vincent De Coninck, Olivier Traxer, Asaf Shvero, Nir Kleinmann, Scott G. Hubosky, Steeve Doizi, Thomas J. Hardacker, Demetrius H. Bagley, and Maryann Sonzogni-Cella

Abbreviations

AUA	American Urologic Association
CIRF	Clinically insignificant residual fragments
CSD	Cumulative stone diameter
CT	Computerized tomography
EAU	European Association of Urology
ESWL	Extra shockwave lithotripsy
KUB	Kidney, ureter, and bladder
NICE	National Institute for Health and Care Excellence
PCNL	Percutaneous nephrolithotomy
RIRS	Retrograde intrarenal surgery

E. X. Keller · V. De Coninck · O. Traxer (✉) · S. Doizi
Sorbonne Université, GRC n°20, Groupe de Recherche Clinique sur la Lithiase Urinaire, Hôpital Tenon, Paris, France
e-mail: olivier.traxer@aphp.fr

A. Shvero · S. G. Hubosky · T. J. Hardacker
Department of Urology, Sidney Kimmel Medical College at Thomas Jefferson University Hospital, Philadelphia, PA, USA
e-mail: Asaf.shvero@jefferson.edu; Scott.Hubosky@jefferson.edu; Thomas.hardacker@jefferson.edu

D. H. Bagley
Department of Urology and Radiology, Sidney Kimmel Medical College at Thomas Jefferson University Hospital, Philadelphia, PA, USA
e-mail: Demetrius.BagleyJr@jefferson.edu

N. Kleinmann
Department of Urology, Sheba Medical Center, Tel-Hashomer, Israel

M. Sonzogni-Cella
Department of Nursing, Thomas Jefferson University Hospital, Philadelphia, PA, USA

© Springer Nature Switzerland AG 2022
S. G. Hubosky et al. (eds.), *Advanced Ureteroscopy*,
https://doi.org/10.1007/978-3-030-82351-1_5

RUS   Renal ultrasound
SFR   Stone-free rate
URS   Ureteroscopy

Ureteral Stone Treatment

Etienne Xavier Keller, Vincent De Coninck, and Olivier Traxer

Introduction

Urolithiasis is a widespread disease with a high associated morbidity and therefore represents a major burden for the healthcare system. In industrialized countries, the prevalence of urolithiasis is about 10%, with an incidence of symptomatic stone events of about 0.1–0.4% and a recurrence rate of >50% within 10 years [1].

Ureteral stones typically become symptomatic because of impaction in the ureteral mucosa at a site of relative narrowing, causing a urinary outflow obstruction with consecutive increase of intrarenal pressure, finally leading to colicky flank pain [2]. In contrast, renal stones may remain asymptomatic over many years and only become symptomatic because of migration to the ureter, retainment at the ureteropelvic junction, or super-imposed infection.

Over the past decades, ureteroscopes (URS) and their ancillary devices have undergone continuous technological improvements and have now become a major player in surgical treatment of ureteral stones. This chapter provides a brief overview of the various treatment alternatives available for ureteral stones and will focus on modern ureteroscopic management of ureteral stones in light of technological advancements.

Indications and Treatment Alternatives

The appropriate choice of treatment for ureteral stones is driven by safety, patient preference, and cost-efficiency. These parameters are reflected by the complication rate and stone-free rate of any available treatment approach and form the basis of international recommendations [3–7]. The determinants of these recommendations are mainly based on stone location and stone size. Treatment alternatives include conservative management, extracorporeal shockwave lithotripsy (ESWL), and ureteroscopy (URS). Of note, endourological approaches have nearly replaced laparoscopic and open surgical approaches to ureteral stones. Percutaneous antegrade approaches (Chap. 9) are typically reserved for special conditions such as impacted proximal ureteral stones or urinary diversions not amenable to retrograde manipulation [8, 9].

Table 5.1 presents an overview of current international guidelines for ureteral stone treatment. Conservative management is recommended for ureteral stones <6–10 mm, and α-blockers may be offered as a medical expulsive therapy, especially for distal ureteral stones. Regular follow-up is recommended, and active treatment should be considered in the absence of spontaneous stone passage after 4–6 weeks. For distal ureteral stones <10 mm, URS and ESWL may be equally offered. For proximal ureteral stones <10 mm, AUA/ES and EAU guidelines agree that URS is the treatment of choice, whereas the SIU/ICUD recommends ESWL as a first choice, provided that the stone can be localized during ESWL. For stones >10 mm, conservative management is not indicated. For distal ureteral stones >10 mm, URS is the treatment of choice. For proximal ureteral stones >10 mm, ESWL may be equally offered under the prerequisite that patients are informed about the lower stone-free rate in a single ESWL procedure compared to URS.

The aforementioned guidelines cannot be applied to several peculiar conditions where case-by-case evaluation is necessary: persistent pain, kidney function impairment, signs of infection, solitary kidney, simultaneous bilateral ureteral stones, and anatomical abnormalities such as urinary diversion, ureterocele, ectopic ureter, or megaureter.

Another condition that is not yet covered by any guideline is URS for ureteral stones in emergency situations. Recent literature revealed high stone-free rates and low complication rates, particularly for distal ureteral stones [10–12]. The role of emergency URS shall be evaluated in future multi-centric prospective randomized studies.

Techniques, Tips, and Tricks

Anesthesia

Ureteroscopic treatment of ureteral stones can be performed both under general and spinal anesthesia. For proximal ureteral stones, general anesthesia offers the advantage to regulate respiratory excursions and allows intermittent apnea, if needed.

Table 5.1 International recommendations for the management or ureteral stones

	AUA/ES recommendations [3, 4]	LoE	Grade of recommendation	EAU recommendations [5]	LoE	Grade of recommendation	SIU/ICUD recommendations [6]	LoE	Grade of recommendation
Conservative management of ureteral stones	Observation is possible for uncomplicated ureteral stones <10 mm	B	Strong	Observation is possible for newly diagnosed stones ≤6 mm	1a	A	Intervention should be undertaken when stones are larger than 7 mm	–	–
	For distal stones, add MET (α-blockers)	B	Strong	Offer α-blockers as MET as one of the treatment options, in particular for (distal) ureteral stones >5 mm	1a	A			
	Maximal duration of conservative management is 4–6 weeks	C	Moderate	Follow up after short periods (but no specific time period is suggested)	4	A*			
Surgical management of distal ureteral stones	**>10 mm** 1. URS 2. ESWL	B	Strong	**>10 mm** 1. URS 2. ESWL	–	A*	**>10 mm** 1. URS 2. ESWL	–	A
	<10 mm 1. URS 2. ESWL	B	Strong	**<10 mm**		A*	**<10 mm** URS **or** ESWL	–	A
	URS for cystine or uric acid ureteral stones	–	Expert opinion	URS or ESWL	–				

Surgical management of proximal ureteral stones	>10 mm 1. URS *patients should be Informed that ESWL is the procedure with the least morbidity and lowest complication rate, but URS has a greater stone-free rate in a single procedure	B	Strong	>10 mm 1. URS 2. ESWL	–	A*	>10 mm URS or ESWL	–	A
				<10 mm 1. URS 2. ESWL	–	A*	<10 mm 1. ESWL 2. URS	–	A
				For severe obesity, URS is a more promising option than ESWL	2b	–			
	<10 mm 1. URS	B	Strong	Use PCNL for ureteral stones as an alternative when ESWL is not indicated or has failed or when URS is impossible	–	A			

AUA American Urological Association, *ES* Endourological Society, *LoE* level of evidence, *EAU* European Association Urology, *SIU* Société Internationale d'Urologie, *ICUD* International Consultation on Urology Disease, *MET* medical expulsive therapy, *URS* ureteroscopy, *ESWL* extracorporeal shockwave lithotripsy

Intravenous sedation for URS has been reported with high success rates and seems especially feasible for distal ureteral stones in females [13].

Antibiotic Prophylaxis

All current international guidelines recommend to perform urine analysis before URS and recommend to exclude or treat any urinary tract infection [3, 5, 6]. Antibiotic prophylaxis according to the local patterns of bacterial resistance to antibiotics is recommended in all guidelines. The possibility to send a stone fragment for bacterial analysis has also been described [7].

Patient Positioning and Set-Up

Whenever possible, the patient should be in a dorsal lithotomy position. Great care must be taken to protect pressure points in order to avoid regrettable complications such as nerve palsy and lower extremity compartment syndrome. Fluoroscopy shall be available and should be able to cover an area ranging from the pubic bone up to the kidney.

Anatomical Considerations

Conventionally, the ureter is divided into three distinct sections: proximal, middle, and distal ureter. The proximal ureter ranges from the ureteropelvic junction until the superior crest of the sacroiliac joint. The mid-ureter ranges from the superior to inferior crest of the sacroiliac joint, and from there, the distal ureter merges into the bladder (Fig. 5.1).

Based on radiographical analyses, the native human ureteral lumen has a diameter of about 6–9 Fr [14]. Three places of relative ureteral narrowing may preclude stone migration toward the bladder: at the level of the ureteropelvic junction, crossing iliac vessels, and the intramural ureter through the bladder detrusor.

Proximal Ureteral Stones

Lithotripsy of ureteral stones should follow two distinct and consecutive aims: first of all, the ureter needs to be unobstructed and only thereafter should follow a phase of stone clearance. This principle is particularly important for treatment of proximal

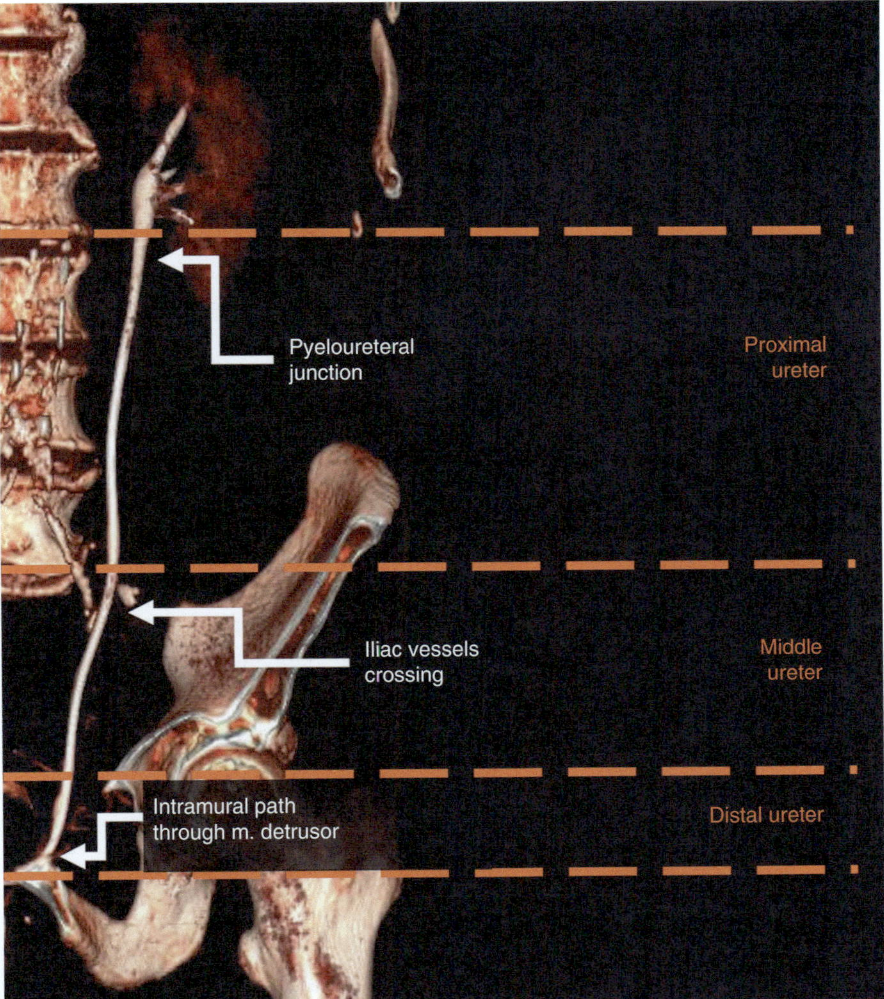

Fig. 5.1 Ureteral path with its section and relative narrowing

ureter stones. Indeed, an instrument may be easily passed beyond a partially obstructed ureter, only to become entrapped by residual fragments at the time of instrument retraction. In such conditions, there is a risk of ureteral avulsion, considering that the ureteropelvic junction is the least resistant part of the ureter against longitudinal traction. Therefore, a laser setting favoring stone fragmentation (high-energy pulses) should be selected, and stone fragments may be flushed toward the pyelocaliceal cavities, in order to ensure free passage of instruments. Clearance of any displaced fragments can thereafter be undertaken under safe conditions.

Mid-ureteral Stones

Mid-ureteral stones are typically trapped proximal to the crossing iliac vessels. Any retrograde instrumentation must be made with the care to avoid any hazardous damage to these vessels. It is thus advisable to push the stone back proximally to a wider and non-edematous section of the ureter before lithotripsy.

Distal Ureteral Stones

In a retrograde view, the distal ureter follows C-shaped path and is prone to ureteral perforation, particularly when an edematous stone bed is present. The site of perforation is typically medio-dorsal: at 6 to 9 o'clock for the left ureter and 3 to 6 o'clock for the right ureter (Fig. 5.2). Noteworthy, the distal ureter is particularly prone to iatrogenic injury, including during ureteroscopic stone removal [15, 16]. Such lesions may result in ureteral strictures. This should be kept in mind when a stone is located a few centimeters proximally to the ureteral meatus on imaging.

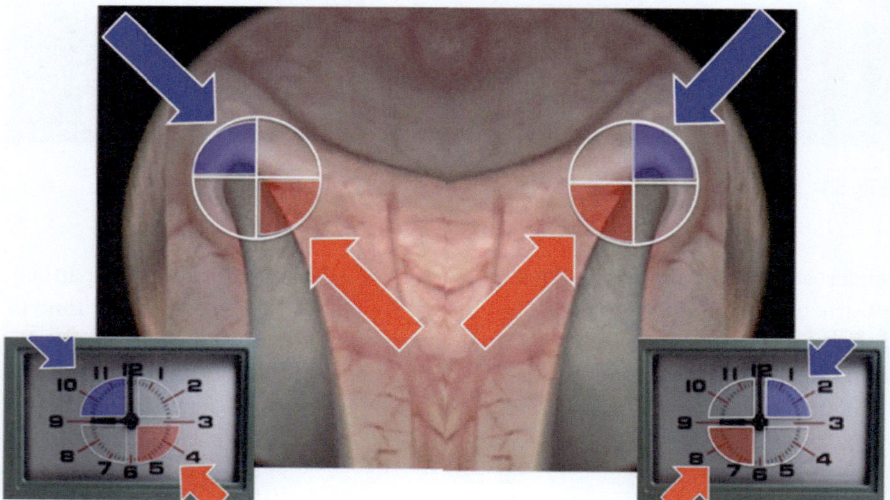

Fig. 5.2 Endoscopic view of the left and right ureteral orifices with marks for the typical place of perforation (red quadrants and arrows)

Flexible Versus Semi-rigid URS

Originally, ureteroscopes capable of transmitting an image of sufficient quality were based on the rod-lens system developed by Harold Horace Hopkins, a British physicist. The Hopkins rod-lens system uses glass columns with refraction in intervening air lenses for light and image transmission. This rod-lens system required the ureteroscope to be rigid and was therefore not well adapted to accommodate angulations of the ureter. It was not until sufficient development of bundled fibers that semi-rigid ureteroscopes (sr-URS) capable of bending up to 2 cm from their axis appeared. From there, development of miniaturized f-URS with optimized durometer and enhanced tip deflection is nearly supplanting semi-rigid URS (sr-URS). The advantages of f-URS particularly become evident for treatment of proximal ureteral stones, because f-URS are able to accommodate to the angulations of the ureter and tip deflection allows for a continuous visual control of the ureteral lumen. Consequently, lower failure and retreatment rates can be achieved by f-URS compared to sr-URS for proximal ureteral stones [17].

One remaining advantage of sr-URS over f-URS lies within its relative ease of manipulation. The conjunction of pivot-like movements centered on the bladder neck and the possibility of a pendular camera view make it relatively easy to pass sr-URS into the ureteral orifice, when compared to f-URS. Overall, the place of sr-URS in the endourological armamentarium is becoming somewhat less popular and might be reserved for the treatment of impacted distal ureteral stones or in situations where a f-URS is ineffective due to bucking of the most distal portion of its shaft.

Ureteral Dilation and Pre-stenting

Ureteral narrowing as well as edematous mucosa around the stone bed can impede endoscopic access to the stone and consequently impact on the stone-free and complication rates. Owing to the lack of sufficient evidence, the advantages and risks of active ureteral dilation (tapered coaxial dilators and balloon dilators) over passive ureteral dilation (ureteral stenting and postponed URS, commonly called "pre-stenting") are the object of an ongoing debate [18]. Comparatively, it may be favorable to stent the ureter and allow passive dilation rather than use active dilation, because the latter typically disrupts the physiologic ureteral wall arrangement, puts the ureteral at risk of ischemia, and therefore may lead to ureteral stricture.

Safety Guidewire

Facilitating urine transport from the kidney to the bladder is the primary aim whenever a ureter wall injury occurs during ureteroscopy, irrespective of the mechanism. Ureteral patency can be ensured with the placement of a safety guidewire (SG) ahead of the insertion of any instrument into the ureter [19]. Its use is recommended by international guidelines based on expert opinion and is subject to some debate simply due to the lack of data evaluating its advantages and limitations. The impact of SG on tensile forces during ureteral access sheath (UAS) placement is minimal [20]. Another advantage of the safety guidewire is that it opens the ureteral meatus, thus facilitating endoscope insertion. We thus recommend systematic use of a SG, especially in urology residency training programs (for complete discussion, see Chapter 3C).

Laser Lithotripsy of Ureteral Stones

The laser fiber tip should always point at the middle of the stone during laser lithotripsy of ureteral stones (Fig. 5.3). This is in contrast to dusting techniques of renal stones, where the fiber tip is typically moved from periphery to the center of the stone. If the ureteral lumen is sufficiently wide, laser lithotripsy may be completed in situ. Alternatively, the stone fragments may be extracted with a basket. Respecting our recommendation, one may avoid potential risks of ureteral wall injury and ureteral stricture formation that are reported in recent literature [21].

Ureteral Access Sheath

Ureteral access sheaths (UASs) facilitate multiple URS passages and increase visibility during lithotripsy by increasing irrigation outflow. While UASs lower intrarenal pressure during renal stone treatment, this advantage appears less important in treatment of ureteral stones [22]. Of note, ureteroscopic evaluation of the ureter

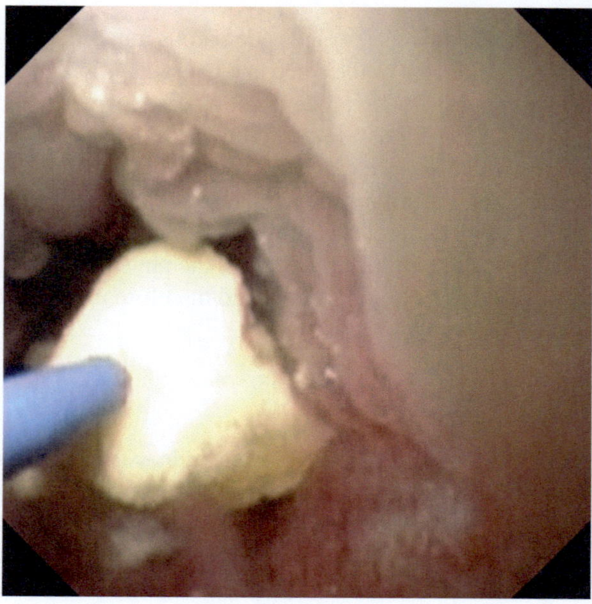

Fig. 5.3 Endoscopic view of a stone in the ureter with the laser fiber tip pointing at the middle of the stone

should always be considered prior to insertion of any UAS, in order to evaluate for possible downward migration of stone.

Basketing: The Trapped Stone

In the event that a stone or fragments have been secured in a basket and a ureteral narrowing hinders retraction of the basket, one should refrain to add longitudinal traction because of the risk of ureteral avulsion (Chap. 10). Releasing trapped stone or fragments (TSF) does not always require cumbersome dismantlement of the basket handle. By putting the basket in a fully open configuration and then pushing the basket shaft in a retrograde fashion, the nitinol wires may disengage the TSF. The basket can then be fully closed and retracted. If this method is not successful, a laser fiber can be inserted in the working channel of the URS parallel to the basket (Fig. 5.4a). Hereby, the TSF can be fragmented within the basket (Fig. 5.4b–c) until the latter can be fully closed and retracted. The combination of a basket and a laser fiber is possible for all currently available f-URS, provided that appropriate device diameters are selected. This technique can also be used to avoid retrograde migration of fragments during lithotripsy.

Pregnancy

Incidence of symptomatic urolithiasis during pregnancy is similar to the non-pregnant population [23]. Symptoms may be rather non-specific, but flank pain or abdominal complaints are present in 85 to 100% of all symptomatic cases [24]. Physiologic hydronephrosis may be found in up to 90% right-sided and 67% left-sided kidneys in pregnant women, and ureteral dilation is typically found proximally from the pelvic organs [25]. This is supposed to be associated with mechanical ureteral compression and relaxing effect of circulating progesterone on the ureteral wall tonus [26]. That state of physiologic dilation may explain why up to 60–80% of all

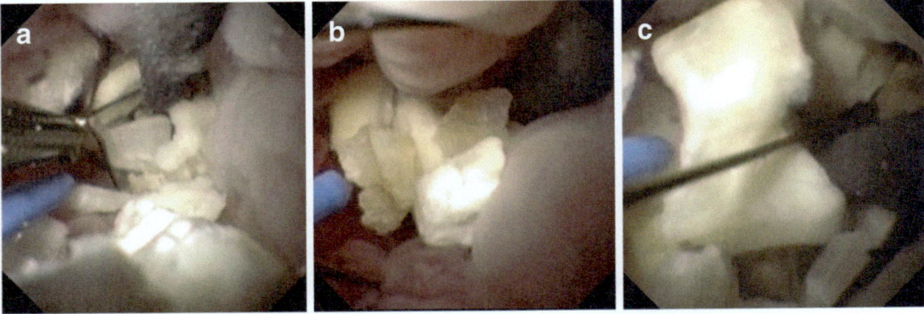

Fig. 5.4 (**a**) Endoscopic view of a laser fiber (273 μm) inserted parallel to a basket (1.9 Fr). (**b**) A ureteral narrowing hinders retraction of the basket. (**c**) Fragments are released by in situ laser lithotripsy

stones pass spontaneously during pregnancy [27]. Diagnostic and therapeutic imaging modalities are limited by the potentially deleterious effect of X-rays on the fetus.

Whenever possible, conservative management should be encouraged. In case of sustained pain, infection, or renal function impairment, active treatment can be offered. The optimal choice of therapy is subject to an ongoing debate beyond the scope of this chapter. Active treatment includes percutaneous and retrograde drainage, as well as emergency ureteroscopy [24]. In case of emergency URS, lithotripsy should only be performed by means of laser energy and not with any of pneumatic, electrohydraulic, and ultrasonic lithotripters, because they may induce premature labor or eventually bear a direct hazard for the fetus [24]. Noteworthy, ureteral stents are prone to encrustation because of gestational hyperuricosuria and hypercalciuria, and therefore regular exchange of percutaneous drains or ureteral stents is required, if definitive treatment is not offered initially [28].

Pediatrics

During childhood, the ureter is more compliant and capable to tolerate large stone fragments compared to adults. This particularity allows for high stone fragment clearance rates after ESWL, even for stones larger than 10 mm [29]. It was not until technological advances allowing for miniaturization of instruments that URS became popular in pediatric urology. Authors tend to agree that ureteral access sheaths are currently not adapted to children and that balloon dilation is best avoided because of the risk for ureteral wall ischemia and stricture [30].

The Narrow Ureteral Meatus: "Tent" Sign

When facing a narrow ureteral meatus, an indirect method to evaluate ease of instrument insertion is to use a stiff guidewire and observe whether the meatus widens up like a tent or not (Fig. 5.5). If the meatus remains round and narrow around the guide wire, no ureteral access sheath should be inserted, and ureteral pre-stenting or a sheathless technique should be pursued.

Conclusions

Ureteroscopy has undergone tremendous technological advances over the last decades and has undoubtedly established itself a treatment of choice for active ureteral stone clearance. Although potentially more morbid compared to ESWL for ureteral stone treatment, URS tends to be more efficacious, requires less secondary procedures, and is independent of stone density or skin-to-stone distance. Strict adherence to fundamental operative techniques will promote favorable results with minimal complications.

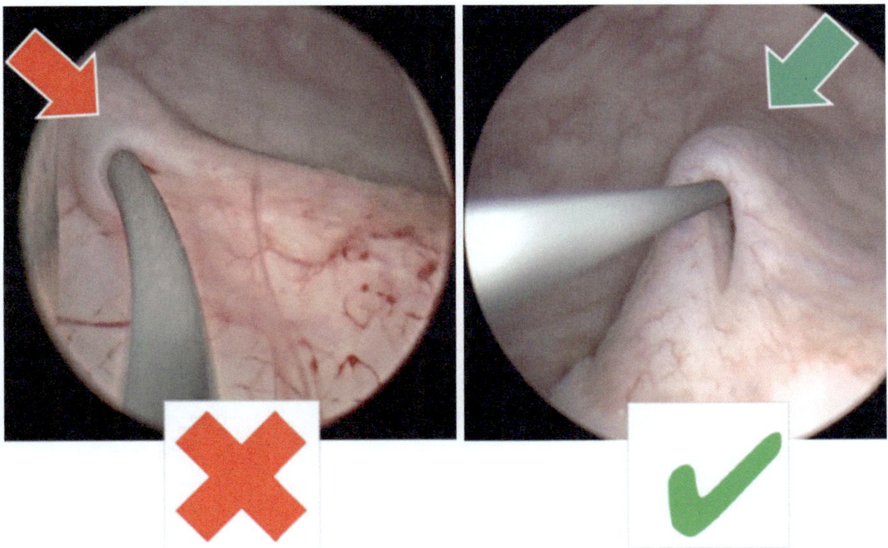

Fig. 5.5 The "tent" sign predicts instrument insertion success

Flexible Ureteroscopic Treatment of Renal Stones

Asaf Shvero, Nir Kleinmann, and Scott G. Hubosky

Indication/Guidelines

The role of retrograde flexible ureteroscopy (URS), or "retrograde intrarenal surgery" (RIRS), in the treatment of urolithiasis continues to expand due to improved surgical outcomes compared to extra-corporal shockwave lithotripsy (ESWL) and a low complication rate compared to percutaneous nephrolithotomy (PCNL) [31, 32]. According to a contemporary study of case logs submitted to the American Board of Urology (ABU), ureteroscopy has surpassed ESWL as the most commonly performed surgical treatment for upper urinary tract stones both among newly trained and senior urologists [33]. Advancement in ureteroscopic technology, including digital cameras, endoscope miniaturization, and improved deflection mechanisms, combined with the growing surgical experience, has placed ureteroscopy at the heart of kidney stone treatment guidelines. In the EAU guidelines on urolithiasis published in 2020, URS for kidney stones is considered as a first-line treatment option for renal stones in all locations and compositions, apart from stones with a diameter larger than 2 cm in which it is considered second-line (Fig. 5.6) [34]. In the most recent AUA guidelines published in 2016, URS is considered first-line for non-lower-pole stones <20 mm and lower-pole stones <10 mm. For lower-pole stones between 10 mm and 20 mm, URS is considered a viable option due to lower complication rate than PCNL, although stone-free rate (SFR) for PCNL is higher.

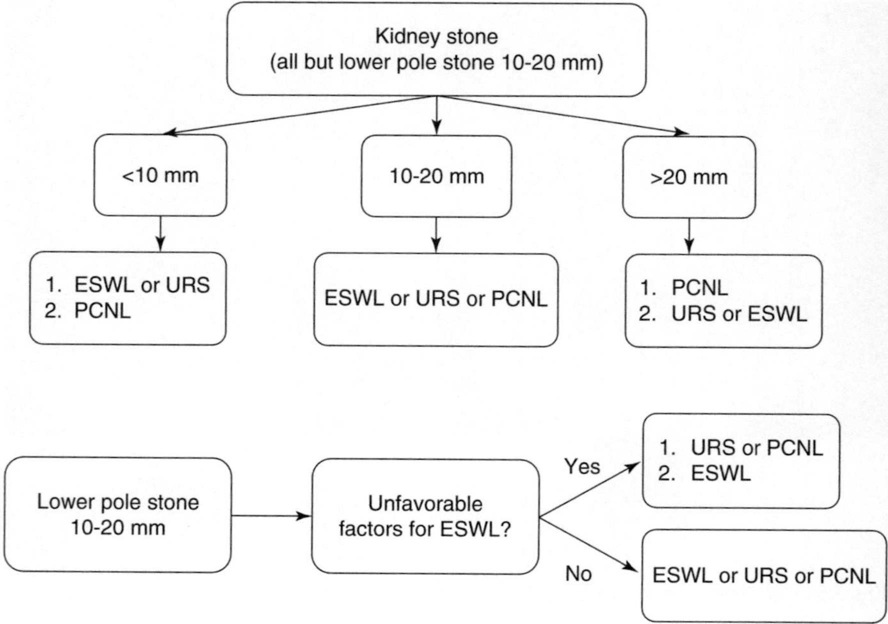

Fig. 5.6 Treatment algorithm for renal stones. (Adapted from [34] Guidelines on Urolithiasis. European association of urology 2020 and [3] AUA/Endourological Society Guidelines for Surgical Management of Stones. 2016)

For renal stones >2 cm, PCNL is considered the first-line treatment [3]. Nevertheless, for stones >2 cm, a staged URS is often feasible and in many cases is preferred by patients because of the less-invasive nature of the procedure.

Stone-Free Rate (SFR)

SFR is the main measure for success of kidney stone surgery. SFR is defined as the percentage of patients that are without evidence of stones or without evidence of significant stone fragments, as viewed by an image modality after surgery. This definition is not uniform among different publications and varies in terms of resultant fragment size and post-surgical imaging modality. The most common definition for "clinically insignificant residual fragments" (CIRF) (a.k.a. stone-free status) is the absence of stone fragments larger than 4 mm regardless of image modality or time of image after surgery [35, 36]. The different imaging modalities (RUS, KUB, and CT) have different sensitivity and specificity for stone fragments and therefore will yield different stone-free rates. The sensitivity and specificity for detection of renal stones of RUS, KUB, and CT are 54% and 91%, 57% and 76%, and 98% and 99%, respectively [37, 38]. While RUS is an attractive modality due to its availability and lack of ionizing radiation, it can lead to over- and underestimation of stone size in 22% of cases and lead to inappropriate decision-making. When critically assessing treatment results of ureteroscopy and laser lithotripsy, it is essential to know how SFR was measured [39]. CT scan is often considered the gold standard but subjects the patient to potentially unnecessary radiation exposure for study purposes.

Measurement of Stone Burden

The choice of treatment modality is set by the characteristics of the patient and the existing stone(s). Perhaps the most important stone characteristic is stone burden. Stone burden is determined by the number of stones and stone sizes. The current EAU, AUA, and NICE guidelines determine stone size to be the largest diameter that can be measured in a preoperative imaging test [3, 34, 40]. However, a luminal stone is a three-dimensional object, and many times it is not conveniently shaped as a sphere or cube but can be branched with variable dimensions throughout. The mere linear length of the stone can greatly underestimate the true stone burden. For example, a 2.0 × 1.0 × 1.0 cm stone (which is considered a "2-cm stone") can yield 2000 1 mm stone fragments, but a 2.0 × 2.0 × 2.0 cm stone (which is also considered a "2-cm stone") can yield 8000 1 mm stone fragments – with an actual stone burden that is four times larger (Fig. 5.7). Using this reasoning, the "ideal 2 cm stone" for URS is long but thin, such that it is only 2 cm in one of three dimensions (Fig. 5.8).

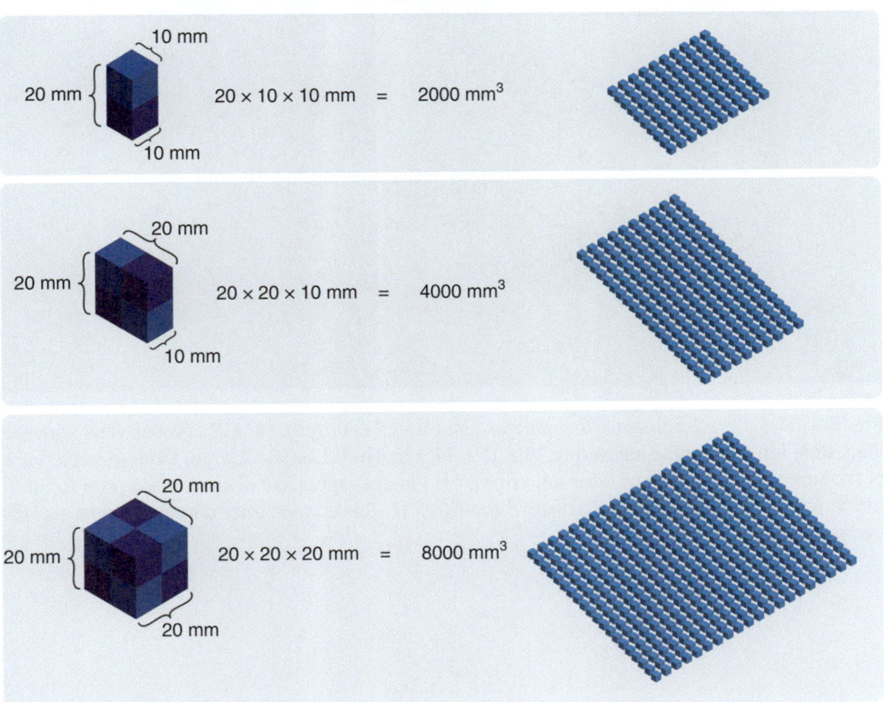

Fig. 5.7 Actual stone volume versus stone diameter. The true stone burden is best quantified when considering all three dimensions

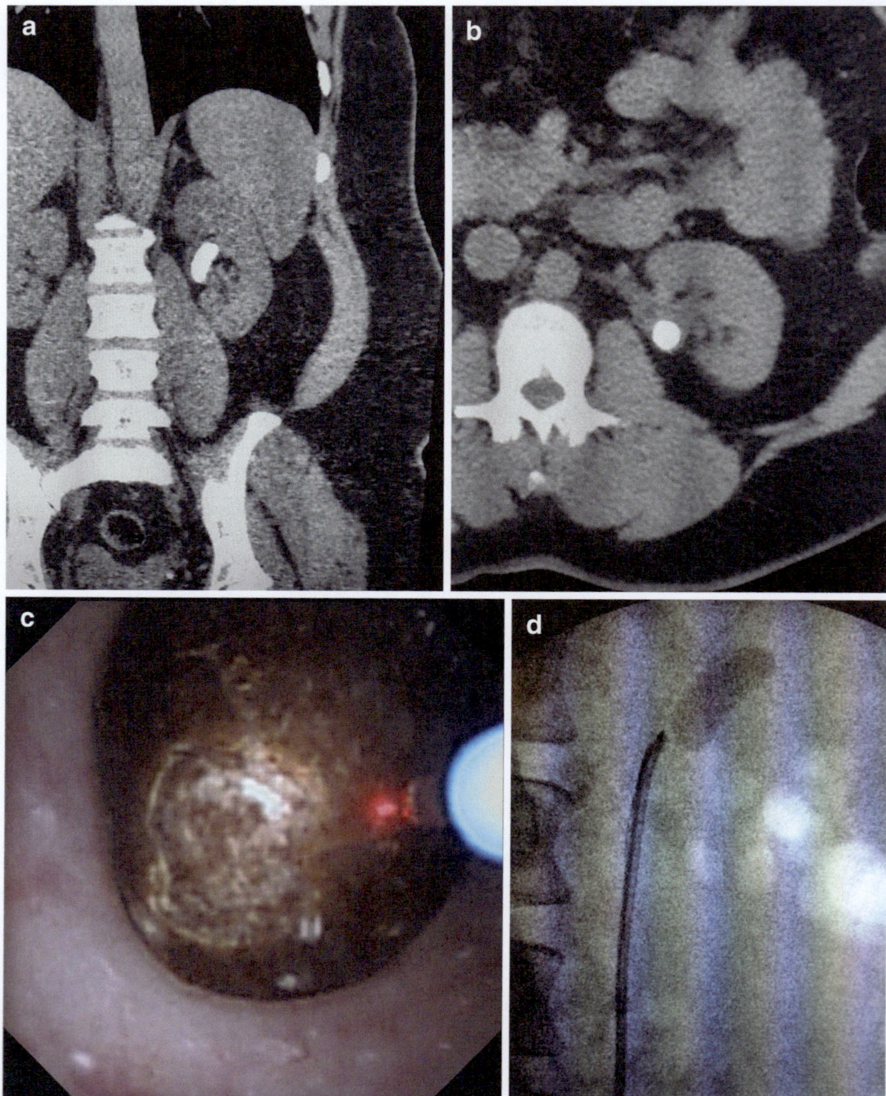

Fig. 5.8 The ideal 2-cm stone for ureteroscopic laser lithotripsy. (**a**) CT coronal view shows a long, thin, left renal stone measuring 20 x 15 x 11 mm. (**b**) CT axial view. (**c**) Ureteroscopic view of the stone with initiation of laser lithotripsy. (**d**) Fluoroscopic view of same stone prior to lithotripsy. (**e**) Same stone after partial laser lithotripsy. (**f**) Same stone after complete ureteroscopic treatment with laser lithotripsy

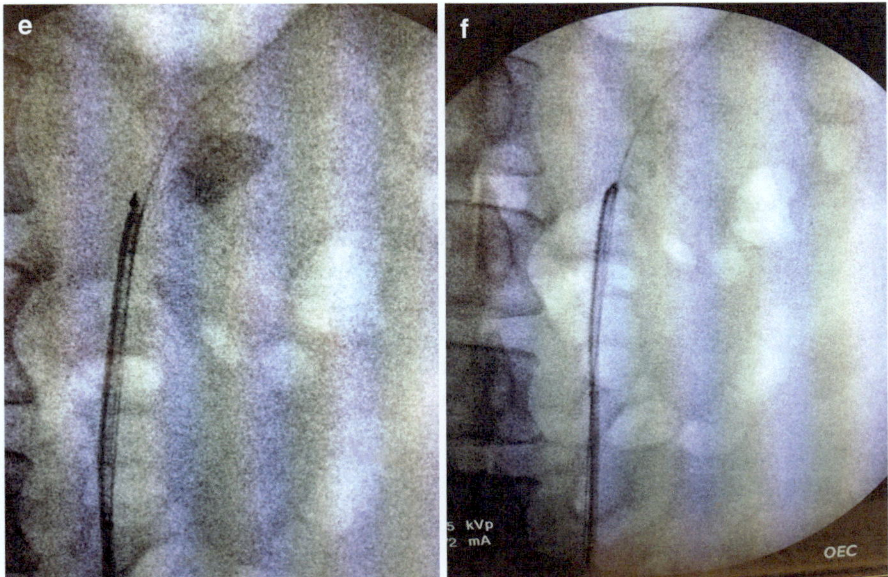

Fig. 5.8 (continued)

The different stone size measurements (linear diameter, volume, surface area, etc.), stone density, collecting system shape, and the different imaging modalities utilized can create heterogeneity in the reporting of outcomes, which is imperative to consider when evaluating reports on stone treatment [41].

Technique

Today, the mainstay of treatment for kidney stones via ureteroscopy utilizes laser energy. The two main techniques for laser lithotripsy are dusting of the stone with high-frequency/low-power laser followed by postoperative spontaneous passage of the small residual stone fragments and fragmentation of the stone with high-power/low-frequency laser followed by active removal of the fragments usually with a retrieval device. In a recent prospective study, Humphreys et al. found no difference in SFR between the two methods among 159 patients [42]. Still, there is usually a personal preference for every surgeon on the method of choice.

Results

Stones >2 cm

As mentioned above, current guidelines consider PCNL as the first-line treatment option for stones with a diameter of 2 cm or greater, with URS as a second-line option for those patients deemed poor candidates for PCNL for reasons such as inability to stop anticoagulants, medical comorbidities, or anatomic considerations [3, 34]. However, there are reports demonstrating good results when using ureteroscopy for large stones, conceding that multiple procedures are required at times (Table 5.2). In a review of 12 studies and 651 patients, URS with laser lithotripsy for stones larger than 2 cm had a mean SFR of 91% and 1.45 procedures per case. Complication rate was 8.6%, among them 4.5% major complications but no deaths. Stone-free definition was not uniform among these studies and varied between no fragments at all and with fragments of up to 4 mm [43]. Usually, larger stones should be dusted and not fragmented, because of the technical challenge of actively removing a large number of fragments with a retrieval device. Multiple procedures are sometimes needed to achieve stone-free status. Hyams et al. found a 63% SFR for single-staged URS among 120 patients with kidney stones larger than 2 cm (SFR defined as fragments $\leq$2 mm). The majority of patients however (84%) underwent one procedure [44].

Table 5.2 Ureteroscopy and laser lithotripsy for stones >2 cm

Series	N	Stone size (cm)	OR time (min)	Mean stages	SFR	Postop evaluation
Grasso 1998 [57]	45	2.6	< 180	1.2	76% (1) 91% (2) 93% (3)	KUB RUS Second URS
El-Anany 2001 [58]	23 7	2–3 >3	70 135	1.0	87% 42%	
Mariani 2008 [59]	63	4.4	49	1.7	95%	KUB, CT, IVP, second URS
Breda 2008 [60]	15	2.2	83	2.3	60% (1) 87% (2) 93% (3)	2nd URS
Hyams 2010 [44]	120	2.4	74	1.0	47% (TSF) 66% (< 2 mm) 83% (<4 mm)	RUS, CT KUB
Al-Qahtani 2012 [61]	120	2.63	89	1.6	58% (1) 87% (2) 96% (3)	KUB, CT
Cohen 2012 [62]	132	3.0	–	1.6	87%	KUB, RUS
Miernik 2013 [63]	38	2.71	95	1.1	82%	RUS, CT
Pieras 2017 [64]	54	2.51	93	1.2	76%	KUB, RUS
Huang 2020 [65]	251	2.7	126	1.4	61.9% (1) 82.9% (2) 89.5% (3)	KUB / RUS

Lower-Pole Stones

Lower-pole stones are often the most challenging targets for retrograde ureteroscopic laser lithotripsy, and achieving stone-free status can be difficult. There are multiple technical reasons for this observation: (1) The limitation of ureteroscope deflection, which makes the stones more difficult to reach and treat, (2) the potential damage to the ureteroscope after enduring long periods of maximal deflection, and (3) the limited spontaneous expulsion of residual fragments from the lower pole. With the growing experience in working with flexible devices, to encounter a difficult-to-reach anatomical location is not common. But, with repeated use, flexible ureteroscopes lose part of their ability to deflect as much. One of the parameters used to predict potential difficulty in reaching a lower-pole stone is the infundibulo-pelvic angle (IPA), which lies at the intersection of the ureteropelvic axis and the central axis of the lower-pole infundibulum in question. This angle is best measured with retrograde pyelogram or intravenous pyelogram. A steep angle <30–90° has been associated with lower SFR with ureteroscopic laser lithotripsy [45, 46]. Several strategies have been developed to overcome these difficulties, including advancements in deflection mechanisms, use of single-use ureteroscopes with "fresh" deflection capabilities, and displacement of stones from the lower pole before laser lithotripsy [47]. SFR after URS for lower-pole stones has been reported to be 59%–82.1% [45, 46, 48].

Multiple Stones

The current EAU, AUA, and NICE guidelines set their recommendations on stone size, with no reference to stone number [3, 34, 40]. As long as the parameter used is stone diameter and not stone volume, the definition of "stone size" will be vague in cases involving multiple stones and may not represent stone burden accurately. Most define "stone size" to be a summation of sizes of all stones (cumulative stone diameter – CSD). This difference between CSD and total volume is more significant in larger stone burdens and with greater number of stones [49]. However, stone number has been incorporated into scoring systems to predict treatment success and risk of complication of URS and PCNL, such as the Resorlu-Unsal score, STONE, and CROES nephrolithometry scores [50–52]. Zetumer et al. analyzed 125 patients with multiple renal stones and noted that a CSD >20 mm did not necessarily favor PCNL over URS as a treatment choice. In fact, patients with more than three stones were much more likely to have undergone URS relative to PCNL. Further examination of the data showed that a total stone burden of ≥35 mm was more impactful on decision-making than the mere number of stones involved. According to the data, 89% of patients with stone burden ≥35 mm had PCNL performed, regardless of stone number. For patients with total stone burden <35 mm, those with fewer number of stones (2–3) were nearly evenly split between URS and PCNL, 48% and 52%, respectively. Conversely, in those patients with stone burden <35 mm but with more than three stones, URS was performed in 91%. SFR were similar in both groups (URS versus PCNL) [53].

Stones in Caliceal Diverticula

Caliceal diverticula are relatively rare and by definition are cystic cavities lined with non-secretory urothelium, which communicate with the remainder of the intrarenal luminal collecting system by way of a narrow ostium. In 40% they can be symptomatic, and in up to 50%, there are stones in the diverticula thought to form due to relatively static urine [54, 55]. Treatment options for symptomatic diverticula depend on the location of the diverticula and the stone burden. Ureteroscopy is an appealing approach especially in middle and upper pole diverticula where access is relatively easier and anterior calyces where percutaneous access is difficult. Posterior diverticula, especially in the lower pole or with relatively large stone burdens, are best accessed percutaneously.

From a technical standpoint, the ostium of the diverticula can be difficult to identify in some cases. If so, it is possible to use a refluxing technique with injecting methylene blue next to the presumed location of the ostium. Then saline irrigation is continued until the dye is cleared from the system. Refluxing of the methylene blue will mark the ostium of the diverticula. After identification of the ostium, a safety wire may be inserted into the diverticulum, and if needed, its neck can be incised with a laser or dilated to enable access. Stones should be treated with laser lithotripsy. When the stone burden is cleared, consideration must be given to ablation of the mucosal surface lining which can be coagulated with laser or electrocautery. In a systematic review, which included 19 retrospective studies and 757 patients, the stone-free rate for URS was 61.4% with 67.9% symptom-free rate. SFR was 83% and only 21.3% for PCNL and ESWL, respectfully. The complication rate was relatively low for URS at 3.3% but 11.9% for PCNL [56].

Conclusion

According to multiple stone treatment guidelines, URS is a first-line option for non-lower-pole stones less than 20 mm in greatest diameter and lower-pole stones less than 10 mm in diameter. Stones greater than 2 cm can be treated with URS, but patients should be counseled that more than one procedure might be necessary. The versatility of URS allows for adaptability and application to other situations including patients with multiple renal stones and select cases in which there is a stone in a calyceal diverticulum.

Post Ureteroscopic Evaluation: Short and Long Term

Etienne Xavier Keller, Vincent De Coninck, Steeve Doizi and Olivier Traxer

Short Term

Patient Monitoring

The basic protocol for monitoring of short-term complications after ureteroscopy (URS) includes vital sign parameter monitoring (heart rate, blood pressure, respiratory rate, and temperature), pain evaluation, and visual inspection of urine. In the absence of bladder catheterization or in case of early catheter withdrawal, proper spontaneous micturition needs to be ensured. Unrecognized gross hematuria puts the patient at risk of delayed blood loss identification and at risk of acute urinary retention due to retained intravesical blood clots.

Outpatient Clinic or Overnight Stay

First reports of URS on an outpatient basis came in the early 1990s [66]. This strategy seems feasible without complications for up to 78% of all patients [67]. Patient selection is generally based on comorbidities, operative complexity, and social factors. Predictors in favor of post-procedural pain and same-day hospital readmission include extended operative time, ureteral stenting, bilateral procedures, as well as any stone location other than the distal ureter [67–69]. Noteworthy, the most lethal threat to the patient after ureteroscopy is potential systemic inflammatory response syndrome (SIRS) [70]. Patients who are suspected to be at high risk for SIRS after URS should be carefully monitored, and overnight stay should be considered.

SIRS and Sepsis

SIRS results from the systemic release of inflammatory cytokines by the immune system, inducing a cascade of events typically leading to fever, tachycardia, tachypnea, white blood cell release, and eventual life-threatening organ dysfunction. As for URS, SIRS is usually a consequence of an infectious insult, which in turn defines sepsis. Up to 3.4% of all patients undergoing URS may have an unplanned hospital readmission for a genitourinary infection, which seems associated with preoperative stenting and operative time [71]. Notably, an unrecognized colonization of the upper tract might be present at the time of URS, despite having obtained negative mid-stream urine cultures [72].

Urologists have to feel confident with the definition of SIRS and sepsis in order to detect signs and symptoms ensuring timely treatment of such conditions. Until recently, sepsis was defined by the presence of at least two out of four SIRS criteria, with a confirmed or suspected infection [73, 74]. In 2016, an updated definition of sepsis had been proposed in a consensus article, abandoning the use of SIRS criteria [75]. This new proposal presupposes a life-threatening organ dysfunction to be present and follows a Sequential Organ Failure Assessment (SOFA) scoring. This updated definition had a superior predictive validity over SIRS criteria for mortality [76]. A major limitation to the SOFA scoring is the complexity of parameter retrieval, which may lead to delayed identification of sepsis. Therefore, a "quick SOFA" scoring (qSOFA) has been proposed. Table 5.3 offers a comparative overview of SIRS criteria, SOFA, and qSOFA scoring.

Post-Procedural Stenting

Urine transport from the kidney to the bladder may be compromised by eventual ureteral wall edema caused by mechanical stress during URS. This may result in pain, infection, unplanned hospital readmission, and emergency operative decompression. Short-term ureteral stenting has therefore become a common routine after

Table 5.3 Comparison of sepsis criteria

	Systemic inflammatory response syndrome (SIRS)	Sequential Organ Failure Assessment (SOFA)	Quick Sequential Organ Failure Assessment (qSOFA)
Score range	0–4 criteria	0–24 points (0–4 points per variable)	0–3 points (1 point per variable)
Definitions	*SIRS:* Two or more criteria *Sepsis:* + confirmed or suspected infection *Severe sepsis:* + organ failure	*Sepsis:* life-threatening organ dysfunction in response to infection *Organ dysfunction:* acute change in total SOFA score ≥2 points consequent to infection	Bedside criteria to identify adult patients with suspected infection who are likely to have poor outcomes if ≥2 points
Vital parameters	Temperature >38 °C or <36 °C	Glasgow coma scale	Altered mentation
	Heart rate >90/min	Mean arterial pressure, +/− concomitant administration of vasopressors	Systolic blood pressure ≤100 mmHg
	Respiratory rate >20/min	Urine output/24 h	Respiratory rate ≥22/min
Laboratory tests	$PaCO_2$ <32 mmHg	PaO_2/FiO_2 ratio	
	White blood cell count >12,000/mm³, <4000/mm³, or >10% immature band forms	Platelet count	
		Bilirubin	
		Serum creatinine	
References	Bone et al. [73]	Singer et al. [75]	Singer et al. [75]

URS, but patient selection is not well established [77]. Currently available evidence suggests past history of urolithiasis as well as recent or recurrent infection as strong predictors of morbidity after URS without a stent [77].

Most of the body of evidence on benefits and drawbacks of ureteral stenting arises from studies on ureteral access sheaths (UASs). The discrepancy between the UAS outer diameter (11.5–18 Fr) and native ureter diameter (6–9 Fr) explains the propensity of UAS for ureteral wall edema, which seems most pronounced at 72 hours postoperatively [14, 78]. Ureteral stenting after the use of a UAS is associated with lower overall pain score and re-intervention rates [79, 80]. A recent meta-analysis on URS confirmed a significantly lower risk of unplanned medical visit for patients with post-procedural stenting [81]. Duration of post-procedural stenting is not well established, but 85% of the responders to a worldwide questionnaire study would remove the stent within 7 days [82]. Post-procedural stenting is associated with a higher risk for irritative urinary symptoms and hematuria [83]. Many efforts have been put toward reducing morbidity associated with ureteral stents, but neither material proprieties, geometry, length, nor catheter coating variations have been successful [84, 85]. Recent reports suggest alpha-blockers, anti-cholinergics or a combination of both for an adequate reduction of irritative urinary symptoms [86, 87].

Rather than questioning the benefit of post-procedural stenting, future studies should examine which risk factors might predict the need for re-intervention following URS when a stent is omitted. Attention should be directed to scoring the severity of ureteral wall insult following ureteroscopic manipulation and using this as a possible predictor of when a post-procedural stent is truly indicated [88, 89].

Long Term

Assessment and Management of Residual Stone Disease

Clearance of all stones and fragments shall be the aim of any active stone treatment. However, there is no consensus on the definition of clinically insignificant residual fragments (RFs). Also, imaging modality and exact time after the procedure to detect them are subject to ongoing debate.

Historically, RFs of <4 mm following extracorporeal shockwave lithotripsy were accepted as clinically insignificant, considering their potential ability to pass spontaneously [90]. In long-term studies, it became apparent that RFs were prone to re-growth and to re-intervention [91, 92]. A recent multi-center analysis revealed a re-intervention rate of 29% and an overall complication rate of 44% within 17 months for patients diagnosed with RF of any size after URS.

Computed tomography (CT) is the current gold standard for post-procedural evaluation, owing to a sensitivity of almost 100% for RF, when compared to 71% for kidney-ureter-bladder (KUB) plain X-ray and 53% for ultrasonography (US)

[93]. The downside of CT is a rather low specificity of 62%, caused by false-positive interpretation of Randall's plaques and intraparenchymal calcifications [94].

Based on the currently available evidence, one may propose an active re-intervention for any remaining renal fragments of >4 mm, based on the association with stone re-growth, complications, and re-interventions [35].

Ureteral Strictures

Prevalence and incidence of ureteral strictures in modern URS is not well established, and currently available evidence is based on few studies where earlier generation devices were used. Predictors for post-procedural ureteral stricture include impacted edematous ureteral stones and ureteral perforation, with the impacted stone being a frequently reported risk factor for ureteral perforation [95, 96]. A recent meta-analysis suggests a higher risk for ureteral stricture formation after holmium:yttrium-aluminum-garnet (Ho:YAG) laser lithotripsy, when compared to pneumatic lithotripsy [21]. One explanation may be the potential thermal injury to the ureteral wall from Ho:YAG lithotripsy [97]. Concerning UAS, the risk for ureteral stricture formation has not been well established to date but may be associated with increasing outer diameter of UASs [98].

Because the time between stricture formation and the appearance of clinical signs resulting from urine transport impairment can be highly variable, routine clinical and sonographic evaluation is recommended postoperatively [37]. Also, patients should be well informed to consider medical consultation in case of prolonged flank pain after URS, which may be a symptom of hydronephrosis.

Metabolic Evaluation

Indications and benefits of metabolic evaluation are subject to another chapter of this book and are therefore not further detailed here.

Conclusions

Ureteroscopic approach to stone disease includes responsible post-procedural care to patients. Any urologist performing URS must feel comfortable with all aspects of post-procedural short- and long-term evaluation. The approach will maximize outcomes and minimize morbidity.

Techniques for Ureteroscopic Holmium Laser Lithotripsy

Thomas J. Hardacker and Scott G. Hubosky

Introduction

Holmium:yttrium aluminum garnet (Ho:YAG) lasers, coupled with increasingly refined small-caliber flexible ureteroscopes, have made accessing and fragmenting stones throughout the entirety of the genitourinary tract feasible. At a wavelength of 2120 nm, holmium laser energy can fragment any composition of urinary tract stone and has been shown to produce relatively smaller stone fragments compared to other modalities, such as electrohydraulic lithotripsy (EHL) [99]. Holmium lasers induce stone fragmentation primarily by a photothermal mechanism, by which photons are transferred through the laser fiber to water within the stone, where they are absorbed and energy is ultimately released as heat [100, 101]. Laser fibers are available in varying sizes, typically ranging from 200 to 365 μm for ureteroscopic procedures. While typically more expensive, 200 μm fibers allow for enhanced irrigant flow leading to potentially better visualization. Furthermore, smaller diameter fibers allow for less inhibition of maximal ureteroscope deflection, which is particularly useful when treating lower-pole stones.

After safely deploying a semi-rigid or flexible ureteroscope into the ureter or renal pelvis, a laser fiber is placed through the working channel and positioned such that the tip is easily visible beyond the ureteroscope tip. Holmium laser energy functions optimally when the tip of the laser fiber is in contact with the stone when activated, resulting in efficient transfer of energy manifesting in stone fragmentation. The resultant effect of the laser on stone treatment is a function of two variables, the energy (J) and frequency (Hz). Each can be adjusted depending on the overall intent of fragmentation and has resulted in the description of two distinct but not mutually exclusive methods of treatment – dusting (lower-power, high-frequency settings) and fragmentation with extraction (high-power, low-frequency settings). Benefits of dusting potentially include decreased operative time, lower cost, and decreased ureteral trauma as it avoids multiple basketing attempts to remove all stone fragments from the collecting system [35, 42, 102]. Fragmentation with stone extraction demonstrates benefits including a higher stone-free rate and potentially fewer stone events following treatment with ureteroscopy. Furthermore, it allows for stone analysis, guiding metabolic prevention in the future [35].

Dusting

Dusting technique utilizes fine movements of the ureteroscope tip to systematically ablate the periphery of the stone. In doing this, the goal is to produce fine particles that resemble dust and will pass spontaneously after the procedure (Fig. 5.9). This

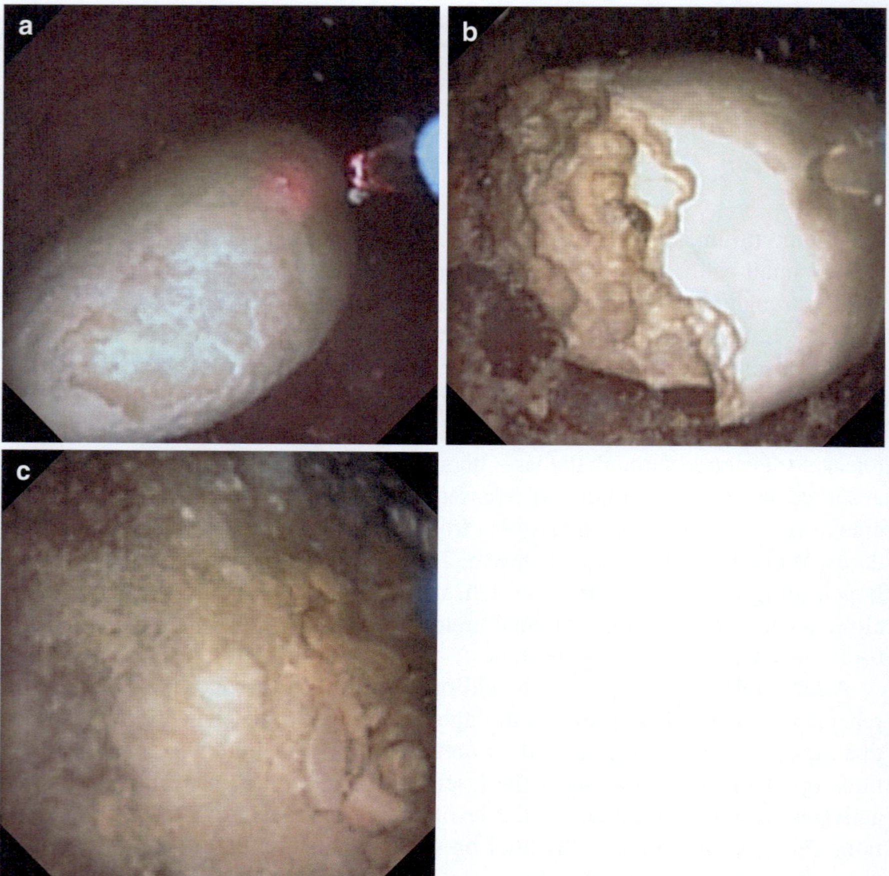

Fig. 5.9 Dusting technique for a 2-cm renal stone. (**a**) Stone prior to treatment with laser fiber at the ready. (**b**) Painting the periphery of the stone demonstrates methodical fragmentation. (**c**) Small resultant fragments relative to a 365-micron laser fiber (right)

strategy utilizes low-power and high-frequency laser settings for optimal results, typically 0.2–0.4 J and 20–80 Hz [103]. These settings, coupled with a long pulse width, decrease retropulsion, resulting in smaller resultant fragments [42, 104]. Production of fine resultant particles that will pass spontaneously reduces potential ureteral trauma from repeated basketing attempts and theoretically decreases associated operative time.

As the stone is progressively reduced in size, the energy delivered will eventually exceed that of the remaining calculus, resulting in increased stone motion. This remaining piece can either be fragmented and extracted or further reduced using other techniques, such as "popcorning." "Popcorning" is a technique in which multiple stone fragments are treated within a confined calyx with laser settings of 1.0 J and 20 Hz [105]. The laser fiber is activated while several millimeters away from the fragments, causing the calculi to bounce rapidly and come in contact with the fiber, resulting in further fragmentation. An equally important advantage of the popcorn setting is that it scatters the smallest resultant stone fragments, which can coalesce in a calyx, making it easier to detect fragments still in need of further refinement. Commonly, resultant stone fragments smaller than 3–4 mm are deemed sufficient for spontaneous passage. Several techniques can be employed in order to gauge the size of remaining stone fragments after treatment. Primarily, the surgeon can visually measure any resultant fragments against the size of the laser fiber or safety wire in use. Secondly, if any fragments are basketed and removed, these can be measured after extraction, giving a general sense of remaining fragment size [102]. Ongoing research involving novel software to accurately measure stone fragments during ureteroscopy has been shown to be accurate within 0.2 mm and has the potential to aid in objective intraoperative stone size assessment [106].

Fragmentation and Extraction

The aim of fragmentation and extraction is to create resultant pieces of stone that are small enough to safely remove with a basket or grasper. In practice, the goal is to completely remove all stone fragments, so as to leave the patient with no nidus for future stone growth, nor with any particles to potentially cause pain or necessitate re-intervention during spontaneous passage. Holmium laser settings are typically between 0.6–1.0 J and 6–10 Hz, with the surgeon beginning at a lower energy and frequency and increasing if necessary, depending on stone characteristics. These settings have been shown to cause larger stone fragmentation size, which is ideal for extraction [107]. The center of the stone is targeted, using the laser fiber to pin the calculus against the urothelial wall with the aim of creating successive halves that can then be extracted [108]. Depending on stone size, ureteral access sheaths (UASs) are deployed in order to aid with multiple basketing attempts required to clear remaining stone burden (Fig. 5.10).

Fragmentation and stone extraction are beneficial in that it confers a higher stone-free rate compared to dusting, which has several advantages. First, any remaining stone fragments can serve as a nidus for future stone growth, and this is avoided by this method. Second, stone particles remaining within the collecting system can cause pain and occasionally need for re-intervention during spontaneous passage. Furthermore, the removal of stone fragments allows for metabolic analysis, which can be beneficial when counseling patients on future stone preventive measures. Despite these advantages, this technique can result in increased operative time as a result of multiple basketing attempts, particularly in cases with large stone burden.

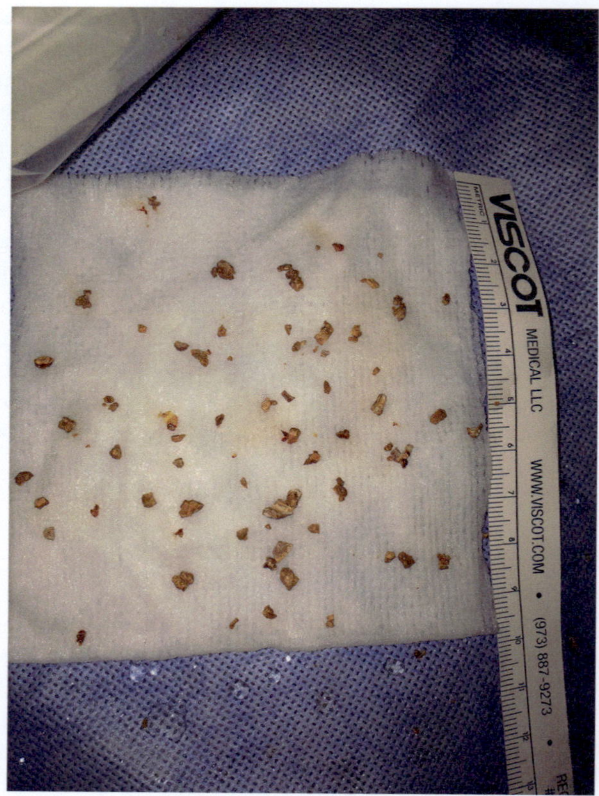

Fig. 5.10 Laser fragmentation with resultant fragments between 3 and 4 mm removed with basket extraction

Conclusions

Several studies have examined stone-free rates when comparing dusting and fragmentation techniques [42, 109]. One retrospective review found an increased rate of unplanned medical visits in the dusting group as compared to fragmentation, though this only included ureteral stones, and postoperative stents were not routinely placed [109]. In the more recent prospective, multi-institutional study, the stone-free rate between the two techniques did not differ significantly on multivariate analysis despite larger stone size in the dusting group, nor did postoperative complications, including symptoms or need for re-intervention [42]. Furthermore, dusting resulted in a 44% reduction in OR time – approximately 38 minutes – as compared to fragmentation. In addition, ureteral access sheaths (UASs) are optional when dusting, which is an added benefit, since UAS placement is not completely innocuous and leads to violation of ureteral wall smooth muscle layers in up to 13% of cases [88].

Clearly, each technique has its own individual benefits and risks. Fragmentation with stone extraction appears more efficient for smaller stones, particularly those in the ureter in which all fragments can be safely removed with limited basketing attempts. This yields a lower future risk of stone formation, as all fragments are removed from the collecting system leaving no nidus for future stone growth. Furthermore, this may result in fewer postoperative symptoms and unplanned medical visits, as suggested by some studies [109]. Dusting appears more efficient for larger stones, in which removal of all fragments would require significant basketing and increased operative time. This technique would allow for efficient stone ablation with apparently similar stone-free rates as compared to fragmentation [42]. Ultimately, both methods have utility in the treatment of urinary calculi and should not be considered as mutually exclusive but rather as complimentary, depending on the particular situation. Newer laser generators are now manufactured with features such as dual control pedals (Fig. 5.11), allowing the surgeon to seamlessly switch between dusting and fragmenting settings as appropriate.

Selection and Need for Metabolic Evaluation

Vincent De Coninck, Etienne Xavier Keller, and Olivier Traxer

Introduction

The main aim of performing a metabolic evaluation is discovering underlying causes and diseases responsible for stone formation. Generally, stratification is based on standard history, physical examination, basic urinary and blood analysis, radiological examination, and stone analysis. In the absence of overt risk factors, empiric preventative measures including appropriate fluid intake, balanced diet, and lifestyle advice are sufficient for relatively low-risk patients. Low-risk individuals are first-time stone formers, who present in adulthood with a single stone and no other risk factors. In the presence of risk factors, a specific metabolic evaluation with two 24-hour urine collections is recommended [110] in order to exclude underlying diseases and to tailor an individualized stone prevention strategy. High-risk individuals are repeat stone formers, patients presenting with multiple stones, positive family history of stones, pediatric patients, or those with other lithogenic conditions such as enteric hyperoxaluria, gout, metabolic syndrome, cystinuria, distal renal tubule acidosis, or hyperparathyroidism, to name a few.

Standard History and Physical Examination

A thorough medical history and physical examination are necessary for getting a simple perspective for a patient's stone risk. It may spare certain portions of the work-up when patients are, for example, at risk for low urinary volumes (e.g., athletes, teachers, drivers, or people living or working in hot environments). Just increasing fluid intake may prevent stone formation for these patients. Further, it

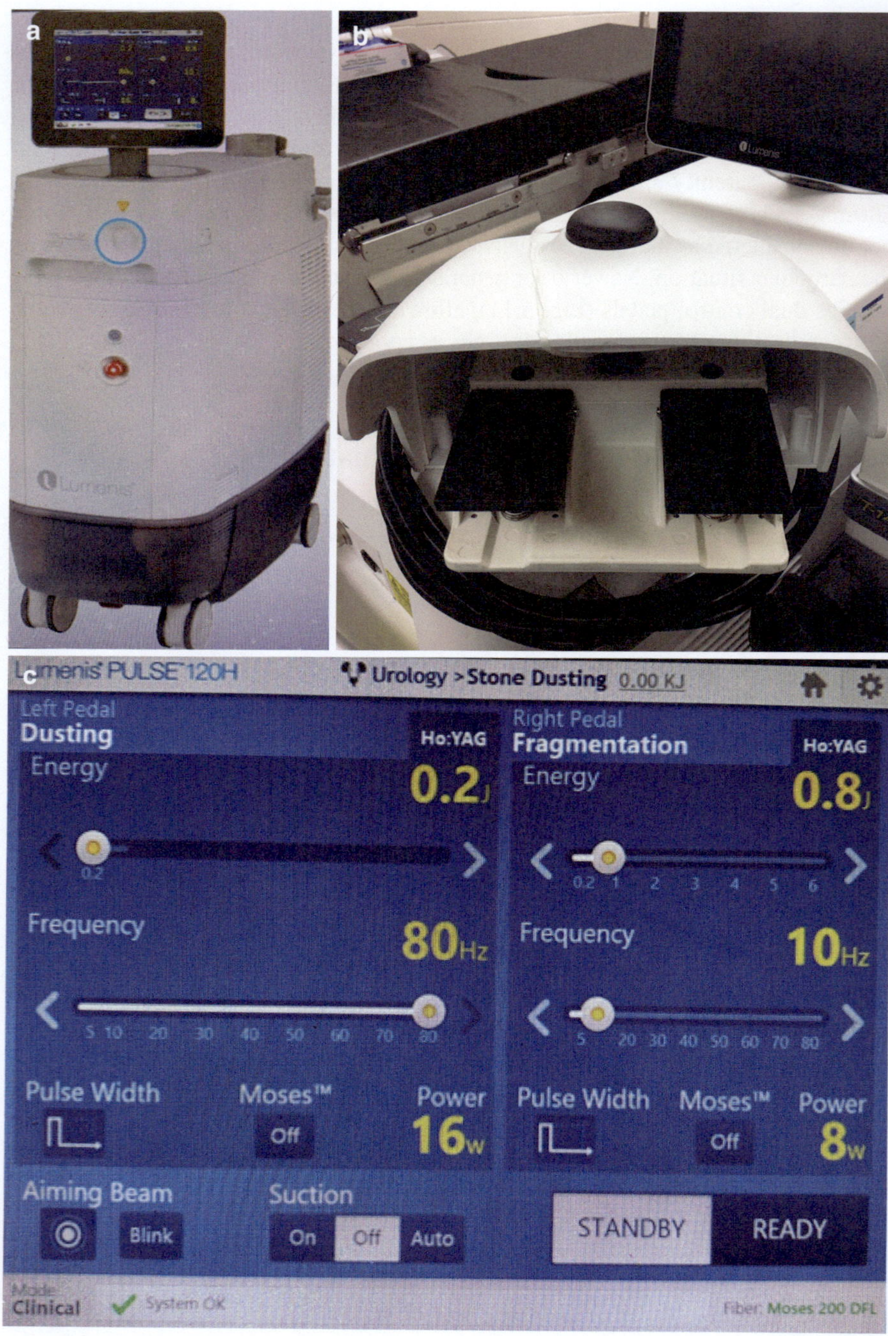

Fig. 5.11 One hundred twenty-watt holmium:YAG laser generator (Lumenis, Yokneam, Israel). (**a**) High-powered 120-watt laser unit. (**b**) Dual pedals allow the surgeon to alternate between preset laser dosimetry settings. (**c**) Unit console shows dusting settings for the left pedal and fragmenting settings for the right pedal

involves questioning about age of first stone diagnosis, medical (e.g., urinary tract infections, diarrhea, gout, diabetes, inflammatory bowel disease) and surgical (e.g., fracture, bariatric surgery, bowel resection) history, and medication (e.g., protease inhibitors, carbonic anhydrase inhibitors, supplements of vitamins, or calcium) [111]. Dietary evaluation should include the quantity of intake of fluid (including type of fluids), calcium (including over-the-counter antacids), animal proteins, purines, sodium, and oxalate. During physical examination, obesity, hypertension, and scars related to surgery should not be overlooked.

Basic Urinary and Blood Analysis

Each patient with urolithiasis needs a succinct blood and urine analysis to identify biochemical causes of stone formation [3, 5]. Blood analysis should include glucose, creatinine, uric acid, sodium, potassium, and calcium. Consideration should also be given to the parathyroid hormone level and serum urate. Occasionally, urolithiasis may represent initial manifestation of diabetes (hyperglycemia), primary hyperparathyroidism, or sarcoidosis (hypercalcemia). Urinalysis includes red and white blood cells, nitrite, pH, and culture. Urinary pH levels constantly above 5.8 in the day profile should give cause for measuring serum bicarbonate. When the latter is low, renal tubular acidosis may be identified, leading to calcium phosphate stone formation.

Radiology

Ultrasound, plain abdominal film, and (low-dose) computed tomography disclose information about stone characteristics, including the number of stones, size, morphology, and radiopacity. Nephrocalcinosis and anatomical anomalies favoring stones like medullary sponge kidney, calyceal diverticula ureteropelvic junction obstructions, and horseshoe kidney can also be found.

Stone Examination

After ureteroscopy, the stone or fragments of the stone of every patient should be sent for determination of composition by X-ray diffraction or infrared spectroscopy. However, stone characterization can already be performed during ureteroscopy [112]. Surface characterization is based on the color, size, pattern and aspect of crystals, and morphological particularities (like papillary umbilication with Randall's plaque) (Table 5.4). During lithotripsy, internal features like concentric, radial, compact, or loose structure and the organization of alternating layers can

Table 5.4 Morphological classification of urinary calculi

Type	Subtype	Composition	Frequency	Surface	Section	Etiology
I	Ia	Whewellite	45	Brown; smooth, mammillary, or mulberry shaped; frequent umbilication	Brown; compact, concentric structure, radial crystallization	Diet hyperoxaluria
	Ib	Whewellite	7	Beige to dark brown; mammillary and rough	Dark brown; compact with some gaps, unorganized	Stasis, conversion
	Ic	Whewellite	0.4	Cream to light brown; smooth or granular	Beige; compact, finely granular, unorganized	Primary hyperoxaluria
	Id	Whewellite	1.6	Pale brown; smooth	Beige; compact, microcrystalline structure, thin concentric layers	Malformative uropathy, stasis, multiple stones
	Ie	Whewellite	0.5	Beige; mammillary or granular	Beige; powdery, unorganized	Enteric hyperoxaluria, short bowel
II	IIa	Weddellite	30	Yellowish-brown; spiculate, entanglement of bipyramidal crystals	Yellowish-brown; crystalline, radial crystallization	Hypercalciuria
	IIb	Weddellite ± whewellite	22	Yellowish-brown; spiculate, entangled pyramidal crystals, blunt edges	Yellowish-brown; compact, crystalline, unorganized	Hypercalciuria ± hyperoxaluria, stasis
	IIc	Weddellite	0.1	Gray-beige to dark yellow-brown; rough, microcrystalline	Dark yellow-brown; peripheral diffuse concentric, core loose unorganized	Hypercalciuria, stasis, multiple stones
III	IIIa	Anhydrous uric acid	2	Ochre or gray-beige; homogeneous, crystalline, smooth, or slightly embossed	Ochre; compact concentric structure, radial crystallization	Hyperuricosuria, acid pH, stasis
	IIIb	Dihydrate uric acid ± anhydrous	9	Whitish to brownish-red; heterogeneous, locally crystalline, rough, or porous	Orange; compact or loosely crystalline, unorganized structure, porous areas	Hyperuricosuria, metabolic syndrome, diabetes, candidosis
	IIIc	Various urates	1.1	Whitish to gray-brown; heterogeneous, rough, locally porous, microcrystalline	Grey-brown; compact, microcrystalline, unorganized	Hyperuricosuria, alkaline pH (iatrogenic, UTI)
	IIId	Ammonium urate	0.2	Grayish to brown; heterogeneous, microcrystalline, rough, and extensively porous	Grey-brown; heterogeneous, loose concentric layers (thick brown/thin beige), locally porous	Hyperuricosuria, diarrhea, malnutrition

Table 5.4 (continued)

Type	Subtype	Composition	Frequency	Surface	Section	Etiology
IV	IVa1	Carbapatite	30	Whitish to beige; homogeneous, crystalline, rough, finely embossed	Beige; homogeneous, microcrystalline, crumbly ± concentric structure	UTI
	IVa2	Carbapatite	1.6	Brown-yellow; heterogeneous embossed, crystalline, glazed, irregular shape	Heterogeneous concentric foliated. Thick brown-yellow layers and thin microcrystalline beige layers	Distal renal tubular acidosis, UTI
	IVb	Carbapatite ± struvite	6	Whitish to brown; heterogeneous, both rough and embossed	Heterogeneous concentric with thick whitish and thin brown-yellow layers	UTI, primary hyperparathyroidism
	IVc	Struvite	2.5	White; homogeneous, crystalline, amalgamate crystals with blunt edges	White; loose, radial crystallization, sometimes diffuse concentric organization	UTI
	IVd	Brushite	1.7	Whitish to beige; homogeneous, crystalline, finely rough or dappled, slightly translucent	White-beige; compact concentric layers with radial crystallization	Hypercalciuria and hyperphosphaturia, primary hyperparathyroidism
V	Va	Cystine	1.1	Brown-yellow; homogeneous, crystalline, granular or embossed, waxy aspect	Yellow-pale brown; homogeneous, unorganized, diffuse radial crystallization	Cystinuria
	Vb	Cystine	0.2	White, beige, brown-yellow; homogeneous, microcrystalline, smooth	Yellow-brown; homogeneous, compact, whitish thin concentric layers in periphery, unorganized core	Cystinuria with inadequate therapy
VI	VIa	Proteins	0.7	White to pale brown; soft, homogeneous, smooth, unorganized, translucent	White-pale brown; homogeneous, unorganized, foci of secondary mineralization	Chronic pyelonephritis
	VIb	Proteins + medication or metabolic derivatives	5	Brown to black; heterogeneous, irregularly rough, locally scaled	Brown blended with color of associated components; heterogeneous, slightly organized	Proteinuria, clots, drugs
	VIc	Proteins and whewellite	0.1	Brown to black; homogeneous, smooth with clefts and scales	Yellow-brown; homogeneous, unorganized, loose, brown or heterogeneous with brown proteic shield surrounding a loose core	End-stage renal failure
VII		Miscellaneous				

Adapted from [113]

Frequency: cumulative for pure and mixed form

help in determining the stone type. Other important marks for understanding the lithogenic process are the localization of the stone (e.g., diverticulum, bladder), its mounting surface, and its metabolic activity (e.g., grayish layer of crystals covering the stone surface indicating recent episode of hyperoxaluria) [113]. Considering all these parameters will help in the early detection of certain pathologies when blood and urine analysis may initially still be normal.

Calcium oxalate monohydrate or whewellite stones (type I) are associated with hyperoxaluria. This can be caused by extensive oxalate intake or inadequate fluid intake, inflammatory bowel diseases, short bowel syndrome, or genetic disorders. Noticing subtype Ic stones should raise a red flag since they are pathognomonic for primary hyperoxaluria and cause renal failure as early as infancy. A high proportion of calcium oxalate stones are a mixture of whewellite and weddellite (type II) stones. The latter are associated with hypercalciuria. Hyperuricosuria can provoke type III stones. They are subdivided in uric acid stones (type IIIa and IIIb) and urate stones (type IIIc and IIId). Patients diagnosed with type IIId stones should be suspected for chronic diarrhea with phosphorus deficiency and malnutrition. Type IVa carbapatite stones are frequently found in patients with chronic urinary tract infections. Other causes include renal tubular acidosis (type IVa2) or primary hyperparathyroidism (type IVd, or type IIa or b with IVa1). When smelling sulfide and seeing white bubbles during lithotripsy, diagnosis of cystinuria (type V) is made intraoperatively (Figs. 5.12, 5.13, 5.14, 5.15, 5.16, and 5.17).

Since less than 10% of stones are pure, it is important to identify the composition during ureteroscopy when only a couple of fragments are sent for analysis. Frequent stone associations are Ia or Ib + IIa or IIb in case of intermittent hyperoxaluria and hypercalciuria, IIa or IIb + IVa1 in case of absorptive or resorptive hypercalciuria, and Ia + IIIb in case of metabolic syndrome and/or type 2 diabetes with hyperoxaluria.

Twenty-Four-Hour Urine Collection and Early Morning Urine

Twenty-four-hour urine analysis should include total volume, creatinine, calcium, sodium, urea, and uric acid. Early morning urine includes pH and osmolality. These tests are performed at least 1 month after surgery when the patient is on a self-determined diet under normal daily conditions. However, it is widely discussed if these collections should be part of a basic assessment or not. The advantages of these cheap exams are the additional value in diagnosing underlying diseases, understanding lithogenic processes, and monitoring patients during follow-up. Intake of fluid (including dispersion), salt, and animal proteins is easily recorded, and the hypocalciuric effect of thiazides can be followed up.

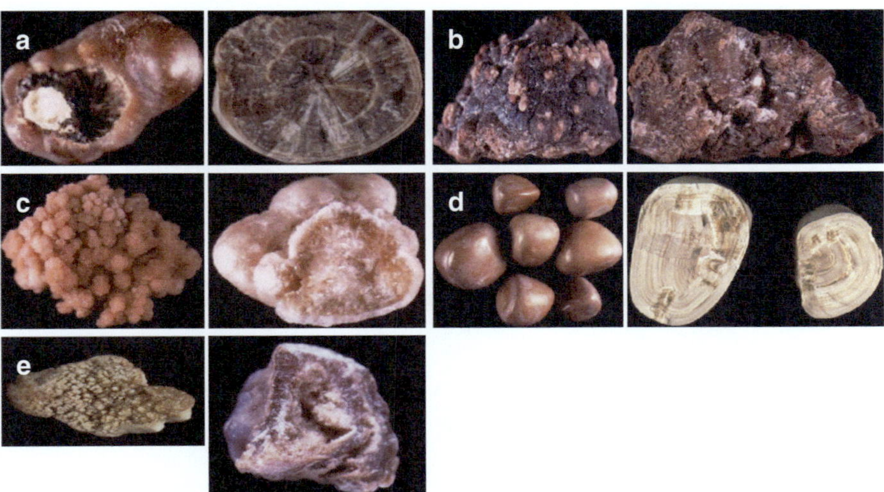

Fig. 5.12 Stone type I: Main morphological stone surface characteristics. Stone subtype Ia (upper left), Ib (upper right), Ic (middle left), Id (middle right), Ie (bottom left)

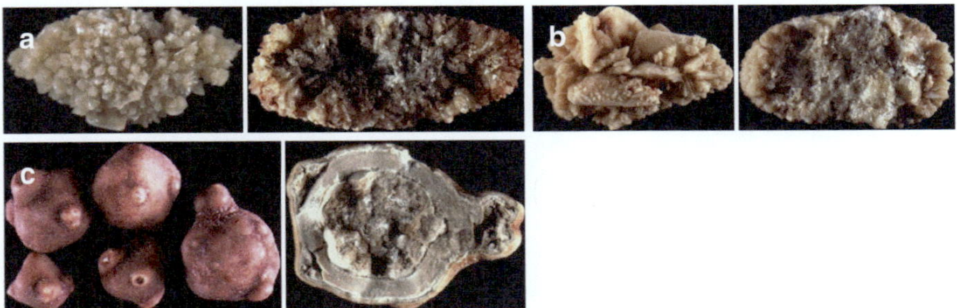

Fig. 5.13 Stone type II: Main morphological stone surface characteristics. Stone subtype IIa (upper left), IIb (upper right), IIc (bottom left)

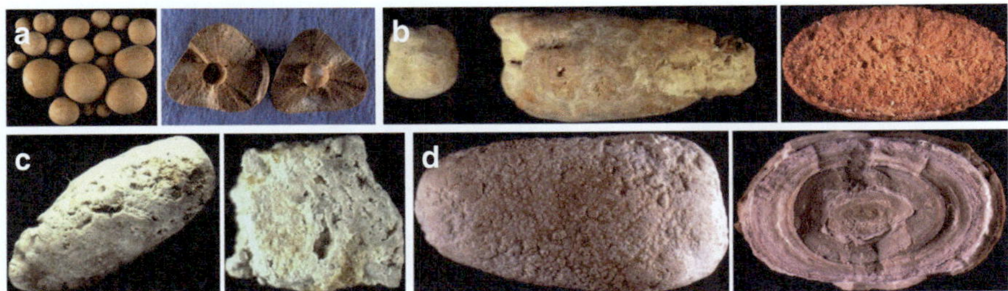

Fig. 5.14 Stone type III: Main morphological stone surface characteristics. Stone subtype IIIa (upper left), IIIb (upper right), IIIc (bottom left), IIId (bottom right)

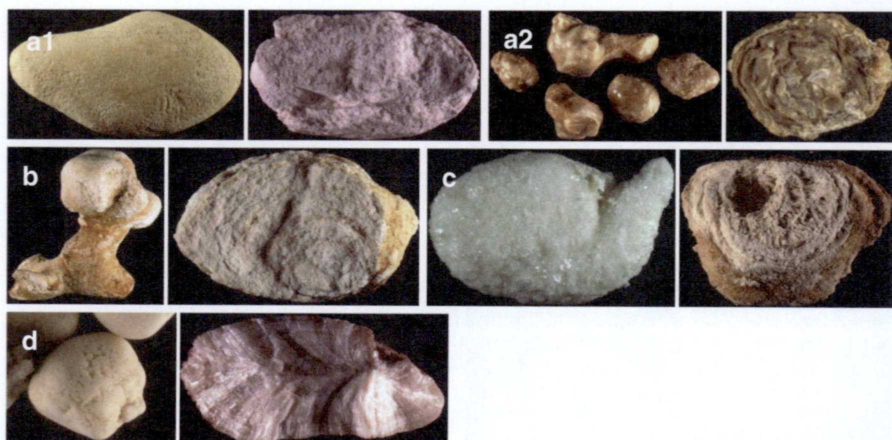

Fig. 5.15 Stone type IV: Main morphological stone surface characteristics. Stone subtype IVa1 (upper left), IVa2 (upper right), IVb (middle left), IVc (middle right), IVd (bottom left)

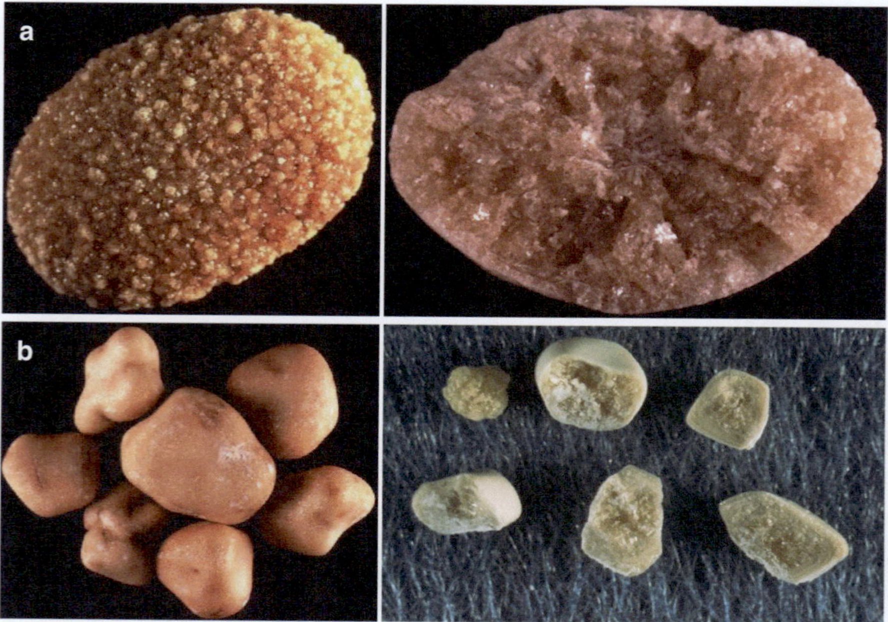

Fig. 5.16 Stone type V: Main morphological stone surface characteristics. Stone subtype Va (up), Vb (down)

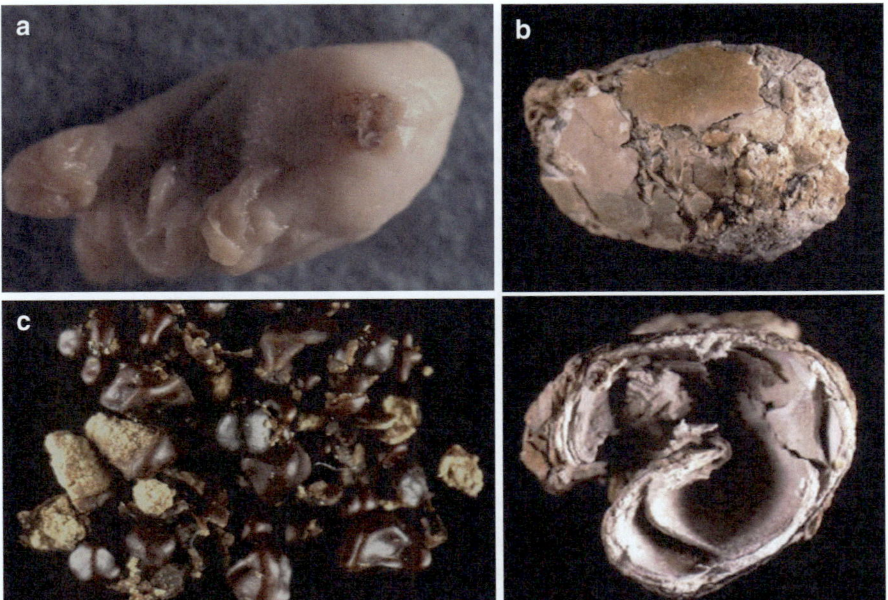

Fig. 5.17 Stone type VI: Main morphological stone section characteristics. Stone subtype VIa (upper left), VIb (upper right and bottom left)

Selection for Further Metabolic Evaluation

Selecting patients for further metabolic evaluation should be individualized. It is based on standard history, physical examination, urinary and blood analysis, radiological examination, and stone analysis. Even if more than 50% of all recurrent stone formers have only one recurrence during their lives [114], it is important to understand the lithogenic process to exclude underlying diseases. All patients with other stones than type Ia, Ib, IIa, or IIb should be selected for further metabolic evaluation after the initial stone episode. Preventive general measures may be sufficient for patients with type Ia, Ib, IIa, and IIb stones, unless in case of early onset of stone formation, multiple stones, stone recurrence, underlying metabolic disorder, drug-induced stone formation, diseases or environmental factors associated with stone formation, genetically determined stone formation, anatomical abnormalities associated with stone formation, solitary kidney, or stones of unknown composition. These patients should undergo a specific metabolic evaluation and stone-specific recurrence prevention.

Conclusion

At least half of all stone-forming patients will have a recurrent stone within 10 years of initial presentation. Developing a preventative plan is essential and starts with risk stratification. The work-up always includes medical history, physical exam, UA, serum studies, stone composition analysis, radiographic studies, and in high-risk individuals 24-hour urine collection to study urinary parameters.

Positioning for Ureteroscopy

Demetrius Bagley, Maryann Sogzoni-Cella, and Scott G. Hubosky

Introduction

Positioning of a patient for an endoscopic procedure must be designed to give optimal access for the urologist and the anesthesiologist with the greatest safety for the patient. The needs will vary with the intended procedure, the type of anesthesia, and the individual patient. Discussion is limited to ureteroscopy as the sole primary procedure or in combination with other procedures.

There are many patient factors beyond the disease being treated that affect the positioning. These include external genitalia and urethra, body weight and habitus, and mobility of the patient's limbs. The genitalia defines the position and accessibility of the urethral meatus. For example, in a male patient, the urethra is readily accessible even in the supine position for flexible endoscopy. In the female, the urethra is readily accessible only with abduction of the legs and is best in lithotomy. A patient with severe contractures of the extremities presents unique limitations in the options for positioning. It may be helpful to position these patients before induction of any anesthesia so that they can recognize and verbalize any discomfort related to position. Body weight at either the high or low end of the normal range demands specific handling for positioning.

Safety of the patient remains foremost as the guide for positioning. Three subjects must be considered when placing the patient in any position for an endoscopic or operative procedure. These points are considered in the description of each specific position.

1. The patient's limbs and body should remain in as natural and neutral position as possible.
2. Safely secure the patient to the bed or operative table in accordance with the individual facility's policy to avoid any change in position during the procedure and to eliminate any risk of falling.
3. To prevent patients from developing a pressure injury, all potential pressure points should be identified and protected with appropriate cushioning throughout the length of the procedure.

Lithotomy Position

The standard lithotomy position is the first choice when ureteroscopy, rigid or flexible, is the primary or sole intended procedure in patients either of sex or of nearly any body weight. Patients are initially placed supine on the endoscopy table with their legs subsequently elevated, abducted, and supported by stirrups. The foot end of the table is then either removed or lowered toward the floor depending on the design in order to free the area between the legs and near the perineum for access to the urethra. Specific care must be taken to avoid over-abduction of the legs, rotation of the leg, or excessive flexion of the hip or knee, and the legs must remain safely secured in the stirrups at all times.

There are several types of stirrups designed to support the legs. The simplest are the candy cane and the knee crutches. The candy cane is placed at the bottom of the shortened table with a simple dual strap placed on the foot and ankle to support the leg. Since there is a risk of the leg pressing laterally against the shaft of the stirrup, it must be carefully padded to avoid nerve compression. The knee crutch, also placed at the end of the shortened table, supports the leg under the knee. It requires considerable cushioning to avoid compression of the vessels and nerves at the knee. These designs are acceptable only for short procedures, preferably when the patient is awake and can potentially recognize discomfort from pressure. They are more commonly seen in the outpatient area where there are shorter procedures and where

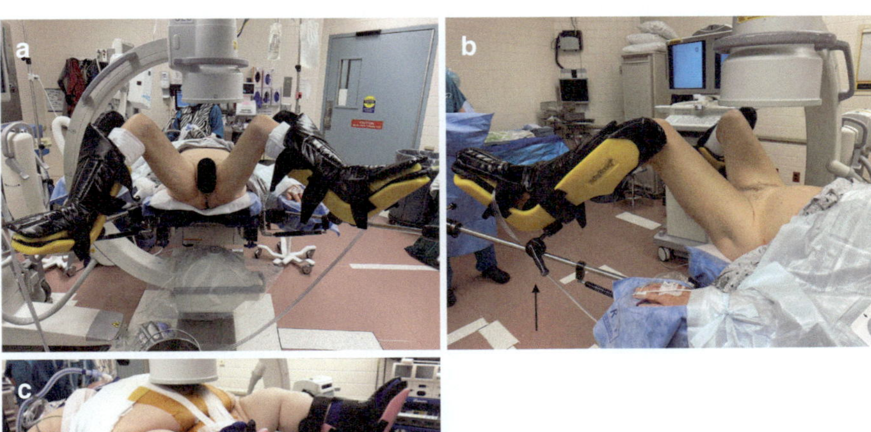

Fig. 5.18 Dorsal lithotomy with Allen Stirrups. (**a**) Allen stirrups (yellow) facilitate dorsal lithotomy position. (**b**) Adjustments can be made to optimize knee flexion depending on the height of the patient (black arrow). (**c**) Hip abduction can be adjusted with single-handed control handle (black arrow). Pink stirrups better accommodate obese patients

general or regional anesthesia is less common. They also have the benefit of a lower cost than more advanced stirrup models [115].

The Allen stirrup design has become the standard for urologic procedures requiring the lithotomy position (Fig. 5.18). It provides support for the foot and ankle or lower leg with extensive padding in those areas. The stirrups can be elevated distally to promote venous drainage. The position of the stirrup and leg can be changed with single-handed release of the control handle. Care must be taken to avoid angulation of the proximal portion of the leg support to avoid compression against the posterior leg.

The patient should be secured to the table to minimize movement by the patient or if changing the position of the table. The patient's trunk is secured with a strap. The legs are secured when the Allen style stirrups are used. Thigh straps can also be used, particularly while caring for a patient with obesity. If the Trendelenburg position is anticipated during the procedure, then shoulder holders are placed. Earlier during the development of ureteroscopy, there was support for different versions described with elevation or abduction of the ipsilateral or contralateral leg. More recently it has become clear with the availability of boot or Allen-style stirrups that modifications can be made as necessary during treatment.

After positioning, the genitalia and perineum are prepared with the prep solutions of choice. Although it was once popular, shaving or clipping of the genital and perineal hair is not necessary. Drapes are placed allowing access to the urethra while covering the legs and abdomen.

Modifications of Lithotomy

As noted above, there can be minor modifications with changes in the position of the patient's legs. As an example, access with a rigid endoscope into one ureter may require abduction of the contralateral leg or possibly abduction and elevation of that leg. With a flexible endoscope, this is usually not necessary.

During treatment, it may be useful to change the position of the entire endoscopic table. For example, steep Trendelenburg will promote movement of stones or fragments of stones into the upper infundibula from the pelvis or lower pole within the kidney. Elevation of the ipsilateral flank with rotation of the table promotes movement of fragments from the lateral calyces into the renal pelvis. Various combinations of these maneuvers can be used to advantage. With these maneuvers, it is essential to confirm the stability of the patient on the operative table and within the stirrups.

Reverse Lithotomy

Some of the major variations of lithotomy have been designed to permit simultaneous ureteroscopic and percutaneous access to the kidney and ureter. One of the earliest modifications was described as reverse lithotomy. Limitations of instrumentation at the time necessitated a specific positioning for simultaneous endoscopic procedures. The patient was placed prone on the operating table, and the lower portion of the table placed fully down toward the floor. The patient's knees were supported in special angled crutches which were slightly abducted and which were attached at the end of the table. In the three female patients described, the urethra and distal ureter became available to a rigid ureteroscope. Simultaneously direct access is provided through the standard posterior nephrostomy site for rigid and flexible nephroscopes [116].

Lithotomy with Flank Roll

Another modification is more useful for patients of either sex. The lithotomy position is modified by elevating the ipsilateral flank on a roll placed inferior to the nephrostomy site giving the flank roll version (Fig. 5.19). Retrograde ureteral endoscopy has nearly standard access, while the nephrostomy site, particularly those located slightly more laterally, is accessible from the side of the table. Access for the anesthesiologist has similar benefits of the supine position. The patient's ipsilateral arm is placed across the chest or on a stand over the chest with appropriate cushioning to maintain skin integrity and prevent the nerve damage. It is necessary to use great care in positioning the patient's lateral flank. If it is too far to the side of the table, the metal support in the table itself will obscure the fluoroscopic image. If it is too far medially, it will be very difficult to reach the kidney with the rigid endoscope. Here again appropriate considerations and interventions are needed at any pressure points. This position can be used with the standard operating/endoscopy table without a special design [117].

This position is similar to the Valdivia or modified Valdivia position which has been used for lateral percutaneous access to the kidney with the patient in the supine position. It offers the same advantages as a flank roll with the addition of better access to the nephrostomy site [118–120].

Prone Split Leg

The prone split leg position gives excellent access to a nephrostomy site placed in the prone position and for flexible retrograde ureteroscopy in patients of either sex. Anesthesia is induced in the supine position, and the patient is then carefully placed

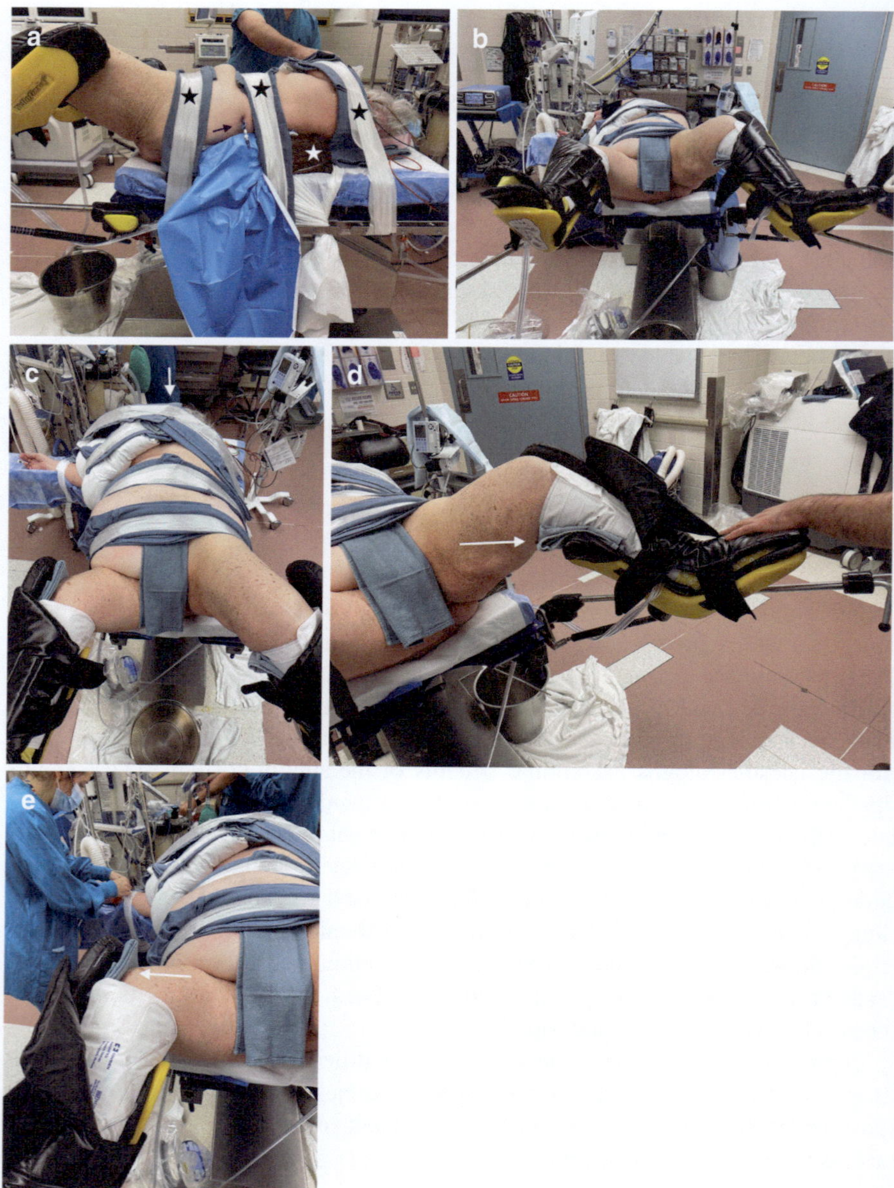

Fig. 5.19 Lithotomy with flank roll. (**a**) Note the gel-roll (white star) under the ipsilateral flank, which extends from the left shoulder to the left hip. This allows access to the left PCN tube (black arrow). The patient is secured to the bed in three spots with 3-inch tape (black stars). (**b**) Note the shift in the patient's hips, placing pressure on the right buttock. (**c**) The ipsilateral (left) arm is brought across the torso, padded and taped (white arrow). (**d**) Extra padding is placed at the medial aspect of the ipsilateral knee (white arrow). (**e**) Extra padding is placed at the lateral aspect of the contralateral knee (while arrow)

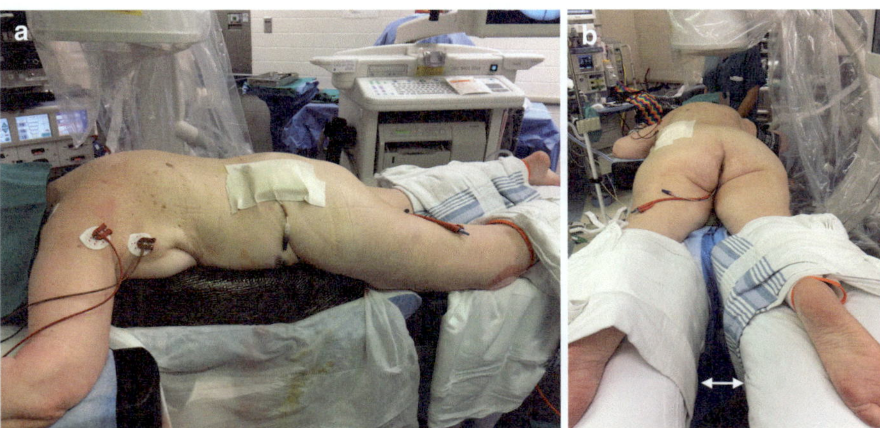

Fig. 5.20 Prone split leg position. (**a**) The patient in prone position, supported by gel-rolls. (**b**) Legs are split on separate individual leg supports, which can be pulled apart in order to abduct the legs and give access to the perineum (white double arrow). Note the Foley catheter and retrograde ureteral catheter

into the prone position on the appropriate operating table by the surgical team. The table must be specifically equipped with movable leg supports. The prone position requires special consideration for pressure points, and positioning aids should be decided upon prior to positioning the patient. Specifically in our practice, the patient is anesthetized in the supine position on the stretcher. A ureteral guidewire or catheter is placed with a flexible cystoscope in that position. It is easier in that way than when the male patient is prone. A Foley catheter with a hole punched in the tip or a council-tip catheter is also placed. A wire can be placed through the catheter to be available to guide a flexible cystoscope into the bladder when in the prone position. The surgical team then rolls the patient into the prone position on the appropriate operative table. The patient's genitalia are placed at the lower margin of the table for urethral access in that position. Each leg is separately secured to the ipsilateral split leg support (Fig. 5.20). They can then be abducted without being flexed. Each operative area is prepped and draped separately [121, 122].

Conclusions

The most commonly used position for ureteroscopy is lithotomy or a modified version. The prone split leg position is now commonly used for combined percutaneous and urethral access. It is extremely important to maintain patient safety during the procedure with appropriate cushioning and neutral positions.

Disclosures Financial Disclosure: Prof. Olivier Traxer is a consultant for Coloplast, Rocamed, Olympus, EMS, and Boston Scientific.

Funding Support: Dr. Etienne Xavier Keller is supported by a travel grant from the University Hospital Zurich and by a grant from the Kurt and Senta Herrmann Foundation. Dr. Vincent De Coninck is supported by a EUSP scholarship from the European Association of Urology and by a grant from the Belgische Vereniging voor Urologie (BVU).

References

Ureteral Stone Treatment

1. Hesse A, Brändle E, Wilbert D, Köhrmann KU, Alken P. Study on the prevalence and incidence of urolithiasis in Germany comparing the years 1979 vs. 2000. Eur Urol. 2003;44:709–13.
2. Teichman JM. Clinical practice. Acute renal colic from ureteral calculus. N Engl J Med. 2004;350:684–93.
3. Assimos D, Krambeck A, Miller NL, Monga M, Murad MH, Nelson CP, et al. Surgical management of stones: American Urological Association/Endourological Society guideline, part I. J Urol. 2016;196:1153–60.
4. Assimos D, Krambeck A, Miller NL, Monga M, Murad MH, Nelson CP, et al. Surgical management of stones: American Urological Association/Endourological Society guideline, part II. J Urol. 2016;196:1161–9.
5. Türk C, Petřík A, Sarica K, Seitz C, Skolarikos A, Straub M, et al. EAU guidelines on interventional treatment for urolithiasis. Eur Urol. 2016;69:475–82.
6. Cloutier J, Anson K, Giusti G, Grasso M, Kamphuis G, Lahme S, et al. Update of the ICUD-SIU consultation on stone technology behind ureteroscopy. World J Urol. 2017;35:1353–9.
7. Pradére B, Doizi S, Proietti S, Brachlow J, Traxer O. Evaluation of guidelines for surgical management of urolithiasis. J Urol. 2018;199:1267–71.
8. Sun X, Xia S, Lu J, Liu H, Han B, Li W. Treatment of large impacted proximal ureteral stones: randomized comparison of percutaneous antegrade ureterolithotripsy versus retrograde ureterolithotripsy. J Endourol. 2008;22:913–7.
9. El-Nahas AR, Eraky I, el-Assmy AM, Shoma AM, el-Kenawy MR, Abdel-Latif M, et al. Percutaneous treatment of large upper tract stones after urinary diversion. Urology. 2006;68:500–4.
10. Guercio S, Ambu A, Mangione F, Mari M, Vacca F, Bellina M. Randomized prospective trial comparing immediate versus delayed ureteroscopy for patients with ureteral calculi and normal renal function who present to the emergency department. J Endourol. 2011;25:1137–41.
11. Sarica K, Tarhan F, Erdem K, Sevinc AH, Guzel R, Eryidirum B. Functional and morphological recovery of solitary kidneys after drainage. Double J stent placement vs emergency ureteroscopy: which one is reasonable? Urolithiasis. 2018;46:479–84.

12. Zargar-Shoshtari K, Anderson W, Rice M. Role of emergency ureteroscopy in the management of ureteric stones: analysis of 394 cases. BJU Int. 2015;115:946–50.
13. Park HK, Paick SH, Oh SJ, Kim HH. Ureteroscopic lithotripsy under local anesthesia: analysis of the effectiveness and patient tolerability. Eur Urol. 2004;45:670–3.
14. Zelenko N, Coll D, Rosenfeld AT, Smith RC. Normal ureter size on unenhanced helical CT. Am J Roentgenol. 2004;182:1039–41.
15. Janssen PF, Brölmann HA, Huirne JA. Causes and prevention of laparoscopic ureter injuries: an analysis of 31 cases during laparoscopic hysterectomy in the Netherlands. Surg Endosc. 2013;27:946–56.
16. Elliott SP, McAninch JW. Ureteral injuries: external and iatrogenic. Urol Clin North Am. 2006;33:55–66.
17. Perez Castro E, Osther PJS, Jinga V, Razvi H, Stravodimos KG, Parikh K, et al. Differences in ureteroscopic stone treatment and outcomes for distal, mid-, proximal, or multiple ureteral locations: the Clinical Research Office of the Endourological Society ureteroscopy global study. Eur Urol. 2014;66:102–9.
18. Rodrigues Netto N Jr, Caserta Lemos G, Levi D'Ancona CA, Ikari O, Ferreira U, Francisco de Almeida J. Is routine dilation of the ureter necessary for ureteroscopy? Eur Urol. 1990;17:269–72.
19. Doizi S, Herrmann T, Traxer O. Death of the safety guidewire. J Endourol. 2017;31:619–20.
20. Graversen JA, Valderrama OM, Korets R, Mues AC, Landman J, Badani KK, et al. The effect of extralumenal safety wires on ureteral injury and insertion force of ureteral access sheaths: evaluation using an ex vivo porcine model. Urology. 2012;79:1011–4.
21. Chen S, Zhou L, Wei T, Luo D, Jin T, Li H, et al. Comparison of holmium: YAG laser and pneumatic lithotripsy in the treatment of ureteral stones: an update meta-analysis. Urol Int. 2017;98:125–33.
22. Rehman J, Monga M, Landman J, Lee DI, Felfela T, Conradie MC, et al. Characterization of intrapelvic pressure during ureteropyeloscopy with ureteral access sheaths. Urology. 2003;61:713–8.
23. Coe FL, Parks JH, Lindheimer MD. Nephrolithiasis during pregnancy. N Engl J Med. 1978;298:324–6.
24. Srirangam SJ, Hickerton B, Van Cleynenbreugel B. Management of urinary calculi in pregnancy: a review. J Endourol. 2008;22:867–75.
25. Peake SL, Roxburgh HB, Langlois SL. Ultrasonic assessment of hydronephrosis of pregnancy. Radiology. 1983;146:167–70.
26. Rajaei Isfahani M, Haghighat M. Measurable changes in hydronephrosis during pregnancy induced by positional changes: ultrasonic assessment and its diagnostic implication. Urol J. 2005;2:97–101.
27. Parulkar BG, Hopkins TB, Wollin MR, Howard PJ, Lal A. Renal colic during pregnancy: a case for conservative treatment. J Urol. 1998;159:365–8.
28. Smith CL, Kristensen C, Davis M, Abraham PA. An evaluation of the physicochemical risk for renal stone disease during pregnancy. Clin Nephrol. 2001;55:205–11.
29. Gofrit ON, Pode D, Meretyk S, Katz G, Shapiro A, Golijanin D, et al. Is the pediatric ureter as efficient as the adult ureter in transporting fragments following extracorporeal shock wave lithotripsy for renal calculi larger than 10 mm.? J Urol. 2001;166:1862–4.
30. Smaldone MC, Corcoran AT, Docimo SG, Ost MC. Endourological management of pediatric stone disease: present status. J Urol. 2009;181:17–28.

Flexible Ureteroscopic Treatment of Renal Stones

31. Donaldson JF, Lardas M, Scrimgeour D, Stewart F, MacLennan S, Lam TBL, et al. Systematic review and meta-analysis of the clinical effectiveness of shock wave lithotripsy, retrograde intrarenal surgery, and percutaneous nephrolithotomy for lower-pole renal stones. Eur Urol. 2015;67:612–6.

32. Bozkurt OF, Resorlu B, Yildiz Y, Can CE, Unsal A. Retrograde intrarenal surgery versus percutaneous nephrolithotomy in the management of lower-pole renal stones with a diameter of 15 to 20 mm. J Endourol. 2011;25:1131–5.
33. Oberlin DT, Flum AS, Bachrach L, Matulewicz RS, Flury SC. Contemporary surgical trends in the management of upper tract calculi. J Urol. 2014;193:880–4.
34. Türk C, Neisius A, Petrik A, Seitz C, Skolarikos A, Somani B, et al. Guidelines on Urolithiasis. European association of urology. 2020. Retrieved from https://uroweb.org/guideline/urolithiasis/ Accessed 29 May 2021.
35. Chew BH, Brotherhood HL, Sur RL, Wang AQ, Knudsen BR, Yong C, et al. Natural history, complications and re-intervention rates of asymptomatic residual stone fragments after ureteroscopy: a report from the EDGE research consortium. J Urol. 2016;195:982–6.
36. Rebuck DA, Macejko A, Bhalani V, Ramos P, Nadler RB. The natural history of renal stone fragments following Ureteroscopy. Urology. 2011;77:564–8.
37. Fulgham PF, Assimos DG, Pearle MS, Preminger GM. Clinical effectiveness protocols for imaging in the management of ureteral calculous disease: AUA technology assessment. J Urol. 2013;189:1203–13.
38. Ganesan V, De S, Greene D, Torricelli FCM. Accuracy of ultrasonography for renal stone detection and size determination: is it good enough for management decisions? BJU Int. 2017;119:464–9.
39. Ulvik Ø, Harneshaug JR, Gjengstø P. What do we mean by "stone free", and how accurate are urologists in predicting stone free status following ureteroscopy? J Endourol. 2021; https://doi.org/10.1089/end.2020.0933. Online ahead of print.
40. Renal and ureteric stones: assessment and management. NICE guideline 2019. Retrieved from www.nice.org.uk/guidance/ng118, Accessed 29 May 2021.
41. Hyams ES, Bruhn A, Lipkin M, Shah O. Heterogeneity in the reporting of disease characteristics and treatment outcomes in studies evaluating treatments for nephrolithiasis. J Endourol. 2010;24:1411–4.
42. Humphreys MR, Shah OD, Monga M, Chang YH, Krambeck AE, Sur RL, et al. Dusting versus basketing during ureteroscopy-which technique is more efficacious? A prospective multicenter trial from the EDGE research consortium. J Urol. 2018;199:1272–6.
43. Geraghty R, Abourmarzouk O, Rai B, Biyani CS, Rukin NJ, Somani BK. Evidence for ureterorenoscopy and laser fragmentation (URSL) for large renal stones in the modern era. Curr Urol Rep. 2015;16:54.
44. Hyams ES, Munver R, Bird VG, Uberoi J, Shah O. Flexible ureterorenoscopy and holmium laser lithotripsy for the management of renal stone burdens that measure 2 to 3 cm: a multi-institutional experience. J Endourol. 2010;24:1583–8.
45. Dresner SL, Iremashvili V, Best SL, Hedican SP, Nakada SY. Influence of lower pole infundibulopelvic angle on success of retrograde flexible ureteroscopy and laser lithotripsy for the treatment of renal stones. J Endourol. 2020;34:655–60.
46. Inoue T, Murota T, Okada S, Hamamoto S, Muguruma K, Kinoshita H, et al. SMART Study Group. Influence of pelvicaliceal anatomy on stone clearance after flexible ureteroscopy and holmium laser lithotripsy for large renal stones. J Endourol. 2015;29:998–1005.
47. Auge BK, Dahm P, Wu NZ, Preminger GM. Ureteroscopic management of lower-pole renal calculi: technique of calculus displacement. J Endourol. 2001;15:835–8.
48. Bozzini G, Verze P, Arcaniolo D, Piaz OD, Buffi NM, Guazzoni G, et al. A prospective randomized comparison among SWL, PCNL and RIRS for lower calyceal stones less than 2 cm: a multicenter experience: a better understanding on the treatment options for lower pole stones. World J Urol. 2017;35:1967–75.
49. Ito H, Kawahara T, Terao H, Ogawa T, Yao M, Kubota Y, et al. Utility and limitation of cumulative stone diameter in predicting urinary stone burden at flexible ureteroscopy with holmium laser lithotripsy: a single-center experience. PLoS One. 2013;8:e65060.

50. Okhunov Z, Friedlander JI, George AK, Duty BD, Moreira DM, Srinivasan AK, et al. S.T.O.N.E. nephrolithometry: novel surgical classification system for kidney calculi. Urology. 2013;81:1154–9.
51. Smith A, Averch TD, Shahrour K, Opondo D, Daels FPJ, Labate G, et al. CROES PCNL study group. A nephrolithometric nomogram to predict treatment success of percutaneous nephrolithotomy. J Urol. 2013;190:149–56.
52. Resorlu B, Unsal A, Gulec H, Oztuna D. A new scoring system for predicting stone-free rate after retrograde intrarenal surgery: the "resorlu-unsal stone score". Urology. 2012;80:512–8.
53. Zetumer S, Wiener S, Bayne DB, Armas-Phan M, Washington SL, Tzou DT, et al. The impact of stone multiplicity on surgical decisions for patients with large stone burden: results from ReSKU. J Endourol. 2019;33:742–9.
54. Waingankar N, Hayek S, Smith AD, Okeke Z. Calyceal diverticula: a comprehensive review. Rev Urol. 2014;16:29–43.
55. Krambeck AE, Lingeman JE. Percutaneous management of caliceal diverticuli. J Endourol. 2009;23:1723–9.
56. Ito H, Aboumarzouk OM, Abushamma F, Keeley FX. Systematic review of caliceal diverticulum. J Endourol. 2018;32:961–72.
57. Grasso M, Conlin M, Bagley D. Retrograde ureteropyeloscopic treatment of 2 cm or greater upper urinary tract and minor staghorn calculi. J Urol. 1998;160:346–51.
58. El-Anany FG, Hammouda HM, Maghraby HA, Elakkad MA. Retrograde ureteropyeloscopic holmium laser lithotripsy for large renal calculi. BJU Int. 2001;88:850–3.
59. Mariani AJ. Combined electrohydraulic and holmium: YAG laser ureteroscopic nephrolithotripsy of large (>2 cm) renal calculi. Indian J Urol. 2008;24:521–5.
60. Breda A, Ogunyemi O, Leppert JT, Lam JS, Schulam PG. Flexible ureteroscopy and laser lithotripsy for single intrarenal stones 2 cm or greater—is this the new frontier? J Urol. 2008;179:981–4.
61. Al-Qahtani SM, Gil-Deiz-de-Medina S, Traxer O. Predictors of clinical outcomes of flexible ureterorenoscopy with holmium laser for renal stone greater than 2 cm. Adv Urol. 2012;2012:543537. https://doi.org/10.1155/2012/543537.
62. Cohen J, Cohen S, Grasso M. Ureteropyeloscopic treatment of large, complex intrarenal and proximal ureteral calculi. BJU Int. 2012;111:127–31.
63. Miernik A, Schoenthaler M, Wilhelm K, Wetterauer U, Zyczkowski M, Paradysz A, et al. Combined semirigid and flexible ureterorenoscopy via a large ureteral access sheath for kidney stones >2 cm: a bicentric prospective assessment. World J Urol. 2014;32:697–702.
64. Pieras E, Tubau V, Brugarolas X, Ferrutxe J, Pizá P. Comparative analysis between percutaneous nephrolithotomy and flexible ureteroscopy in kidney stones of 2-3cm. Actas Urol Esp. 2017;41:194–9.
65. Huang JS, Xie J, Huang XJ, Yuan Q, Jiang HT, Xiao KF. Flexible ureteroscopy and laser lithotripsy for renal stones 2 cm or greater, a single institutional experience. Medicine (Baltimore). 2020;99:e22704.

Post Ureteroscopic Evaluation: Short and Long Term

66. Wills TE, Burns JR. Ureteroscopy: an outpatient procedure? J Urol. 1994;151:1185–7.
67. Ghosh A, Oliver R, Way C, White L, Somani BK. Results of day-case ureterorenoscopy (DC-URS) for stone disease: prospective outcomes over 4.5 years. World J Urol. 2017;35:1757–64.
68. Cheung MC, Lee F, Leung YL, Wong BB, Chu SM, Tam PC. Outpatient ureteroscopy: predictive factors for postoperative events. Urology. 2001;58:914–8.
69. Tan HJ, Strope SA, He C, Roberts WW, Faerber GJ, Wolf JS. Immediate unplanned hospital admission after outpatient ureteroscopy for stone disease. J Urol. 2011;185:2181–5.

70. Zhong W, Letto G, Wang L, Zeng G. Systemic inflammatory response syndrome after flexible ureteroscopic lithotripsy: a study of risk factors. J Endourol. 2015;29:25–8.
71. Moses RA, Ghali FM, Pais VM, Hyams ES. Unplanned hospital return for infection following ureteroscopy-can we identify modifiable risk factors? J Urol. 2016;195:931–6.
72. Mariappan P, Loong CW. Midstream urine culture and sensitivity test is a poor predictor of infected urine proximal to the obstructing ureteral stone or infected stones: a prospective clinical study. J Urol. 2004;171:2142–5.
73. Bone RC, Balk RA, Cerra FB, Dellinger RP, Felin AM, Knaus WA, et al. Definitions for sepsis and organ failure and guidelines for the use of innovative therapies in sepsis. The ACCP/SCCM Consensus Conference Committee. American College of Chest Physicians/Society of Critical Care Medicine. Chest. 1992;101:1644–55.
74. Levy MM, Fink MP, Marshall JC, Abraham E, Angus D, Cook D, et al. 2001 SCCM/ESICM/ACCP/ATS/SIS international Sepsis definitions conference. Crit Care Med. 2003;31:1250–6.
75. Singer M, Deutschman CS, Seymour CW, Shankar-Hari M, Annane D, Bauer M, et al. The third international consensus definitions for Sepsis and septic shock (Sepsis-3). JAMA. 2016;315:801–10.
76. Seymour CW, Liu VX, Iwashyna TJ, Brunkhorst FM, Rea TD, Scherag A, et al. Assessment of clinical criteria for Sepsis: for the third international consensus definitions for Sepsis and septic shock (Sepsis-3). JAMA. 2016;315:762–74.
77. Hollenbeck BK, Schuster TG, Seifman BD, Faerber GJ, Wolf JS. Identifying patients who are suitable for stentless ureteroscopy following treatment of urolithiasis. J Urol. 2003;170:103–6.
78. Lallas CD, Auge BK, Raj GV, Santa-Cruz R, Madden JF, Preminger GM. Laser Doppler flowmetric determination of ureteral blood flow after ureteral access sheath placement. J Endourol. 2002;16:583–90.
79. Rapoport D, Perks AE, Teichman JMH. Ureteral access sheath use and stenting in ureteroscopy: effect on unplanned emergency room visits and cost. J Endourol. 2007;21:993–7.
80. Torricelli FC, De S, Hinck B, Noble M, Monga M. Flexible ureteroscopy with a ureteral access sheath: when to stent? Urology. 2014;83:278–81.
81. Pais VM, Smith RE, Stedina EA, Rissman CM. Does omission of ureteral stents increase risk of unplanned return visit? A systematic review and meta-analysis. J Urol. 2016;196:1458–66.
82. Auge BK, Sarvis JA, L'esperance JO, Preminger GM. Practice patterns of ureteral stenting after routine ureteroscopic stone surgery: a survey of practicing urologists. J Endourol. 2007;21:1287–91.
83. Wang H, Man L, Li G, Huang G, Liu N, Wang J. Meta-analysis of stenting versus non-stenting for the treatment of ureteral stones. PLoS One. 2017;12:e0167670.
84. Joshi HB, Chitale SV, Nagarajan M, Irving SO, Browning AJ, Biyani CS, et al. A prospective randomized single-blind comparison of ureteral stents composed of firm and soft polymer. J Urol. 2005;174:2303–6.
85. Lingeman JE, Preminger GM, Goldfischer ER, Krambeck AE, et al. Assessing the impact of ureteral stent design on patient comfort. J Urol. 2009;181:2581–7.
86. Zhou L, Cai X, Li H, Wang KJ. Effects of alpha-blockers, antimuscarinics, or combination therapy in relieving ureteral stent-related symptoms: a meta-analysis. J Endourol. 2015;29:650–6.
87. Betschart P, Zumstein V, Piller A, Schmid HP, Abt D. Prevention and treatment of symptoms associated with indwelling ureteral stents: a systematic review. Int J Urol. 2017;24:250–9.
88. Traxer O, Thomas A. Prospective evaluation and classification of ureteral wall injuries resulting from insertion of a ureteral access sheath during retrograde intrarenal surgery. J Urol. 2013;189:580–4.
89. Lildal SK, Sørensen FB, Andreassen KH, Christiansen FE, Jung H, Pedersen MR, et al. Histopathological correlations to ureteral lesions visualized during ureteroscopy. World J Urol. 2017;35:1489–96.
90. Delvecchio FC, Preminger GM. Management of residual stones. Urol Clin North Am. 2000;27:347–54.

91. Osman MM, Alfano Y, Kamp S, Haecker A, Alken P, Michel MS, et al. 5-year-follow-up of patients with clinically insignificant residual fragments after extracorporeal shockwave lithotripsy. Eur Urol. 2005;47:860–4.
92. Candau C, Saussine C, Lang H, Roy C, Faure F, Jacqmin D. Natural history of residual renal stone fragments after ESWL. Eur Urol. 2000;37:18–22.
93. Gokce MI, Ozden E, Suer E, Gulpinar B, Gulpinar O, Tangal S. Comparison of imaging modalities for detection of residual fragments and prediction of stone related events following percutaneous nephrolitotomy. Int Braz J Urol. 2015;41:86–90.
94. Pearle MS, Watamull LM, Mullican MA. Sensitivity of noncontrast helical computerized tomography and plain film radiography compared to flexible nephroscopy for detecting residual fragments after percutaneous nephrostolithotomy. J Urol. 1999;162:23–6.
95. Roberts WW, Cadeddu JA, Micali S, Kavoussi LR, Moore RG. Ureteral stricture formation after removal of impacted calculi. J Urol. 1998;159:723–6.
96. Fam XI, Singam P, Ho CC, Sridharan R, Hod R, Bahadzor B, et al. Ureteral stricture formation after ureteroscope treatment of impacted calculi: a prospective study. Korean J Urol. 2015;56:63–7.
97. Li L, Pan Y, Weng Z, Bao W, Yu Z, Wang F. A prospective randomized trial comparing pneumatic lithotripsy and holmium laser for management of middle and distal ureteral calculi. J Endourol. 2015;29:883–7.
98. Delvecchio FC, Auge BK, Brizuela RM, Weizer AZ, Silverstein AD, Lallas CD, et al. Assessment of stricture formation with the ureteral access sheath. Urology. 2003;61:518–22.

Techniques for Ureteroscopic Holmium Laser Lithotripsy

99. Teichman JM, Vassar GJ, Bishoff JT, Bellman GC. Holmium: YAG lithotripsy yields smaller fragments than lithoclast, pulsed dye laser or electrohydraulic lithotripsy. J Urol. 1998;159:17–23.
100. Chan KF, Vassar GJ, Pfefer TJ, Teichman JM, Glickman RE, Weintraub ST, et al. Holmium: YAG laser lithotripsy: a dominant photothermal ablative mechanism with chemical decomposition of urinary calculi. Lasers Surg Med. 1999;25:22–37.
101. Vassar GJ, Chan KF, Teichman JM, Glickman RD, Weintraub ST, Pfefer TJ, et al. Holmium: YAG lithotripsy: photothermal mechanism. J Endourol. 1999;13:181–90.
102. Matlaga BR, Chew B, Eisner B, Humphreys M, Knudsen B, Krambeck A, et al. Ureteroscopic laser lithotripsy: a review of dusting vs. fragmentation with extraction. J Endourol. 2018;32:1–6.
103. Tracey J, Gagin G, Morhardt D, Hollingsworth J, Ghani KR. Ureteroscopic high frequency dusting utilizing a 120-W holmium laser. J Endourol. 2018;32:290–5.
104. White MD, Moran ME, Calvano CJ, Borhan-Manesh A, Mehlhaff BA. Evaluation of retropulsion caused by holmium: YAG laser with various power settings and fibers. J Endourol. 1998;12:183–6.
105. Chawla S, Chang M, Chang A, Lenoir J, Bagley D. Effectiveness of high-frequency holmium: YAG laser stone fragmentation: the "popcorn effect". J Endourol. 2008;22:645–50.
106. Ludwig WW, Lim S, Stoianovici D, Matlaga BR. Endoscopic stone measurement during ureteroscopy. J Endourol. 2018;32:34–9.
107. Sea J, Jonat LM, Chew BH, Qiu J, Wang B, Hoopman J, et al. Optimal power settings for Holmium: YAG lithotripsy. J Urol. 2012;187:914–9.
108. Aldoukhi AH, Black KM, Ghani KR. Emerging laser techniques for the management of stones. Urol Clin N Am. 2019;46:193–205.
109. Schatloff O, Lindner U, Ramon J, Winkler HZ. Randomized trial of stone fragment active retrieval versus spontaneous passage during holmium laser lithotripsy for ureteral stones. J Urol. 2010;183:1031–5.

Selection and Need for Metabolic Evaluation

110. Pearle MS, Goldfarb DS, Assimos DG, Curhan G, Denu-Ciocca CJ, Matlaga BR, et al. Medical management of kidney stones: AUA guideline. J Urol. 2014;192:316–24.
111. Daudon M, Lacour B, Jungers P. Influence of body size on urinary stone composition in men and women. Urol Res. 2006;34:193–9.
112. Cloutier J, Villa L, Traxer O, Daudon M. Kidney stone analysis: "give me your stone, I will tell you who you are!". World J Urol. 2015;33:157–69.
113. Daudon M, Bader CA, Jungers P. Urinary calculi: review of classification methods and correlations with etiology. Scanning Microsc. 1993;7:1081–106.
114. Strohmaier WL. Course of calcium stone disease without treatment. What can we expect? Eur Urol. 2000;37:339–44.

Positioning for Ureteroscopy

115. Gupta A, Meriwether K, Tuller M, Sekula M, Gaskins J, Stewart JR, et al. Candy cane compared with boot stirrups in vaginal surgery: a randomized controlled trial. Obstet Gynecol. 2020;136:333–41.
116. Lehman T, Bagley DH. Reverse lithotomy: modified prone position for simultaneous nephroscopic and ureteroscopic procedures in women. Urology. 1988;32:529–31.
117. Grasso M, Nord R, Bagley DH. Prone split leg and flank roll positioning: simultaneous antegrade and retrograde access to the upper urinary tract. J Endourol. 1993;7:307–10.
118. Valdivia JG, Valer J, Villarroya S, Lopez JA, Bayo A, Lanchares E, et al. Why is percutaneous nephroscopy still performed with the patient prone? J Endourol. 1990;4:269–77.
119. Ibarluzea G, Scoffone CM, Cracco CM, Poggio M, Porpiglia F, Terrone C, et al. Supine Valdivia and modified lithotomy position for simultaneous anterograde and retrograde endourological access. BJU Int. 2007;100:233–6.
120. Scoffone CM, Cracco CM, Cossu M, Grande S, Poggio M, Scarpa RM. Endoscopic combined intrarenal surgery in Galdakao-modified supine Valdivia position: a new standard for percutaneous nephrolithotomy? Eur Urol. 2008;54:1393–403.
121. Nord RG, Goodman AC, Bagley DH. Prone split-leg position for simultaneous retrograde ureteroscopic and percutaneous nephroscopic procedures. J Endourol. 1991;5:13–6.
122. Lezrek M, Ammani A, Bazine K, Assebane M, Kasmaoui el H, Qarro A, et al. The split-leg modified lateral position for percutaneous renal surgery and optimal retrograde access to the upper urinary tract. Urology. 2011;78:217–20.

Chapter 6
Upper Tract Urothelial Carcinoma

Benjamin H. Rudnik, Scott G. Hubosky, Kim HooKim, Demetrius H. Bagley, María Rodríguez-Monsalve, Etienne Xavier Keller, Vincent De Coninck, Olivier Traxer, Michael Grasso III, Nitin Sharma, Andrew I. Fishman, Joseph K. Izes, and Anna W. Komorowski

B. H. Rudnik · S. G. Hubosky (✉) · K. HooKim · J. K. Izes
Department of Urology, Sidney Kimmel Medical College at Thomas Jefferson University Hospital, Philadelphia, PA, USA
e-mail: Benjamin.Rudnick@jefferson.edu; Scott.Hubosky@jefferson.edu; Joseph.Izes@jefferson.edu

K. HooKim
Department of Pathology, Anatomy and Cell Biology, Sidney Kimmel Medical College at Thomas Jefferson University Hospital, Philadelphia, PA, USA
e-mail: Kim.Hookim@jefferson.edu

D. H. Bagley
Department of Urology and Radiology, Sidney Kimmel Medical College at Thomas Jefferson University Hospital, Philadelphia, PA, USA
e-mail: Demetrius.BagleyJr@jefferson.edu

M. Rodríguez-Monsalve
Sorbonne Université, Service d'Urologie, AP-HP, Hôpital Tenon, Paris, France

Sorbonne Université, GRC n°20, Groupe de Recherche Clinique sur la Lithiase Urinaire, Hôpital Tenon, Paris, France

Department of Urology, Hospital universitario Puerta de Hierro, Majadahonda (Madrid), Spain

© Springer Nature Switzerland AG 2022
S. G. Hubosky et al. (eds.), *Advanced Ureteroscopy*,
https://doi.org/10.1007/978-3-030-82351-1_6

E. X. Keller · V. De Coninck · O. Traxer
Sorbonne Université, GRC n°20, Groupe de Recherche Clinique sur la Lithiase Urinaire,
Hôpital Tenon, Paris, France
e-mail: olivier.traxer@aphp.fr

M. Grasso III
Department of Urology, New York Medical College, Valhalla, NY, USA

N. Sharma
Phelps Memorial Hospital, Sleepy Hollow, NY, USA

A. I. Fishman
Department of Urology, New York Medical College, Valhalla, NY, USA

A. W. Komorowski
Department of Medical Oncology, Donald and Barbara Zucker School of Medicine at
Hofstra/Northwell, Hempstead, NY, USA
e-mail: Akomorowski@northwell.edu

Diagnosis of Upper Tract Urothelial Carcinoma

Benjamin H. Rudnik, Scott G. Hubosky, Kim HooKim
and Demetrius H. Bagley

Imaging

Radiographic evaluation plays a critical role in the evaluation of upper tract urothelial
carcinoma (UTUC). Intravenous pyelography was traditionally used as the primary
imaging modality for detecting upper tract lesions; however it has largely been
replaced by intravenous contrast-based computed tomographic urography (CTU).
Radiographic findings on CTU to suggest UTUC most often include a radiolucent
filling defect (Fig. 6.1) but may also manifest as an area of incomplete filling within
the upper urinary tract or an infiltrative process involving the collecting system. The
differential diagnosis of a collecting system filling defect on contrast-based imaging
includes blood clots, radiolucent calculi, sloughed papilla, external compression from
a crossing vessel, or a benign lesion (i.e., a fibroepithelial polyp). Enhancement on
contrast-based imaging is an important finding to differentiate benign and malignant
lesions. That being said, urothelial wall thickening may represent an infiltrating
UTUC or a generally non-specific inflammatory process (e.g., chronic inflammation
in the setting of a previously impacted calculus).

CTU has proven to be both a sensitive and specific modality for detection of UTUC. A
2010 meta-analysis by Chlapoutakis et al. reported a pooled sensitivity and specificity
of 96% and 99%, respectively [1]. Intravenous pyelography, on the other hand, has been
found to detect only 50–60% of upper tract lesions [2, 3]. CTU does inherently carry
increased radiation exposure for patients with approximately 1.5 times the radiation risk
associated with conventional urography [4]. The standard three-phase CT urography

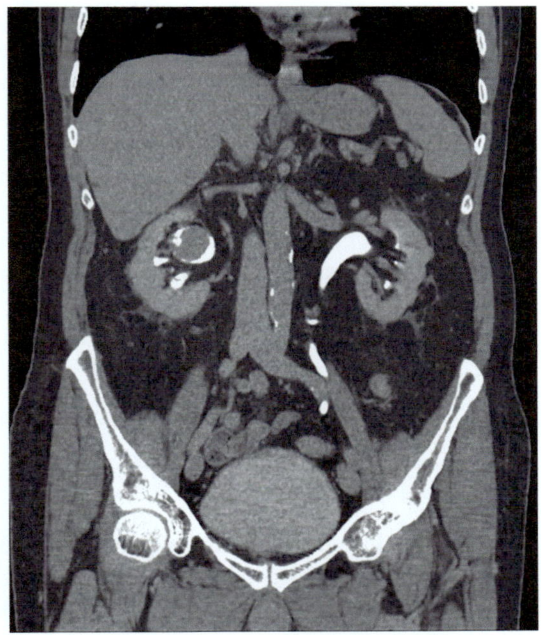

Fig. 6.1 Coronal view of CT Urogram shows a large filling defect in the right renal pelvis

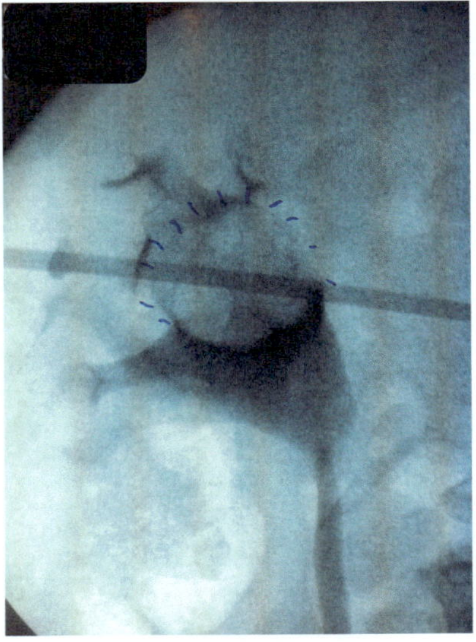

Fig. 6.2 Right retrograde pyelogram shows a large, space-occupying filling defect in the right intrarenal collecting system (outlined in blue dashes)

includes an unenhanced, nephrographic, and excretory phase, which collectively provides the most complete radiographic assessment of the upper urinary tract and bladder. A two-phase CTU protocol may be utilized at some centers to limit radiation exposure; however detection of lesions and ureteral opacification may be suboptimal and therefore is only recommended as a screening evaluation for low-risk patients [5].

In patients with a severe contrast allergy or impaired renal function, retrograde ureteropyelography may be indicated (Fig. 6.2). Operator variability and technique can affect the sensitivity and specificity when defining upper tract lesions, often with lack of uniformity in the interpretations of urologist and radiologist [6]. Magnetic resonance urography (MRU) is commonly employed in this setting, with the application of chelated gadolinium-based contrast minimizing risks in patients with renal insufficiency. MRU has been shown to have comparable specificity in detection of UTUC; however its sensitivity might be inferior to CTU with the largest known study of 91 MRU exams reporting a sensitivity of only 69% for upper tract lesions [7].

Renal ultrasound has a limited role in the evaluation of UTUC. Renal ultrasound can detect renal calculi, hydronephrosis, and renal masses with reasonable accuracy; however it has a limited ability to detect urothelial lesions in the upper urinary tract. In the DETECT (Detecting Bladder Cancer Using the UroMark Test) study, the sensitivity of renal and bladder ultrasound to detect UTUC was poor at only 14.3% among 2166 patients examined [8].

Urinary Cytology and Biomarkers

There is a significant interest and research effort being placed in the development of urinary biomarkers to aid in both the diagnosis and surveillance of urothelial carcinoma in the bladder and upper urinary tracts [9]. The goal is to develop less invasive and more cost-effective means to detect urothelial carcinoma and potentially reduce repetitive, expensive endoscopic instrumentation and/or cross-sectional imaging. Biomarkers originating from the urine and serum are being evaluated (Table 6.1),

Table 6.1 Urine-based biomarkers for the diagnosis of upper tract urothelial carcinoma

Test	Marker description	Sensitivity (%)	Specificity (%)	References
Urine cytology	Urinary sediment cell morphology	55–62	91	15, 16
ImmunoCyt/uCyt+	Fluorescent-labeled antibodies targeting tumor-associated antigens M344, LDQ10, and 19A11	75–91	95–100	29
UroVysion	FISH assay to identify aneuploidy of chromosomes 3, 7, and 17 and loss of p16 locus on 9p21	77	95	19
NMP-22	Nuclear matrix protein (reflection of mitotic activity)	44	98	63
BTA stat	Detection of human complement factor H-related protein (CFHrp)	82	89	64
Telomerase reverse transcriptase (TERT) mutation	TERT promoter gene mutation PCR assay	46–90	92–100	27, 65
GDF15, TMEFF2, and VIM methylation	Quantitative DNA methylation changes	91	100	66
CDH1, HSPA2, RASSF1A, TMEFF2, VIM, and GDF15 promoter methylations	Quantitative DNA methylation changes	84	91	67

but thus far large studies with long-term follow-up and validation are lacking. Therefore the gold standard of endoscopic evaluation and cross-sectional imaging has not yet been supplanted.

Urine cytology may be useful in the diagnosis of UTUC, but its utility remains limited by its overall low to moderate sensitivity. Sensitivity of urine cytology is dependent on a number of factors, including specimen source (voided versus upper tract site-specific aspirate), grade of tumor, and the inclusion of "suspicious" or "atypical" specimens versus only those that are overtly positive. The sensitivity of urine cytology for low-grade UTUC ranges from 10% to 20%, likely limited by cellular features similar to that of non-specific reactive atypia. High-grade UTUC lesions, however, demonstrate cytology sensitivity as high as 83%, with specificity that approaches 100% [10, 11].

The method of cytology collection has been shown to improve the quality of the specimen and diagnostic accuracy. Historically, the sensitivity of selective ureteral cytologies has ranged from 43% to 78% with false-negative rates as high as 50% for low-grade lesions [12–14]. A 2016 meta-analysis by Potrezke et al. found selective cytology to have a high-pooled specificity of 91% for detecting UTUC; however sensitivity was modest at 55% [15]. In a cohort of 326 patients who underwent radical nephroureterectomy or distal ureterectomy without a concurrent bladder malignancy, Messer et al. found a positive urine cytology to be a modest predictor of high-grade or invasive UTUC, with a sensitivity of 56% and 62% for high-grade and muscle-invasive UTUC, respectively [16]. When limited to only patients with selective upper tract cytologies, sensitivity for both high-grade disease and muscle-invasive UTUC improved to 71% and 78%, respectively.

Selective ureteral catheterization is often indicated in patients with a positive voided cytology without a tumor identified on cystoscopy and normal upper tract imaging. Fluoroscopically guided brush biopsy has been historically performed as well (i.e., Gill Brush) [17]. Although it has demonstrated superior sensitivity to selective ureteral catheterization, significant complications have been described including exacerbation of hematuria [18]. Compared to these procedural methods in obtaining site-specific cytology, contemporary ureteroscopic evaluation is preferred since it offers more in terms of diagnostic yield.

Fluorescence in situ hybridization (FISH) may also be useful in the detection of UTUC. FISH uses a multi-target assay to identify aneuploidy of chromosomes 3, 7, and 17, as well as loss of the p16 locus at 9p21. When compared to cytology, it has shown increased sensitivity, but differences have not been statistically significant in larger series [19, 20]. FISH may provide increased detection of UTUC when used in conjunction with cytology [21]. As seen with urine cytology, the sensitivity of FISH to detect UTUC is dependent on tumor grade [22]. Of note, FISH does add significant cost burden in cancer detection [23].

The role of epigenetic changes in UTUC has been investigated in recent years as well. In a study by Xiong et al., the methylation status of multiple genes including BRCA1, CDH1, HSPA2, RASSF1A, GDF15, THBS1, and TMEFF2 was found to be significantly associated with tumor stage, tumor grade, and lymph node status in patients with UTUC [24]. When this same group evaluated the methylation status of these genes in voided urine specimens from 98 patients, they found a sensitivity of 82% and specificity of 68% for detection of UTUC [25].

The unique genomic factors associated with UTUC have also been investigated as potential diagnostic targets. In the largest genomic study of UTUC to date, Sfakianos and colleagues found that genes FGFR3, CDKN2B, and HRAS were associated with high-grade UTUC [26]. One study that investigated FGFR3 and telomerase reverse transcriptase (TERT) as potential diagnostic biomarkers for UTUC found that when combined with cytology, they yielded a sensitivity and specificity of 78.6% and 96%, respectively [27].

Other novel tumor markers including nuclear matrix protein 22 (NMP22) and ImmunoCyt/uCyt+ have demonstrated improved sensitivity in the diagnosis of UTUC, but studies remain limited to date [28, 29]. Further research is required to better understand their role in the evaluation of UTUC moving forward.

Ureteroscopic Biopsy Technique

Endoscopic evaluation for suspected UTUC begins with thorough cystoscopy using both 30-degree and 70-degree telescopes in a rigid endoscope or a flexible cysto-scope to assess for concomitant bladder pathology. A urine cytology specimen is collected upon evaluation of the bladder, and bilateral retrograde ureteropyelograms are performed using an 8F cone-tip catheter. Initial ureteral catheterization should be avoided to limit trauma to the upper urinary tract urothelium.

The suspected upper tract is then directly examined using a "no-touch" technique. A small semirigid ureteroscope is introduced into the ureter under direct vision. The use of a guidewire at this point is avoided to limit potential tumor shearing and suboptimal evaluation. The ureteroscope is passed proximally to assess the distal and mid ureter. Once the ureteroscope has reached its most proximal extent, a guidewire is placed to the level of the ureter that has been inspected, and the ureteroscope is removed atraumatically.

The smallest flexible ureteroscope available is then passed over the guidewire, and ureteropyeloscopy is completed. If a flexible ureteroscope can be passed directly into the distal ureter initially, then the use of the semirigid ureteroscope and guidewire as previously described is not necessary. Given the advent of flexible ureteroscopes with greater shaft stiffness and superior tip control in recent years, the use of the semirigid ureteroscope can be avoided in many cases [30]. Pyeloscopy should be carried out in a systematic fashion, beginning with the renal pelvis followed by the upper pole calyces, the mid pole, and lastly the lower pole.

Any lesion encountered during ureteroscopy should be biopsied at that time unless more proximal lesions are suspected based on retrograde ureteropyelogram or preoperative imaging. Prior to biopsy, a cytology washing is collected using the irrigation port of the ureteroscope. Biopsy can be performed using a variety of methods, and technique should be tailored to the appearance of the lesion. A papillary tumor, for instance, can be biopsied using a 2.2F or 2.4F flat-wire basket. In this scenario, the basket is opened adjacent to and then directed around the tumor under direct vision. It should be snug but not so tight that it crushes the tumor. The ureteroscope, basket, and tumor specimen are then removed entirely as a single unit (Fig. 6.3). This technique provides excellent diagnostic results, with a successful cytopathologic diagnosis achieved in 94% of cases [31]. The stainless-steel flat-wire basket or double-snare design is preferred because the basket's more rigid wires offer an edge to hold the tissue. The round and more flexible wires of nitinol baskets tend to slide off the specimen rather than holding it.

To biopsy a sessile or flatter lesion, a 3F cup biopsy forceps is most often employed. Multiple small specimens are removed through the endoscope's working channel and incorporated in a small aliquot of sterile saline of Hank's solution. This biopsy method can suffer from crush artifact and yields smaller, often < 1 mm, specimen; however it still provides acceptable sensitivity with a 74.9–79% diagnostic rate reported [32, 33]. Another device is the BIGopsy® (Cook Urological, Spencer, Indiana), which obtains larger specimens with reported diagnostic rates of 90–100% [32, 33]. It must be back-loaded into the flexible ureteroscope, which in turn must be advanced through a ureteral access sheath. The large 6F tip also significantly reduces the visual field and limits deflection of the ureteroscope [34].

Immediately following tumor biopsy, a barbotage specimen of sterile saline obtained through the ureteroscope's working channel is collected for cytological evaluation. If a lesion is treated endoscopically, an additional final cytology is collected after treatment has been completed, all performed to increase the sensitivity of the cytopathologic grading.

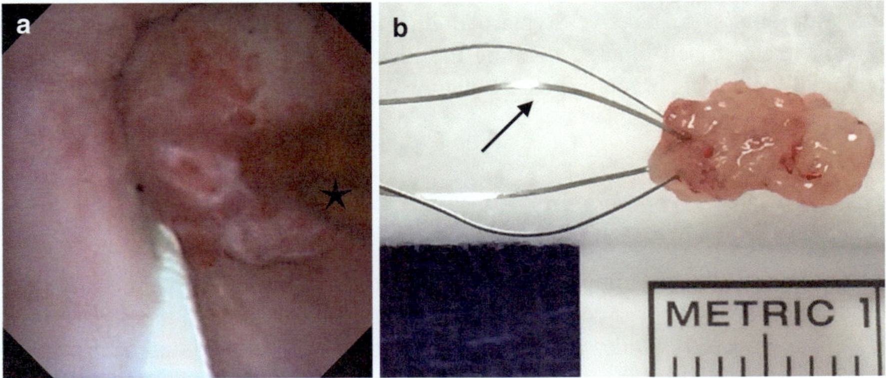

Fig. 6.3 (**a**) Luminal tumor biopsy with stainless steel flat wire basket (star). The tumor is removed en bloc, similar to a stone. (**b**) Flat wires of the stainless steel basket (arrow) are more rigid than nitinol and superior in holding tissue in the angle between the wires with flat edges. Relatively large volume specimens can be sampled

Specimen Processing

Historically, ureteroscopic biopsies processed with standard cassette histopathology had limited diagnostic yield, as many specimens did not survive processing. Therefore, all aspirates and biopsy specimens are sent to cytopathology for processing to help ensure adequacy. Solutions are concentrated by centrifugation into cytospins or by liquid-based technology. Cytospins use a high-speed centrifuge to concentrate cells on a slide in a uniform monolayer 6 mm in diameter, which enhances the morphological appearance of the cells [35]. This technique increased diagnostic yield from 42.9% to 97.2% [36]. Using a similar technique, Sheridan et al. found that cytologic processing of ureteral biopsies showed superior sensitivity for detecting high-grade UTUC, which they attribute to an increased number of intact urothelial cells [37]. Today, the majority of urinary specimens are processed by liquid-based technology, which concentrates material in a uniform monolayer, reduces obscuring debris, and improves cellular detail and preservation by fixation [38].

Generally, cell blocks may be prepared by a variety of techniques, such as HistoGel (Richard-Allan Scientific Processing Gel, Thermo Fisher Scientific, Kalamazoo, Michigan), plasma-thrombin clot technique, agar gel, Cellient technology (Hologic, Marlborough, Massachusetts), or centrifugation into a pellet. Cell blocks are useful when immunocytochemistry is needed, such as diagnosing non-urothelial malignancies, like metastatic carcinoma, lymphoma/leukemia, or for the detection of polyomavirus. Cell blocks also provide histologic examination of intact tissue fragments for architecture, thickness, and polarity of the urothelium, which are essential in the classification and grading of urothelial neoplasia. This approach is particularly helpful in diagnosing low-grade papillary UTUC in which the architectural abnormalities are not preserved in cytologic preparations and cellular features are similar to reactive atypia. Additionally, subepithelial stroma may also remain intact in cell blocks, enabling the identification of possible invasion and potentially resulting in more accurate staging of advanced tumors.

Grading with Ureteroscopy

Tumor grade is the most important prognosticator when treating upper urinary tract urothelial malignancies. Accurate tumor grading is thus critical in the diagnosis of UTUC as it directly guides clinical management. Histologic grading of urothelial carcinoma has evolved from the original 1973 World Health Organization (WHO) classification, which consisted of a three-tier system of low grade 1, intermediate grade 2, and high grade 3 based on the degree of anaplasia [39]. The parameters for assessing anaplasia are increased cellularity and thickness of the urothelium, loss of polarity and maturation, crowding, nuclear polymorphism, variations in nuclear size, hyperchromasia, abnormal chromatin, and abnormal mitoses (Fig. 6.4). Grade 1 tumors show the least anaplastic features, grade 3 tumors show marked anaplasia,

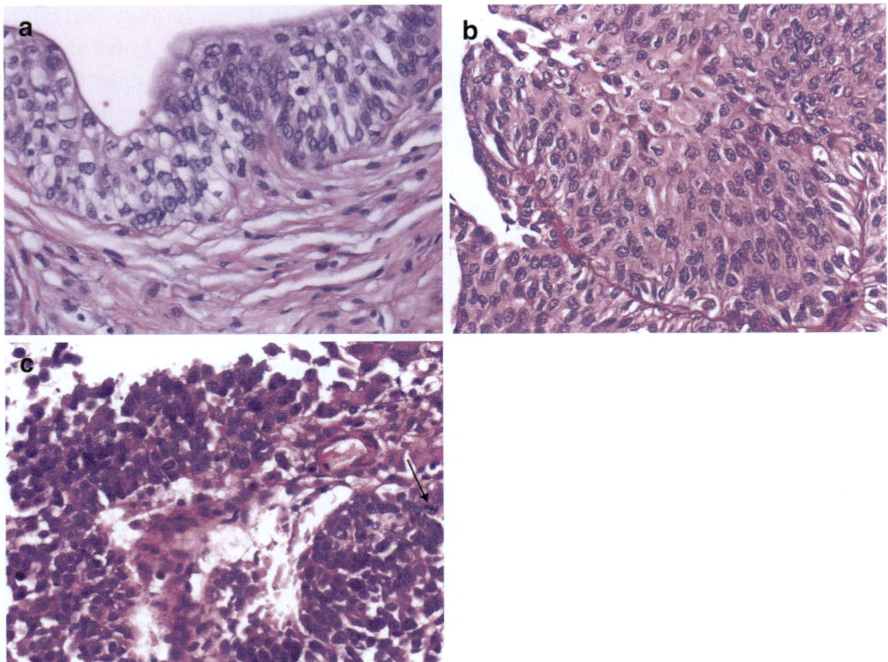

Fig. 6.4 (**a**) Normal ureter: The ureter is lined by transitional epithelium, also known as urothelium. The urothelium is a stratified layer of 3–6 cell layers in thickness. The most superficial layer is scalloped with fuzzy cytoplasm, and contains umbrella cells, which are multinucleated benign urothelial cells. The intermediate layer contains polygonal cells with low nuclear/cytoplasmic ratio and orderly arrangement. The basal layer is more compact with cells arranged perpendicular to the basement membrane. (**b**) Low-grade papillary urothelial carcinoma: The tumor cells contain mildly enlarged nuclei. There is no significant nuclear hyperchromasia or pleomorphism. Note that cellular polarity is maintained. Mitoses are also rare or absent. (**c**) High-grade papillary urothelial carcinoma: The tumor cells are crowded with loss of polarity, severe hyperchromasia, high nuclear/cytoplasmic ratio and course chromatin. Mitoses are seen (black arrow)

and grade 2 tumors are intermediate or moderately anaplastic. Subsequent modified versions include a four-tier scheme (grade 1, grades 2a or 2b, and grade 3) [40] and a five-tier system (grades 1, 2a, 2b, and 3 and grade 4) [41]. These systems aimed to improve grading as a predictor of clinical behavior and outcomes. However, an intermediate-grade UCC might be considered as a low- or high-grade UCC in another system. There was also significant variability in their interpretation and use among pathologists and studies [42]. Therefore, studies utilizing different experts and grading criteria made comparison problematic and confusing.

Consequently, the WHO/International Society of Urological Pathology (ISUP) introduced the 1998 WHO/ISUP grading classification to improve and simplify histologic grading to a two-tier system of low- or high-grade UCC [43]. The 2004 WHO/ISUP and the current 2016 WHO/ISUP grading systems use the 1998 two-tier grading [44]. One of the important features that distinguish the 2016 WHO/ISUP from the 2004 WHO/ISUP is that grading is not only restricted to morphologic features of anaplasia but also correlates with tumor biology and clinical behavior. Following the 2004 WHO/ISUP, several studies have shown that the majority of invasive (T1 or greater) tumors show only focal low-grade features using either 1973 or 2004 WHO/ISUP criteria. More importantly, stage-matched invasive UCCs behaved similarly irrespective of their assigned grade, with no difference in recurrence-free, cancer-free, or overall survival. This is particularly evident in the deceptive nested variants of urothelial carcinoma of the bladder, which have poor prognosis due to extensive invasion despite their low-grade histology. Pursuant to these studies and recommendations by the International Consultation on Urological Diseases (ICUD), all invasive UCCs should be considered as high grade [45].

Despite the various grading systems and their challenges, multiple series of ureteroscopically treated UTUC patients over two decades have demonstrated that ureteroscopic (URS) biopsy provides very good diagnostic accuracy in regard to tumor grade. In 1997, Keeley et al. demonstrated a strong (90%) correlation between ureteroscopic biopsy grade and the final pathological grade seen on nephroureterectomy specimen [36]. Ten years later and in a retrospective review of more patients who had undergone nephroureterectomy for UTUC, Brown et al. found there was tumor grade concordance in 112/119 (94%) patients who had URS biopsy prior to nephroureterectomy [46]. In a study of 137 biopsies in 81 patients with suspected UTUC, Rojas and colleagues found a comparable tumor grade concordance rate of 92.6% [47]. Interestingly, they also showed that the volume of tissue removed at time of URS biopsy did not affect the diagnostic accuracy of tumor grade. In a large multi-institutional cohort of 230 patients undergoing extirpative surgery for UTUC, Clements et al. found that high-grade biopsy pathology had a 92% positive predictive value (PPV) for high-grade pathology at time of definitive surgery; however, low-grade biopsies only had a PPV of 54% [48]. This study was significantly limited; however, in that, biopsy specimens were performed using three different biopsy techniques including brush biopsy, and specimens were interpreted by several different genitourinary pathologists.

The issue of ureteroscopic UTUC biopsy grade discordance to the final pathological NU specimen grade is occasionally reported in the urological literature and deserves mentioning [49, 50]. A 2018 multi-institutional study by Margolin and colleagues that reviewed 314 patients who underwent URS biopsy followed by nephroureterectomy or segmental ureterectomy for UTUC found that 51% of cases of low-grade tumors on biopsy were upgraded at time of surgical resection [49]. The rate of upgrading was slightly lower when baskets were used (45%) compared to biopsy forceps (51%), but this was not statistically significant. Brush biopsies were not included in this cohort. It is critical to note that in this series, pathologic interpretation was performed according to the 1973 and 1998 World Health Organization (WHO) classification systems, depending on time of biopsy, and no central pathology review was performed. Tumors identified as grade 1 or 2 based on the 1973 classification were collectively defined as low grade. As previously mentioned, discordant grading affected tumor grading results, with significant upgrading of up to 50% of grade 2 lesions as defined by the 1973 classification system. These lesions display tumor heterogeneity and would qualify as high-grade lesions according to the updated WHO grading system [51]. Therefore, studies reporting upgrading of ureteroscopic biopsies relative to the final surgical specimens must be interpreted with caution. This is especially the case when more than one pathologic grading system was utilized over the term of the study in the absence of central pathology review. Nevertheless, ureteroscopic biopsy grading should not be utilized in a vacuum for clinical decision making. Cross-sectional imaging characteristics and site-specific cytology, as well as dedicated cytopathologists familiar with the variability associated with specimen collection and treatment effects, are essential, especially in patients on post-treatment surveillance.

Staging of Upper Tract Urothelial Carcinoma

Ureteroscopic biopsy has general limitations in determining tumor stage given the small size of tissue specimens and the thin nature of the upper tract muscularis propria as compared the bladder. Margolin et al. found that the likelihood of missing muscle-invasive disease on URS biopsy was significantly increased when specimens were limited to 1 mm or less in diameter [49]. Contemporary series have demonstrated that staging concordance rates between biopsy specimens and final surgical specimens range from 55% to 66% [49, 52, 53].

Tumor grade, the most important prognosticator, has been found to be associated with pathologic stage in multiple studies; however the degree of its predictive value has varied greatly. Brown et al. found in their 71 patients with high-grade biopsies there was a 66% PPV for pT2 or greater disease and a 42% PPV of pT3 or greater disease [46]. Conversely, in those 48 patients with low-grade biopsies, negative predictive values for pT2 and pT3 disease were 72% and 92%, respectively [46]. In their cohort of 238 patients, Clements et al. found that high-grade biopsy pathology had 60% predictive accuracy for muscle-invasive disease and on multivariate analysis was associated with a fourfold greater risk of pT2 disease [48]. Low-grade biopsies were less predictive of tumor stage, as nearly 30% of patients with low-grade biopsies were ultimately found to have muscle invasion at time of surgical resection [40]. Jeon et al. studied multiple preoperative variables including cross-sectional imaging characteristics and ureteroscopic biopsy information. Although only able to be obtained in about 50% of ureteroscopic biopsies, the presence of lamina propria invasion by tumor was the best predictor of the final pathologic grade $\geq$ pT2 on multivariate analysis with odds ratio of 5.57. Lamina propria invasion on ureteroscopic biopsy with the simultaneous presence of high-grade tumor demonstrated muscle-invasive UTUC on NU specimen in 84% of cases [54]. This represents improved detection compared to ureteroscopic grade alone for prediction of muscle-invasive disease, which historically has been reported by multiple groups to be 66% [36, 46].

Cross-sectional imaging has shown good accuracy in determining regional or distant metastatic UTUC; however its utility in determining local stage has been historically poor. Preoperative axial CT imaging has been shown to accurately stage UTUC in only 52–59% of patients [55, 56]. In a study of 106 patients who underwent radical nephroureterectomy for UTUC, Ng and colleagues did find that hydrone-phrosis on preoperative CT imaging was associated with advanced pathologic stage and a predictor of non-organ-confined disease on the final pathology [57]. Another study by Brien et al. looked at the presence of preoperative hydronephrosis on CT imaging in conjunction with positive urine cytology and high-grade biopsy speci-mens. They found that when all three of these factors were present the PPV was 89% for pT2 or greater disease, and when none were present, the NPV was 100% [58]. Similarly, Faveretto et al. described a model combining cross-sectional imaging with biopsy results that predicts pT2 disease or greater with over 70% accuracy [59].

Other imaging modalities have been explored as potential tools to aid in the stag-ing of UTUC. High-frequency endoluminal ultrasound (ELUS) has been investi-gated with a reported diagnostic accuracy of 63–67% in two series [60, 61]. Experience with ELUS remains limited in scope, and further studies are required before it is incorporated into clinical practice.

In recent years optical coherence tomography (OCT) has been described as a potential UTUC staging tool utilized at time of ureteroscopy. This technology uses a 2.7F intravascular imaging probe introduced through the working channel of a flexible ureteroscope that provides a cross-sectional image at planned biopsy sites. A recent study of 26 patients found an 83% staging concordance rate with a sensitiv-ity and specificity for tumor invasion of 100% and 92%, respectively [62]. It should be noted that OCT is limited in that it provides only a binary classification system (invasive or non-invasive disease) and has a limited imaging depth, making the stag-ing of larger exophytic tumors non-diagnostic. Further studies are required to better appreciate the diagnostic value of OCT for clinicians managing patients with UTUC.

Enhanced Endoscopic Imaging Techniques for Upper Tract Urothelial Carcinoma

María Rodríguez-Monsalve, Etienne Xavier Keller, Vincent De Coninck and Olivier Traxer

Introduction

Diagnosis of upper tract urothelial carcinoma (UTUC) is based on imaging tech-niques, diagnostic ureterorenoscopy (URS) and biopsy. These techniques have some important limitations. Difficulties for diagnosis of upper tract carcinoma in situ (UT-CIS), differentiation of flat malignant lesions from inflammatory tissue, and limitations in biopsy samples for an accurate diagnosis of grading and staging are the most commonly recognized challenges [63, 64].

Conservative endoscopic treatment using URS is a valid option in selected patients with low-grade and low-stage disease, with cancer-specific survival rates

Table 6.2 Characteristics of the new extended imaging techniques in UTUC

	NBI	Image 1-S	PPD	OCT	CLE
Principle	Absorption	Digital image processing	Fluorescence	Scattering	Absorption/ reflection
Field of view	Macroscopic	Macroscopic	Macroscopic	Microscopic	Microscopic
Contrast	No	No	5-ALA, HAL	No	Fluorescein
Depth	Surface	Surface	Surface	2–3 mm	0.4–0.7 μm
Aim	Improving visualization and detection of tumors	Improving visualization and detection of tumors	Improving visualization and detection of tumors	Real-time information on histopathology	Real-time information on histopathology

compared to nephroureterectomy [65]. Given the frequency of local recurrence, regular ureteroscopic surveillance and close follow-up are required for optimal oncologic control in patients undergoing endoscopic treatment for UTUC.

Accurate information regarding not only tumor grade and stage but also local extent is essential in order to select and optimally treat UTUC patients with nephron-sparing ureteroscopic techniques. The development of enhanced imaging modalities to be used with ureteroscopy offer a significant improvement in the detection and management of UTUC, including UT-CIS. In addition, new real-time optical diagnostic techniques are capable of providing instant information about tumor grade and stage, which open the possibility to more expeditiously direct patients to appropriate treatment.

The new imaging technologies are classified depending on the field of view in macroscopic or microscopic imaging modalities (Table 6.2). Macroscopic technologies are similar to white light and provide information about a wide area of urothelium with enhancement, in order to facilitate the localization and delineation of suspicious lesions. Examples of this type of technique are narrow-band imaging (NBI) and Storz Image 1-S technology (formerly Storz professional image enhancement system (SPIES)). Photodynamic diagnosis (PDD) also is included in these macroscopic techniques and is based on fluorescence and the addition of a topical fluorophore. Microscopic technologies confer of a high resolution with important characterization of the tissue related with suspected lesions, giving real-time information on histopathology. The main techniques in this category are optical coherence tomography (OCT) and confocal laser endomicroscopy (CLE).

Image Enhancement Techniques

Narrow-Band Imaging (NBI)

This endoscopic technique has been developed by Olympus®. It is an optical tool that filters white light into two narrow bandwidths of 415 nm and 540 nm that correspond to blue and green light, respectively. It is based on the fact that the depth of light penetration increases with wavelength. These wavelengths are both strongly absorbed by hemoglobin and only minimally penetrate the mucosal surface. This effect creates an enhanced contrast between vascular structures and mucosa. The blue band (415 nm) penetrates the superficial mucosa layers and results in a brown appearance of the more superficial vessels. The green band (540 nm) has a deeper penetration to the submucosal layers and accentuates the vessels with green appearance [66]. In the generated image, the vascularized areas appear in a dark brown/green color in contrast with the pink/white of normal urothelium. The aim of this technology is to help identify hypervascularized areas, highlighting neoangiogenesis of urothelial tumors.

An advantage of this technique is that it does not require administration of exogenous contrast facilitating its applicability. Also, the results from the use of this technique have demonstrated that it does not require a significant learning curve to interpret the findings, with no significant difference between novel and experienced users in terms of detection rates. This technique improved the tumor detection rate by 22.7% according to a study of 27 patients that underwent URS for UTUC, subsequently with white light and NBI by the same urologist, in the same setting. Compared to traditional white light URS, five additional tumors were detected, and three other tumors were noted to have expanded margins, using NBI, which otherwise would have been missed [67]. NBI technology is exclusively integrated to digital flexible ureteroscopes manufactured by Olympus®, including the URF-V, URF-V2, and URF-V3 [68].

Image 1-S Technology (Formerly: Storz Professional Image Enhancement System "SPIES")

This technology developed by Storz® is based on spectral separation. It filters white light images digitally to produce four different contrasts that modify the displayed image.

SPECTRA A is a combination of green and blue signals that highlights the differences between vascular structures and mucosa. SPECTRA B is based on the reduction of red spectral reflection and also helps define a better contrast between tissues and structures. The CLARA mode uses an adaptation of image brightness clarifying the visualization of the darker areas in the image. CHROMA mode intensifies color contrast which is very useful to define the optimal sharpness of the image structures [69]. A study comparing image perception of bladder tumors among urologists showed concordance in the interpretation of the 80 spectral images evaluated. In low agreement cases, CLARA CHROMA and SPECTRA B showed less variations in interpretation than SPECTRA A [70]. The value of this technique in the upper urinary tract is under investigation.

Photodynamic Diagnosis (PDD)

This technique employs fluorescence as a contrast mechanism, based on the interaction between light and increased accumulation of fluorochrome in the malignant tissue. The fluorochrome has the property of absorbing light and re-emitting it in a longer wave than the original one. This is explained by the fact that the absorbed light excites the electrovibrational state of the fluorochrome, so when the molecule relaxes to ground state a photon is emitted to realize the energy difference. This emitted light has a longer wavelength than the illuminated one.

This modality of enhanced imaging uses photosensitive protoporphyrin analogues, so-called fluorochrome agents, combined with blue light to stimulate fluorescence. In the majority of cases, the agents utilized are porphyrin-related fluorochrome 5-aminoaevulinic acid (5-ALA) and its derivate hexaminolevulinate (HAL).

These substances can be administrated as an oral solution or instilled directly by the working channel of ureteroscope. Tumor cells have an important accumulation of photosensitizers 5-ALA and HAL and are visualized red when using blue light (380–470 nm) in contrast with the normal urothelium that has a blue/green coloration. Special endoscopes or filters are needed to illuminate tissue with this blue light. An advantage of this technique is the relatively easy interpretation of images considering red fluorescent areas.

Nevertheless, this technique has several obstacles for a routine use in the upper urinary tract (UUT). Firstly, if a topical instillation of the fluorochrome is proposed, it is more difficult in the UUT than in the bladder because of its anatomical characteristics and accessibility. Secondly, it is important to recognize that the application of light tangential to the mucosa can give false-positive results in up to a 30% of cases. Acquiring a perpendicular viewing angle in the UUT could be challenging especially in the ureter [71, 72].

In the largest study available to date including 106 upper urinary tract units, sensitivity was estimated in 95.6% in the UUT, similar to the 92% reported in the bladder [73, 74]. Several studies have shown a high detection rate, especially for flat lesions or CIS, with PPD-guided URS after oral administration of 5-ALA [75].

A recent systematic review was published. The overall adverse events rate with this technique was 25.8%, all of them minor complications (Clavien I) [76]. The most common complications related to the use of 5-ALA in these studies were hypotension, nausea, increase of liver enzymes, photosensitivity skin reaction, and photodermatosis [77].

Optical Diagnostic Techniques

Optical Coherence Tomography (OCT)

This technique is the optical equivalent of ultrasound imaging, based on the measurement of light reflectivity versus depth instead of using reflected ultrasounds waves like in echography. A 2.7F probe composed of optical fibers with distant rotation light firing at 90° with automatic retrieval over a 5-cm distance is used. Light scattering signal decreases with depth, and its range is limited to a 2-mm depth. The attenuation coefficient μ_{oct} is defined as the rate of OCT signal decreased with depth. Measurement of μ_{oct} is sensitive to the different cell layer organization and can be associated with different grade lesions, creating a cross-sectional image of the tissue. This association of information, real-time high-quality images with digital scopes, and optical attenuation coefficient gives real-time information about tumor grade and stage. This technology can make distinction of the ureteral wall layers and its architecture. This leads to differentiate low- and high-grade lesions.

In a study with 26 patients that underwent diagnostic URS and OCT, the results of OCT were compared with the histopathology of the radical nephroureterectomy or segmental ureter resection. Sensitivity for staging was 83%. For tumor invasion, sensitivity was 100% and specificity 92%. Tumor size >2 cm and inflammation were the main cause of false positives [62].

Disadvantages of this technique are the current limit of lumen imaging with a maximum diameter of 10 mm and its maximal imaging depth hindering assessment about invasiveness of large-volume tumors; hence tumor staging is not feasible when exophytic growth is greater than imaging depth [78]. More clinical experience is required before conclusions on the utility of OCT for UTUC staging can be made.

Confocal Laser Endomicroscopy (CLE)

CLE is an innovative, high-resolution probe imaging technique (3.5 µm) based on the use of fluorescence, allowing imaging of tissue with a maximal depth of 40–70 µm.

This technique uses a 488-nm laser light in combination with fiberoptic in a pinhole to ensure that only light from the focal plane of tissue is collected. The light that is out of focus is rejected by the pinhole, which acts as a diaphragm. The size of the probe is defined by the number of fibers used for the CLE imaging. A 3F-diameter probe is available for ureteroscopic use in the upper urinary tract. This technology requires the use of fluorescein as a luminal contrast agent to highlight microarchitecture and small vessels. Real-time imaging of the cellular and subcellular level is achieved, resulting in differentiation between normal, low-grade, and high-grade tumor tissue [79], in effect, giving a real-time optical biopsy.

For CLE, the definitions of histological architecture in the upper urinary tract are as follows:

- Normal tissue: layers of superficial and polygonal umbrella cells and smaller intermediate cells more deeply.
- Low-grade tumors: organized, densely packed, monomorphic cells, absence of umbrella cells, and papillary structures surrounded by fibrovascular structures.
- High-grade tumors: disorganized, pleomorphic cells without defined borders or cohesion, absence of umbrella cells, and fibrovascular stalks with disorganized structure.

Some drawbacks of this technique have been reported. CLE imaging has significant sensitivity to movement that could lend to motion artifacts and subsequently poor quality images. Also, limited penetration depth and the dependence on the position of the probe to obtain a good quality image have been reported.

Interpretation of the findings requires certain experience; several studies have defined in vivo characteristics of bladder urothelium, and in vivo pilot studies have proven the use of this technique in the upper urinary tract [80, 81]. The use of this system provides dynamic microscopic evaluation of cellular architecture.

A recent study in which 14 flexible ureteroscopies with CLE were performed showed a correspondence between CLE images and the final histopathological result in 100%, and inter-observer agreement was also found between CLE and histological reading ($k = 0,64$) [82].

Conclusions

Enhanced endoscopic imaging techniques exist for better detection, delineation, and diagnostic characterization of UTUC. Existing clinical experience with ureteroscopy is limited, but preliminary studies have demonstrated the feasibility of these various technologies to be applied to the morphologically challenging upper urinary tract. Further prospective analyses are needed to clarify the outcomes of these new diagnostic methods (Fig. 6.5).

Ureteroscopic Treatment of Upper Tract Urothelial Carcinoma

Michael Grasso III, Nitin Sharma, Andrew I. Fishman, Joseph K. Izes, Demetrius H. Bagley and Scott G. Hubosky

Rationale for Nephron-Sparing Approaches

Nephroureterectomy (NU) has been the standard treatment of upper tract urothelial carcinoma (UTUC). In general, the biology of these urothelial tumors is similar to the lower urinary tract, and as such, there is a great interest in treating these lesions ureteroscopically, thus preserving functional renal parenchyma. Ample data exist which tie rates of hospitalization, cardiovascular events, and mortality to incremental decreases in glomerular filtration rate (GFR) [83]. Over-utilization of radical nephrectomy, rather than partial nephrectomy for small renal cortical lesions, has been shown to be an independent risk factor for chronic renal insufficiency [84]. As a result, there has been a shift in the management of lower-risk renal cell carcinoma toward nephron-sparing approaches, especially in those with pre-existing chronic

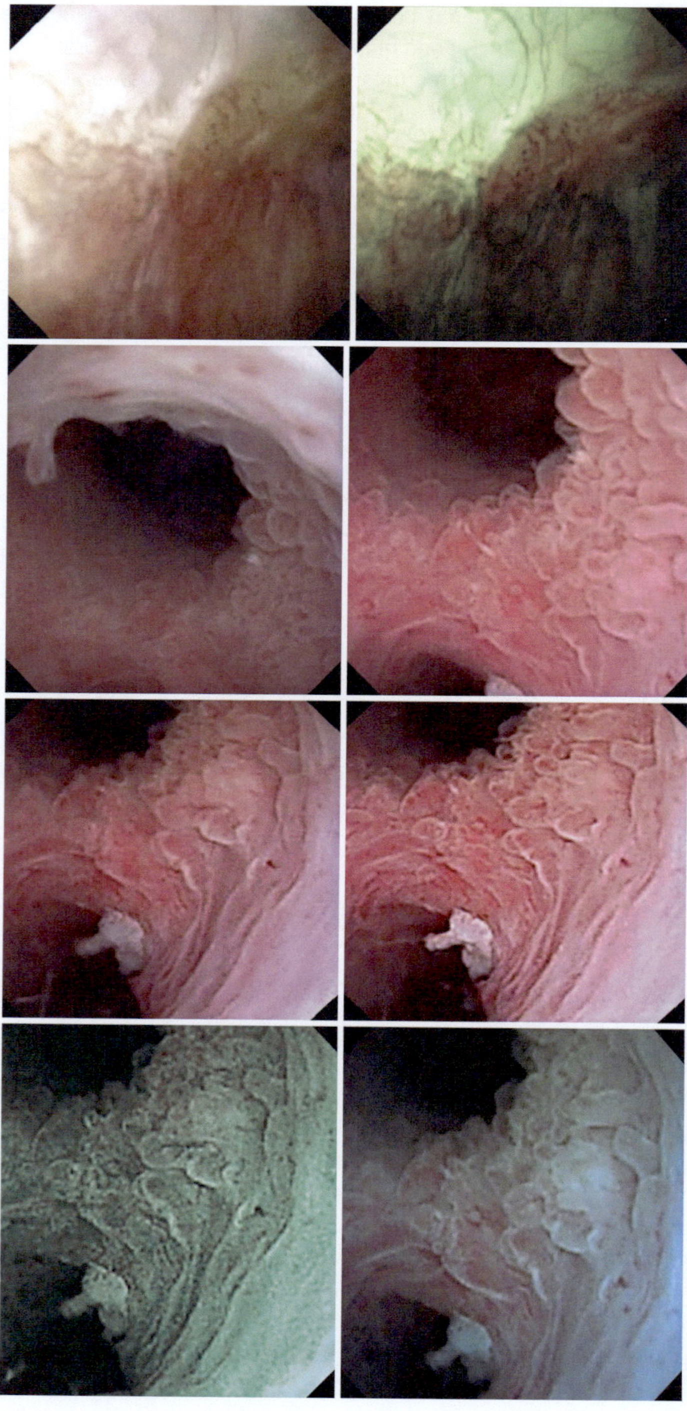

Fig. 6.5 Image of UUT lesion with white light (left) and same lesion with NBI (right)

kidney disease [85]. Since up to 51% of patients presenting with UTUC may have GFR < 60 [86], the same rationale should apply, thus highlighting the importance of effective ureteroscopic treatment as a prime nephron-sparing approach in this vulnerable population. Improvements in instrumentation and deliverable energy sources have facilitated retrograde ureteroscopic therapies. Endoscope downsizing and miniaturization, improved mechanics, and deflectability combined with progressive laser energy sources have made ureteroscopic treatment of UTUC more practical [87, 88]. Due to the rarity of UTUC, no prospective, randomized trials comparing ureteroscopic treatment to radical NU exist, but multiple meta-analyses have been published which support equivalent outcomes in terms of cancer-specific survival (CSS), in carefully selected patients with low-grade, non-invasive UTUC [89, 90].

Patient Selection

Selecting the treatment for UTUC requires balancing adequate oncologic control, preserving renal function, and minimizing morbidity. Ureteroscopic treatment has been employed for UTUC in patients with prohibitive comorbidities associated with nephroureterectomy for well over 30 years. Relative contraindications to nephroureterectomy would include solitary kidney, bilateral tumors, chronic kidney disease, and hereditary predisposition to UTUC such as Lynch syndrome. Favorable treatment outcomes and renal preservation rates have been demonstrated with ureteroscopy in patients with solitary kidneys and renal insufficiency as well as in carefully selected patients with a normal contralateral kidney [91, 92]. As instrumentation and techniques for efficient tumor ablation have improved, endoscopic treatment of low-grade UTUC has become a standard therapy, as detailed in both contemporary European and National Comprehensive Cancer Network (NCCN) guidelines [93, 94].

Although not meant to be considered in isolation, tumor grade is the most important prognosticator when planning treatment for UTUC. Other important variables to consider are baseline renal function, tumor burden, location within the collecting system, multifocality, and a history of prior bladder carcinoma. Pre-intervention risk stratification can be challenging and requires diagnostic ureteroscopy and both tissue sampling and cytologic washing. Tumor grade, based on both histology and cytopathologic evaluation, is by far most the important prognosticator. It is important to remember that the highest-grade flat lesions and carcinoma in situ may have indeterminate results on tissue sampling, while cytology is diagnostic. CIS, for example, on cup biopsy often has fibrous substructure without urothelium, which has peeled off, and so the cytologic washing in that setting is diagnostic. It is also important to note that tumors can be of mixed grade and papillary low grade on biopsy with washings that are high grade. Any parameter that is diagnostic for high grade directs future treatment; thus a high-grade washing with low-grade biopsy is treated as a high-grade presentation.

The European Association of Urology guidelines stratify patients into low risk versus high risk based on clinical, endoscopic, histologic/cytologic, and radiographic factors [93] (Table 6.3).

Patients in the low-risk category should always be considered for a nephron-sparing modality, which includes the ureteroscopic approach. Even low-risk patients, however, need to be well informed about the relatively high rate of local recurrence for low-grade UTUC treated ureteroscopically, which approaches 68–90%, as seen in large series with extended mean follow-up of almost 5 years [95–97]. In general, these locally recurrent lesions are amenable to ureteroscopic treatment but demand high patient compliance with repetitive endoscopic surveillance. It is also important to counsel patients on the rate of progression of low-grade UTUC to high-grade UTUC, which has been defined as about 15% over a mean of about 38 months of follow-up [96], but has been observed to be as high as 31% in patients with higher-volume tumors [98].

Patients with high-grade UTUC should always be counseled to consider radical NU, as long as there is a normal contralateral kidney and the patient is fit for extirpative surgery. Individuals with high-grade UTUC who do not qualify for treatment with NU can undergo ureteroscopic treatment but must be clearly made aware that the expectation is not curative but rather is palliative with the goals of avoiding persistent gross hematuria and upper urinary tract obstruction [96]. These patients may benefit from the addition of adjunctive systemic immunotherapy or chemotherapy.

Biopsy and Physical Removal of Tissue

Several endoscopic techniques for the removal of upper tract urothelial carcinoma have been described, and these include mechanical removal, electrosurgical resection, fulguration, and laser ablative therapies. Endoscopic approaches for lesions localized in the renal collecting system include retrograde (ureteroscopic) and antegrade (percutaneous). Choice of treatment is again influenced by lesion size, location, and the presence of multifocality. Historically, the 12-Fr uretero-resectoscope was employed to treat ureteral tumors, resecting them with a small loop electrode. The only practical indication for this instrument is large-volume distal ureteral lesions in patients who have been pre-stented such that the ureter can accept this

Table 6.3 Low risk and High risk patient's characteristics. Adapted from Roupret et al. [93]

Low risk	High risk
Tumor less than 2 cm	Tumor greater than 2 cm
Unifocal disease	Multifocal disease
Low-grade cytology/biopsy	High-grade cytology/biopsy
Non-invasive disease by imaging	Hydronephrosis or invasive disease by imaging or prior cystectomy

large instrument. Care must be taken not to resect circumferentially; rather staged therapy allowing for ureteral healing will help minimize subsequent stricture disease. Ureteral resectoscopes are generally not available for contemporary use, but lasers with ablative capabilities can be effective for these tumors.

Mechanical removal of tumor utilizes the same previously described techniques used for ureteroscopic biopsy of tumor. Ureteroscopic access should be obtained using a "no-touch" technique to assist in visually differentiating low-grade disease or carcinoma in situ from guidewire trauma [99]. As such, ureteral access sheaths are largely unnecessary, though possibly useful in larger resections after ensuring that no ureteral tumors are present, prior to sheath placement. While intuitively appealing, there is no evidence that ureteral access sheaths reduce the incidence of secondary tumors of the bladder. The approach of diagnostic ureteroscopy and biopsy techniques for UTUC are described in detail in section "Diagnosis of Upper Tract Urothelial Carcinoma".

In section "Enhanced Endoscopic Imaging Techniques for Upper Tract Urothelial Carcinoma" the various optical enhancers available to improve the sensitivity of diagnostic ureteroscopy are presented. A key point is the marked improvement with digital actively deflectable flexible ureteroscopes, with increased sensitivity from 3000- to 10,000-pixel power for the traditional fiberoptic to over 200,000 for the newest digital imagers. A variety of digital enhancers are available with the reusable digital platforms, including narrow-band imaging. Certain enhancers drop out specific spectrum colors, which allow for easier visualization of aberrant vascularity, a trademark of papillary urothelial carcinoma. These technologies are in their infancy, and improvements with regard to defining flat lesions are areas of current research.

Energy Sources Applied for Ureteroscopic Tumor Ablation

Variables that are considered when crafting a treatment plan, beyond tumor grade, include location, multifocality, volume, and vascularity. A spectrum of energy sources, such as lasers and electrocautery, should be available such that intraoperatively encountered variables can be addressed in real time rather than in stages. From a technical standpoint, the operative treatment goal is to eliminate all luminal neoplasm, in as few operative stages as possible, while minimizing the future risk of ureteral or intrarenal stricture. Not surprisingly, maintaining adequate visualization and the ability to ureteroscopically reach all lesions are the operative challenges, which must be met by the advanced ureteroscopist. Understanding the nuances and limitations of both the ureteroscope and ablative energy source is crucial to successful outcomes [68]. Laser light is the most frequent energy source utilized for the ureteroscopic treatment of urothelial lesions. Electrocautery employing the smallest diameter probes also serves a supportive role. The endourologist must be keenly aware of the effects and depth of penetration of the energy sources used and the limitations of each.

Electrocautery was the first available ablative modality for UTUC. This modality serves a secondary role in tumor treatment today, mostly when laser fibers cannot reach a luminal tumor. Flexible Bugbee electrodes from 1.9 to 3.0 F (Greenwald and Olympus Inc.) are the least likely to inhibit the deflectability of ureteroscopes and are useful in peripheral and very dependent calyces. The irrigant required must allow for conduction of current, and so sorbitol, glycine, or small aliquots of sterile water are required. A limitation is that even with low-power setting (10 W), electrocautery tends to char tumor peripherally, often with viable remnants centrally. Once charred other energy sources can be ineffective, and so electrocautery tends to be used toward the end of ureteroscopic treatment to address remaining peripheral tumors, which might be otherwise inaccessible to the relatively stiff laser fibers, known to partially inhibit flexible ureteroscope deflection. In addition, while laser energy is effective only when delivered with a directly forward approach relative to the laser fiber tip, electrocautery applies energy with lateral contact from the electrode. Therefore the Bugbee can be placed adjacent to tumors, which would otherwise be difficult to reach with a direct approach. A key planning therapy, particularly in the ureter, is defining whether the lesion is circumferential. Electrocautery and certain laser energies, for example, Nd:YAG (neodymium) should not be employed circumferentially since this is associated with higher postoperative rates of ureteral stenosis. The same principle applies to infundibula in the intrarenal collecting system.

Laser Energy Techniques

Laser energy can be delivered through low-water-density quartz fibers passed through the working channel of actively deflectable, flexible ureteroscopes. It is used to coagulate and/or ablate urothelial lesions. These fibers range from less than 200 to 400 μm [87]. Larger-diameter laser fibers inhibit ureteroscope deflectability and minimize the volume of cooling sterile saline irrigant that can pass through the single working channel. The first lasers utilized for UTUC therapy were neodymium:YAG (Nd:YAG) and the holmium:YAG. The neodymium:YAG laser was first used for the cystoscopic treatment of bladder tumors. Initial application of this laser to upper tract urothelial carcinoma was performed using open surgical techniques to ablate urothelial carcinoma in the renal pelvis and intrarenal collecting system [100]. The technique was subsequently applied ureteroscopically [101] and was shown to ablate upper tract tumors with a lower rate of ureteral stricture formation than electrocoagulation [102].

The operating surgeon must remain mindful that the neodymium:YAG laser has a significant depth of penetration, which requires careful control. Deep penetration into the surrounding tissue can be achieved after several seconds of exposure. This can be useful for invasive intrarenal lesions to obtain deeper coagulation. To help minimize adjacent tissue thermal damage, the fiber tip is non-contact and moved across the lesion avoiding prolonged exposure. Characteristic blanching is a useful endpoint and should occur within seconds at a continuous setting of 20–30 watts.

The indication is basically for intrarenal lesions, while the application in the ureter is controversial and has been associated with higher stricture rates.

The holmium:YAG laser is the most widely employed for soft tissue application in the upper urinary tract. This is a solid-state pulsed laser that can both fragment calculi and coagulate and ablate tissue. The application of holmium laser energy for upper urinary tract tumor therapy was first reported by two groups, Erhard and Bagley as well as Razvi and Denstedt, in 1995 [103, 104]. Pulsatile delivery and low overall power efficiently cleared low-grade papillary lesions but often was associated with obscuring hematuria. At a wavelength of 2100 nm, this device produces a fiber-tip vaporization bubble, which has a localized effect when applied in saline irrigant. The fiber effect is thus a near-contact laser. Variables including delivered energy, frequency of pulsation, and pulse width can all be applied to obtain a desired tissue effect. Lower settings are better for ablation and to minimize hematuria, starting at 0.6 joules and 5–10 hertz and adjusting accordingly thereafter. Pulse width can be widened to improve coagulation, while tight pulse width and higher frequency are preferred when incising or ablating tissue.

Treated tissue or stone for that matter is disrupted with pulsatile holmium laser energy, producing a cloud of debris. Irrigation is required to clear the optical field of vision. Control of bleeding can be achieved by applying lower energy settings and increased pulse duration and diffusing the laser light spot focus by increasing the distance between the fiber tip and target [105]. The synergistic combination of Nd:YAG applied to devascularize lesions and then holmium as a resecting wavelength applied through the same optical fiber in a stepwise manner is a common technique, which increases the efficiency of tumor therapy (Fig. 6.6).

The newest laser energies employed for tumor therapy include 1470 nm/Raman lasers and the thulium:YAG laser which employs a wavelength of 2013 nm. Both are delivered through the same small caliber fibers employed for ND and holmium:YAG. Unlike Nd:YAG, both do not require a chromophobe to obtain a tissue effect. The 1470 nm/Raman laser can be delivered in a pulsatile or CW mode and is an efficient coagulator and simultaneous ablator of the tissue. The hemostatic effect is superior to holmium, while the surrounding tissue's thermal effect is within a few millimeters of the fiber tip and thus much safer and more precise than Nd:YAG. Thulium:YAG is employed as a tumor resector, delivered in a pulsatile fashion similar to holmium. Recent laser advances allow for the simultaneous delivery of both wavelengths through the same optical fiber (Jena Laser Systems, Germany), thus coagulating and resecting in a clear field with minimal bleeding, maximizing treatment efficiency with minimal debris cloud [106, 107].

Ureteroscopic Treatment of Large Intrarenal Lesions

Large urothelial lesions (i.e., > 2.5 cm), either within the intrarenal collecting system or ureter and those that are circumferential in the ureter are often treated in stages allowing for adjacent tissue healing and sloughing of coagulated tumor.

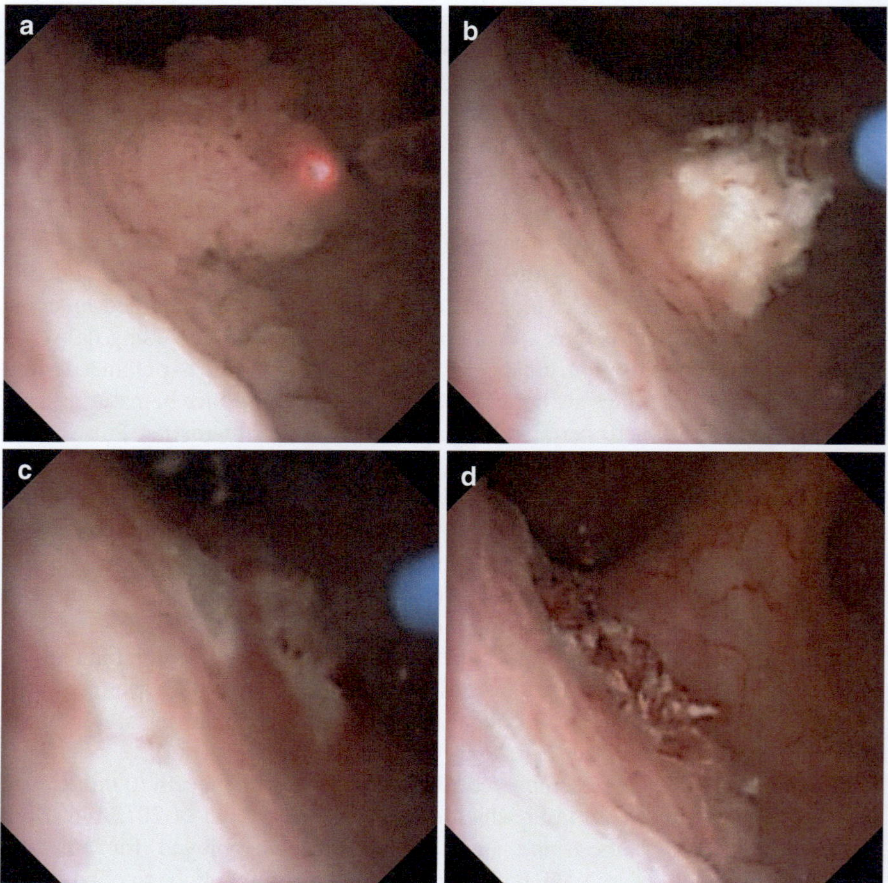

Fig. 6.6 (**a**) Digital ureteroscopic view of a papillary upper urinary tract lesion targeted for laser ablation. (**b**) Neodymium (Nd:YAG) laser coagulates the tumor resulting in a blanched, devascularized appearance (**c**) Holmium laser then ablates the coagulated tissue in a virtually bloodless field. (**d**) Successful tumor resection down to the base of the collecting system surface with excellent hemostasis

Treating a section of the ureteral wall, for example, and then allowing a period of healing with re-epithelialization before completing treatment minimize the risk of stricture associated with thermal energy applied in this way [98]. First-stage ureteroscopic treatment requires interval ureteral stenting, with the patient returning after a period of interval healing (i.e., 3–6 weeks) for additional treatment. Second-look ureteroscopy is also employed after extensive and/or multifocal tumor therapy to ensure complete resection and when visualization is compromised during the initial intervention due to associated hematuria, for example, where the optical field is suboptimal. Using this approach, Villa et al. have demonstrated residual tumor present in 51.2% of UTUC cases treated ureteroscopically with holmium in a series of 41 patients with mean index tumor size of 13 mm [108].

For sizable intrarenal lesions that are particularly vascular, Nd:YAG laser energy can be employed to devascularize the lesion, with holmium laser energy employed immediately thereafter as a resecting wavelength. More recently 1470 nm/Raman laser and thulium has been employed with more efficient clearance of tumor and less associated hematuria. Applying these two laser wavelengths simultaneously can efficiently remove a sizeable lesion. A ureteral stent is regularly placed after the initial treatment, maintaining drainage while tumor sloughs, and edema from thermal therapy resolve. Employing the staged methodology can facilitate clearance of sizable low-grade lesions. Other relative indications for ureteral stenting post-ureteroscopic treatment include a solitary renal unit, tumor multifocality, and tumor that is located in the intra-mural ureter.

At times, extensive low-grade tumors may be found carpeting large surface areas of the upper tract urothelium. These may be the only lesion in the system or may be associated with other large low-grade or even high-grade tumors. It is essentially impossible to aim a laser at each and coagulate or ablate all of them individually. They can be removed effectively by non-contact ablation. The holmium laser is set at a higher energy (1–2 J) and frequency (20–30 hertz) and activated slightly off the surface. The laser is painted over the tumor-bearing area, and the lesions can be seen to disappear without bleeding.

Percutaneous/Antegrade Nephroscopic Approaches

The presentation of antegrade nephroscopic and ureteroscopic therapy is for completeness. The authors prefer a closed system when treating urothelial tumors endoscopically, and by definition percutaneous access has the inherent risk of track seeding and so is employed in very select clinical presentations. Allowing a percutaneous tract to mature before performing endoscopic resection while placing the access in a tumor-free calyx may minimize tract seeding [109].

Indications for an antegrade percutaneous endoscopic treatment include inability to access the collecting system in a retrograde fashion based on prior reconstruction (e.g., urinary diversion, neobladder, etc.) of lower urinary tract pathology prohibiting retrograde access (e.g., concurrent malignancies, prior radiotherapy, severely tortuous ureter) [110]. While historically antegrade endoscopic access was employed for dependent lower pole lesions, improved flexible ureteroscope design with greater mechanical deflectability has basically removed this indication except in very select cases [110–112].

Instrumentation for antegrade endoscopic tumor therapy is similar to retrograde energy sources, with the caveat that larger endoscopes and instrumentation and more irrigant can be employed through the operative sheath. Care must be taken to minimize tissue trauma and thermal effects while treating lesions in the kidney. This is underscored by the higher transfusion rate associated with this intervention.

Outcomes and Recurrence

As UTUC is relatively uncommon, outcome data close to four decades of uretero-scopic treatment of urothelial cancer consists mostly of retrospective non-randomized studies [89, 90, 111]. In 2012, Grasso et al. published a non-randomized, prospectively accrued cohort with a 15-year follow-up of UTUC cases [96]. These results in 2018 were further analyzed with a 20-year follow-up. It illustrates that patients who were treated ureteroscopically for low-grade UTUC had cancer-specific survival outcomes similar to patients treated with radical nephroureterec-tomy (Fig. 6.7).

It was a landmark study validating the change in management of low-grade UTUC using endoscopic techniques. In this study, Grasso et al. defined 2-, 5-, and 10-year cancer-specific survival rates in the low-grade group were 97%, 87%, and 78%, respectively (Fig. 6.7).

On further analysis of those patients treated ureteroscopically with low-grade UTUC, 77% had a recurrence, with the majority being small lesions cleared endo-scopically. It is important to note that over time 15.2% of these patients progressed in grade and required additional therapies (Table 6.4).

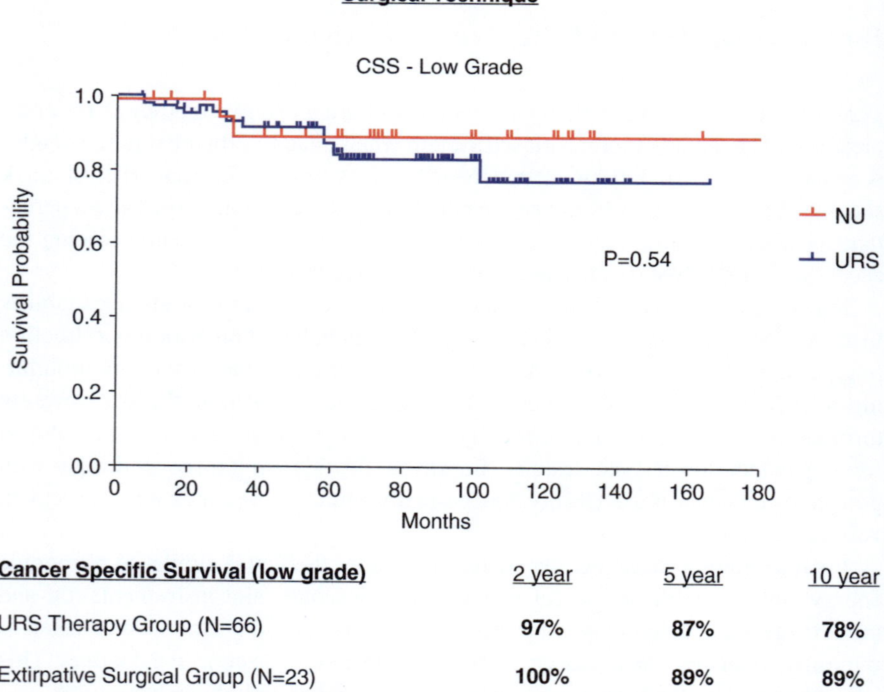

Cancer Specific Survival (low grade)	2 year	5 year	10 year
URS Therapy Group (N=66)	97%	87%	78%
Extirpative Surgical Group (N=23)	100%	89%	89%

Fig. 6.7 Comparison of survival in LG UTUC undergoing ureteroscopy or nephrectomy

Table 6.4 Outcome of ureteroscopy in the low-grade and high-grade UTUC cases

	Gr1 (therapeutic URS)	Gr2 (palliative URS)
No. of patients, n	66	14
Upper tract recurrence	51	14
Progression		
Progression to high grade	10 (15%)	NA
Subsequent nephroureterectomy	11	4
Survival		
Median OS (months)	126.8	29.2
Cancer-related deaths	8	12

Adapted from Grasso et al. [96]

In this study, patients were divided into three groups: Group 1, low-grade treated ureteroscopically; Group 2, high-grade ureteroscopic (palliative), and Group 3, radical nephroureterectomy. Further subgroup survival analysis was performed (Fig. 6.8).

Size, and thus tumor volume, appears to be a prognosticator in patients with low-grade UTUC. Hubosky and Bagley's report on treating large (>2 cm) low-grade lesions ureteroscopically reviewed 80 patients with a mean tumor diameter of 3 cm and mean follow-up of 43.6 months [98]. Ipsilateral recurrence was 90%, while progression in grade on follow-up was higher at 31.7%, with progression noted at a median of 26.3 months. OS was 75%, while CSS was 84% at 5 years. Therefore, grade progression is clearly higher in patients with larger lesions, a finding that needs to be discussed with patients when deciding whether to continue with nephron-sparing treatment or consider NU, depending on the unique individual circumstances.

Alternatively, in those with high-grade disease treated ureteroscopically, this tends to be palliative. In Grasso's series local control was obtained in the majority, while all progressed in stage and succumb to metastatic disease during follow-up [96]. The median survival of patients in this group was 29.2 months, with a 2-year survival rate of 54%. Given the difference in these outcomes between low- and high-grade diseases, it was not surprising that tumor grade was by far the most significant predictor of overall and cancer-specific survival in those patients presenting with upper tract malignancies regardless of surgical intervention (Fig. 6.9). It is in this group that adjuvant chemotherapy and immunotherapy, employing both check point and kinase inhibitors, are being explored.

In general, local recurrence rates and cancer-specific survival are clearly influenced most importantly by tumor grade and volume. In a meta-analysis examining over 20 ureteroscopic series of UTUC treatment involving 736 patients, Cutress et al. reported local ipsilateral upper tract recurrence rates of 52–54% for low- to intermediate-grade tumors and 76% for high-grade tumors with follow-up between 14 and 73 months [111]. The pooled disease-specific mortality was observed to be 9%. In larger, more contemporary series with longer follow-up (range 44–54 months), local recurrence rates range from 68% to 91% with cancer-specific survival rates of

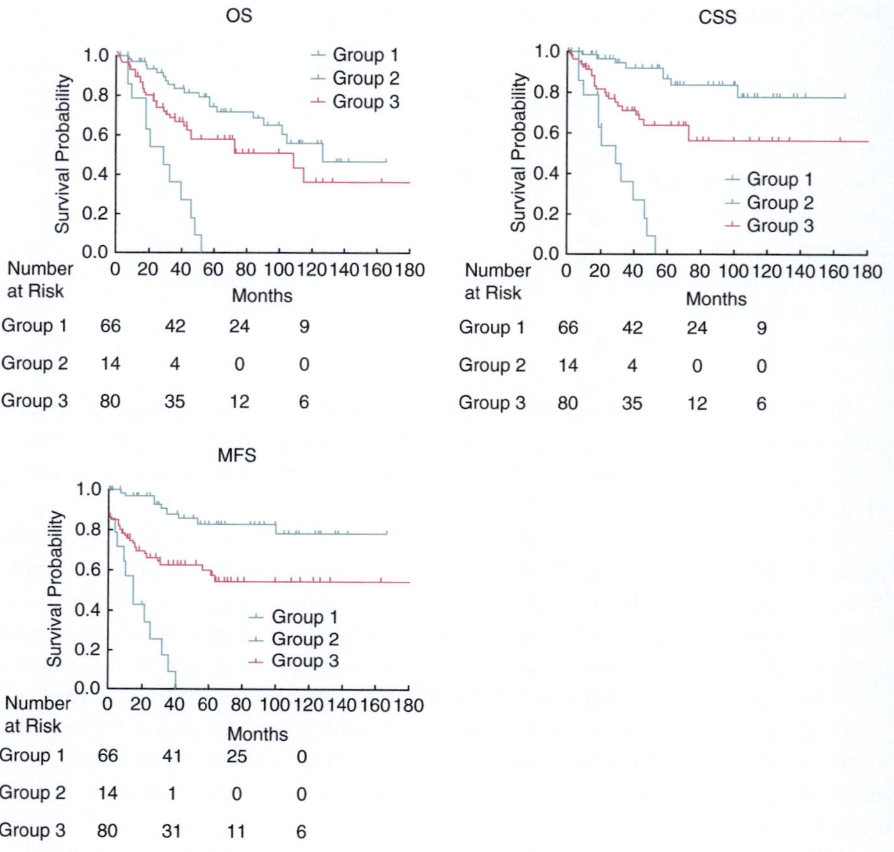

Fig. 6.8 Ureteroscopic and extirpative treatment of upper urinary tract urothelial carcinoma: a 15-year comprehensive review of 160 consecutive patients. Overall survival (OS), cancer-specific survival (CSS), and metastasis-free survival (MFS). (BJU International 110(11):1618–26, First published: 28 March 2012, DOI: (10.1111/j.1464-410X.2012.11066.x)

84–95% [95–98]. In patients with initial low-grade index lesions, progression to high-grade disease can be expected in 15% over time [96] and up to 30% in those presenting with tumor size greater than 2 cm [98]. Careful surveillance is absolutely mandatory, and second-stage evaluations are recommended within 6–8 weeks to treat residual luminal tumor, which has been reported in up to 51.2% following a first-stage procedure [108]. Undergrading of UTUC is also a legitimate concern, and diagnostic accuracy of ureteroscopic biopsy varies considerably in the literature [36, 46, 49, 50]. This is explained not only by various grading systems for UTUC used over time but also by inter-observer variations among cytopathologists and the fact that grade heterogeneity exists in UTUC much like it does in urothelial carcinoma of the bladder [113]. For these reasons, site-specific cytologies [114] should

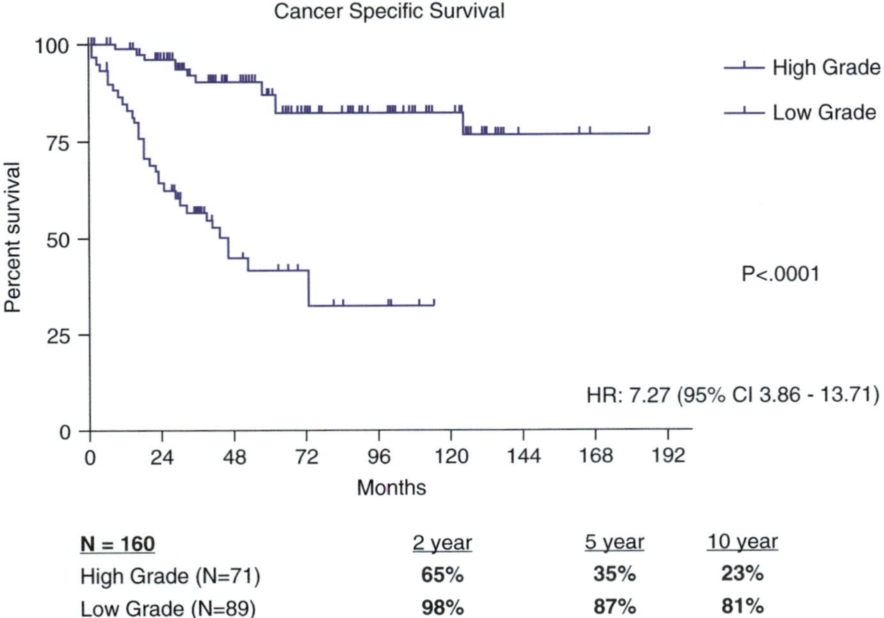

Fig. 6.9 Comparison of survival between high-grade and low-grade UTUC

always be obtained along with biopsies of any local recurrence. Yearly cross-sectional imaging should be obtained in all patients undergoing ureteroscopic treatment for UTUC, as there have been reports of patients developing locally advanced and/or metastatic disease even with low-grade index lesions and good local endoscopic control of luminal tumor [96, 115].

Surveillance cystoscopy is also essential in UTUC patients since development of urothelial carcinoma of the bladder is very common. Individuals with new UTUC and no prior history of bladder cancer have been shown to present with simultaneous bladder tumors 17% of the time [116]. In ureteroscopic series of patients treated for UTUC without prior bladder tumors, the eventual evolution of bladder cancer was noted in 33–34% [117, 118]. It has been noted that 80–90% of bladder tumors in cases such as this will develop within the first 2 years of UTUC diagnosis and will be non-muscle invasive in 88–95% [119, 120]. A series of UTUC patients with extended follow-up show higher rates of eventual bladder tumor development at 42–61% with follow-up of 52–54 months [95, 96]. Risk factors for intravesical recurrence in UTUC patients undergoing NU include tumor multifocality, pathologic staging, and overall tumor size [121] as well as a history of immunosuppression [122]. To help minimize the risk of bladder recurrence, the role of intravesical chemotherapy after diagnostic ureteroscopy is appealing. O'Brien et al. have shown a decrease in bladder tumor development in bladder cancer-naïve UTUC patients undergoing NU and receiving a postoperative single dose of intravesical mitomycin versus those patient who did not. Within the first 12 months of NU, bladder tumor development was 16% in those receiving mitomycin versus 27% in those who did not [123].

Complications

Initial concerns of tumor dissemination following ureteroscopic treatment of UTUC have been alleviated by reported clinical experience. Kulp and Bagley demonstrated no evidence of free tumor cells in the vascular or lymphatic spaces within the submucosal space or renal parenchyma of NU specimens following ureteroscopic evaluation and laser ablation of 13 consecutive patients treated for UTUC [124]. One patient had locally advanced disease, but this was suspected on pre-ureteroscopic imaging. No patient was found to have metastatic disease in follow-up. Later in a larger series of 96 patients undergoing NU for UTUC of which 48 patients had ureteroscopic biopsy and 48 did not, it was noted that there was no difference in rates of metastatic disease (12.6% versus 18.8%) or cancer-specific death (10.4% both groups) [125]. Thus, experiences such as these have shown us over time that the mere performance of ureteroscopy fails to demonstrate a negative impact on long-term or disease-specific survival in patients with UTUC.

The most common complication of ureteroscopic treatment for UTUC is ureteral stricture formation. A recent review of the literature examined 38 published series representing the clinical experience of over 1100 patients and defined a median stricture rate among these series of 10% [126]. This is considerably higher compared to the rates of ureteral stricture formation in patients undergoing ureteroscopy for stone treatment, which is reliably under 1% [127, 128]. Reasons for the higher stricture rate in UTUC patients include primary ureteral tumor location, choice of ablative energy source, need for repetitive surveillance procedures, and potential use of intraluminal chemotherapies. In Lenihan's review of the literature, the highest reported rate of stent-dependent ureteral stricture was 27% (4/15 renal units) [129]. This was a series of UTUC patients with Lynch syndrome, a unique cohort of individuals with upper tract disease in which tumors are more commonly found in the ureter compared to the intrarenal collecting system [130]. Furthermore, these patients often have multiple pelvic malignancies including colorectal and endometrial carcinomas, necessitating frequent pelvic surgery and/or external beam radiation treatment, both potential promoters of ureteral ischemia. Given the potential for metachronous UTUC development in these patients, conservative ureteroscopic treatment is encouraged whenever clinically possible [131]. Thus, Lynch syndrome patients with UTUC, not surprisingly, offer a significant clinical challenge in terms of ureteral stricture development (Fig. 6.10).

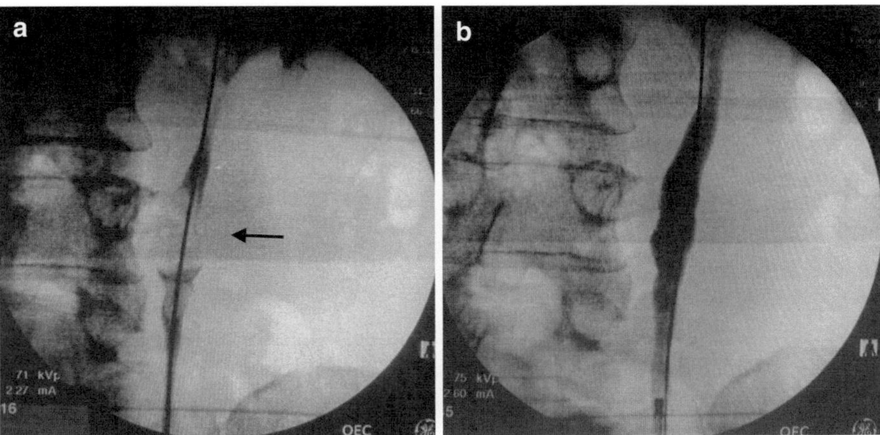

Fig. 6.10 (**a**) Retrograde pyelogram demonstrating long, multi-focal, broad-based proximal ureteral tumor (arrow) in a female patient with Lynch syndrome, history of hysterectomy, and pelvic radiation treatment for endometrial carcinoma. (**b**) Ureteroscopic resection of tumor results in complete resolution of filling defect on retrograde pyelogram. Unfortunately, but not surprisingly, this patient evolved a stent-dependent ureteral stricture but has no evidence of locally advanced or metastatic disease at the time of publication

Conclusion

Ureteroscopic tumor ablation of UTUC is the prime nephron-sparing treatment modality for well-selected, low-risk patients with equivalent cancer-specific survival relative to radical NU. Local ipsilateral upper tract recurrences are common, as are recurrent bladder lesions, and although usually very amenable to further ablative treatment mandate strict lifetime commitment to surveillance. With increasing experience, larger luminal lesions are able to be treated but can manifest with higher rates of local recurrence and grade progression. The ultimate treatment choice for UTUC must consider tumor grade, tumor size/volume, best estimate of clinical stage, baseline renal function, condition of the contralateral renal unit, and fitness for nephroureterectomy.

Adjuvant Treatment for Upper Tract Urothelial Carcinoma: Topical and Systemic

Michael Grasso III, Joseph K. Izes, and Anna W. Komorowski

Adjuvant Topical Treatment

Introduction

In bladder cancer, intravesical installation of topical therapy is well established as an adjuvant therapy for patients with high-risk superficial disease, multifocal disease, and/or carcinoma in situ. These topical treatments have been extended to patients with upper tract urothelial cancer (UTUC). As in treatment of urothelial bladder cancers, several agents including Bacillus Calmette-Guérin (BCG), alpha interferon, mitomycin C, gemcitabine, and valrubicin have been employed topically for UTUC to decrease the rates of recurrence and progression post-endoscopic therapy.

Delivery Routes

The main challenge in instillation of topical therapies into the upper tract is ensuring adequate urothelial contact time/exposure due to lack of storage organ similar to bladder due to the constant flow of urine. The three main delivery methods include [132–134]:

1. Antegrade via a small caliber pigtail nephrostomy catheter.
2. Retrograde via single-pigtail ureteral catheter secured to a Foley bladder drainage catheter.
3. Intravesical instillation with vesico-ureteral reflux via a double- pigtail stent.

Topical agents should be administered under low pressure, preferably with gravity drip. With all the three techniques, intrarenal pressures must be kept low, to prevent pyelovenous or pyelolymphatic back flow. One also must be mindful of the renal pelvic volume, in an undilated system, which can vary between 5 and 15 mL. A variation of the retrograde ureteral catheter is that of Patel and Fuchs, who described placement of a 5Fr single-pigtail catheter by way of a suprapubic route for instillation of topical BCG, therefore bypassing the urethra [135].

Instillation Technique

The application of topical agents in the upper urinary tract requires an externally draining catheter. A single-pigtail ureteral stent of relatively small diameter, most commonly 6 French, is employed which is secured to a bladder drainage catheter during treatment. This ureteral stent can be positioned post-ureteroscopic treatment into the upper urinary tract with the proximal pigtail precisely coiled in a predetermined segment of the intrarenal collecting system, preventing inadvertent instillation into the tissue. By contrast, if an open-ended catheter is placed, the tip may inadvertently penetrate the tissue, increasing the risk of absorption with significant systemic risk. For this reason, as a routine, the pigtail catheter's position should be verified with contrast fluoroscopically before instillation of the topical agent.

A small aliquot of contrast (e.g., 2 to 10 cc based on the volume of the intrarenal collecting system) is employed through the catheter with simultaneous real-time fluoroscopic imaging to obtain a retrograde ureteropyelogram. If significant extravasation is noted at the end of the ureteroscopic procedure during this maneuver, then the application of the topical chemotherapy should be delayed, and the catheter set to gravity until the upper urinary tract seals.

Reflux based on an indwelling ureteral stent failed to facilitate upper tract urothelium coverage with the desired agent in at least 50% of renal units in a porcine model, underscoring the lack of reliability of that technique [136]. Percutaneous nephrostomy application has the inherently greater risk of bleeding and infection associated with initial placement and has the theoretical risk of tract seeding. Allowing the percutaneous tract to mature before infusion is recommended to minimize tissue absorption and to create a closed system.

In an ex vivo porcine model, Pollard et al. measured the percentage of upper tract urothelium stained by continuous infusion over 1 hour of indigo carmine solution via the three methods [137]. An open-ended ureteral catheter resulted in 83.6% of surface area stained versus 65.2% and 66.2% for the nephrostomy and refluxing double-pigtail stent, respectively.

BCG typically requires a course of treatment, mandating either a long-term nephrostomy or repeated insertion of a retrograde catheter or Patel and Fuchs' technique described above [135]. On the other hand, mitomycin C is employed as a single dose immediately after ureteroscopic ablation or on a fixed schedule (e.g., for treatment of CIS) applied via a single-pigtail ureteral catheter. Regardless of the route of administration, dwell time, that is, the duration of contact between active agent and urothelium, is a limiting factor even with slow infusion.

Mitomycin C Treatment

Mitomycin C (MMC) is an alkylating agent, which is used to prevent recurrence of bladder cancer. MMC has been employed most commonly as an adjuvant therapy after ureteroscopic resection of an upper urinary tract urothelial tumor. The application is applied through a single-pigtail stent, infused slowly to allow for prolonged urothelial contact time. It has been used in the adjuvant setting after endoscopic treatment of UTUC at a dose of 40 mg. Martinez-Pineiro et al. treated 14 renal units and demonstrated a recurrence rate of 14% [138]. Keeley and Bagley treated 21 renal units with MMC after endoscopic treatment due to high-risk features including residual luminal tumor (13 cases), multifocal lesions (10 cases), high-grade tumor (3 cases), or history of rapid recurrence after previous endoscopic treatment (2 cases). A complete response was seen in 45% (9/19 cases) and partial response in 37% (7/19 cases) [139]. Aboumarzouk et al. presented 19 patients treated in a retrograde fashion with 65% without recurrence at 20 months, while 15% presented with ureteral stricture disease [140].

Table 6.5 presents various retrospective studies where topical MMC instillation was employed in UTUC (Table 6.5). A recent retrospective review of patients who underwent complete ureteroscopic resection of papillary disease and then received a course of induction therapy via ureteral catheter or percutaneous nephrostomy with mitomycin C showed a 3-year recurrence-free, progression-free, and overall survival rate of 60%, 80%, and 76%, respectively [141]. Of note, 9 of 27 patients in

Table 6.5 Various retrospective trials evaluating role of MMC in UTUC

Author	Year published	Journal	Retrograde or percutaneous	Agent used	Patients (tumors)	Grade/stage	Recurrence rate (%)	Nephroureterectomy (NU) or progression (P)	F/U months (median)
Metcalfe M [141]	2017	*J Endourol*	Retrograde (19) Precut (9)	MMC	27 (28)	HG (25%) LG (75%)	39	NU (5/28) P 5/28	19 m
Gallioli A [142]	2020	*J Endourol*	Retrograde Single J catheter (19) Stent with urethral catheter and bladder instillation (6)	MMC	25 (25)	HG (36%) LG (52%) Not evaluable 12 (%)	32	NU 2/25 P 3/25	18 m
Balasubramaniam [143]	2018	*World J Urol*	Retrograde (8) Nephrostomy (10)	BCG 10 MMC 8	18 (18)	HG 11 LG 7	50	P 3/18 NU 5/18	36.5 m
Keeley [139]	1997	*J Urol*	Retrograde 1–3 days after treatment	MMC (40MG)	19 (21)	G1–G5 G1/G2–G2 G2–G8 G3–G4	54	NU 4/19 P-0	30 m
Easthem [144]	1993	*J Urol*	Percutaneous	MMC (40 MG)	7	G2/G3,ta-3 G2/G3, T1–T3 CIS-1	28.5	Cystectomy-1/7	1–12 m
Goel [145]	2003	*J Urol*	Retrograde or percutaneous	MMC (40 MG)/ epirubicin (50 MG)	24	LG-15 HG-5 SCC-2	50	NU-10 (14) P-2 (8)	64 m
Grasso M			Retrograde	MMC (40MG)	19 (20)	G1/G2 ta-16 G3Ta-2 (1 also with CIS) G3T1–2	35	NU-1 (5) Cystectomy-1(5) P-0	24

this series experienced an intervention-related adverse outcome, but there was no systemic toxicity seen. Gallioli et al. reported an almost 50% reduction in rates of recurrence following a single, immediate postoperative dose of upper urinary tract mitomycin C after therapeutic ureteroscopy for complete endoscopic removal of low-grade lesions [142]. The mean time to local urothelial recurrence in those treated with the single postoperative dose of MMC was 28.8 months compared to 18.8 months in those who did not receive MMC. Balasubramanian et al. demonstrated some success with salvage topical therapy using a variety of agents [143]. In this small study with most patients having a contraindication to NU, there was a 50% overall response rate to second-line treatment. It was observed that 62% (8/13) of patients with clinical Ta to T1 disease responded compared to only 20% (1/5) of patients with upper tract CIS showing a response [143]. Therefore, within the limits of this small study, second-stage topical therapies may serve a palliative role in those with recurrent disease unable to tolerate NU, although those with recurrent upper tract CIS are less likely to benefit.

Complications and side effects MMC is generally well tolerated. Fatal pneumonia has been reported rarely due to agranulocytosis following MMC extravasation [138]. Hence, retrograde pyelogram should be performed after catheter placement to ensure proper positioning without extravasation. Both ureteral stricture and infundibular stenosis have been reported with topical MMC application and may be a product of prolonged contact time [146].

Mitomycin Gel Topical Therapy

The FDA recently approved a sustained release formulation of mitomycin C based on a proprietary thermal-sensitive hydrogel technology for low-grade upper tract urothelial cancer. Marketed as "Jelmyto," this preparation is liquid at cold temperatures and becomes a gel at body temperature. Mitomycin-containing reverse thermal gel (M-CRTG) is slowly dissolved by urine and provides 4–6 hours of contact exposure of the urothelium to mitomycin C when administered through a ureteral catheter (Fig. 6.11). In a porcine model-based study, it was found to be safe with no evidence of sepsis, myelosuppression, or urinary obstruction [147]. In a recent single-arm phase 3 trial, patients with LG UTUC across 24 different centers in the USA and Israel had the agent instilled for chemoablation of luminal index lesions measuring between 5 and 15 mm, with 6 weekly instillations of the gel. Out of 71 patients, who received at least one dose of the gel, 42 (59%) had a complete response at initial primary evaluation performed at 4–6 weeks after completion of therapy (Fig. 6.12) [148]. An important secondary endpoint was durability of response in those patients who achieved initial complete response. At the time of publication, only 20 patients were available for 12-month post-treatment assessment, and 14 (70%) demonstrated no local recurrence. The study lacked a control group. In addition there was a high rate of adverse events: 85% of patients have at least one reported adverse event, and 37% had at least one serious adverse event. The most common adverse events included ureteral stenosis (44%), UTI (32%), and

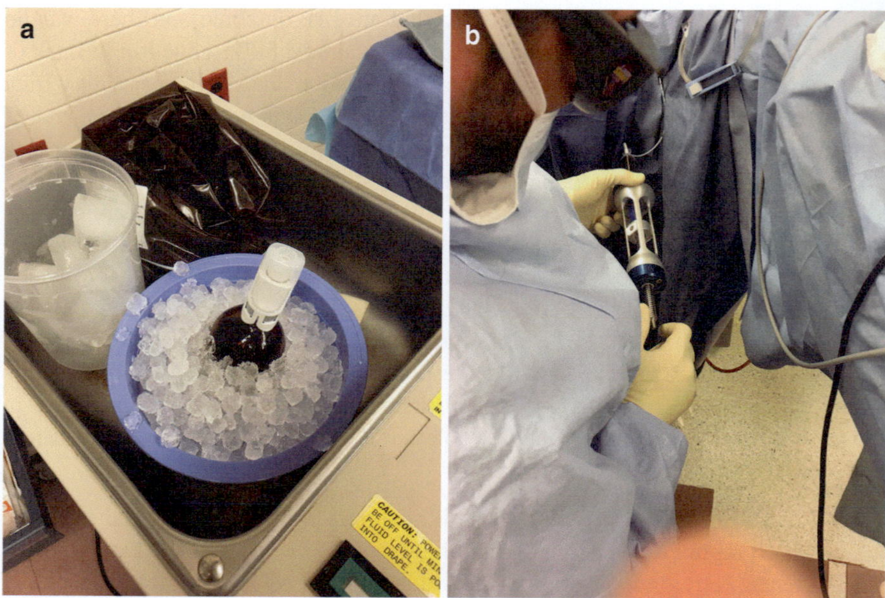

Fig. 6.11 (**a**) Mitomycin-containing reverse thermal gel is liquefied at temperatures between 35 and 46 °F; therefore it is kept at this cold temperature prior to installation. (**b**) While liquefied at cold temperatures, a carefully selected volume of the reverse thermal gel, based on previously obtained volumetric measurements of the individual patient, is administered into the luminal space of the upper urinary tract. This is performed under fluoroscopy, through a ureteral catheter measuring between 5 and 7Fr with a proprietary syringe lever especially designed to deliver the high-viscosity liquefied gel

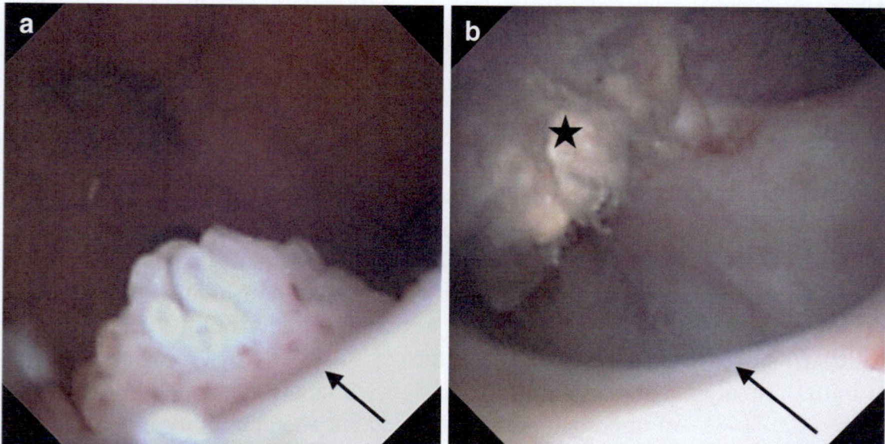

Fig. 6.12 (**a**) Low-grade upper urinary tract index lesion (black arrow) in a position difficult to ablate with flexible ureteroscopy. (**b**) Complete chemoablation of the index lesion after six treatments of mitomycin-containing reverse thermal gel, with former position marked by black arrow. Black star marks necrotic tumor formerly treated with laser coagulation (separate from index lesion)

hematuria (31%). As of publication, there were 11 (15%) patients in whom stents were considered "necessary in the long term" and two patients who underwent NU due to stent-dependent ureteral stricture. Both of these cases demonstrated no residual cancer on the final pathologic assessment. Although not mandating permanent stent dependence, some cases of what can be considered sub-clinical ureteral stenosis can make necessary ureteroscopic surveillance more technically challenging (Fig. 6.13). In summary, early clinical data show a promise for the gel as an adjuvant treatment modality, particularly for low-volume, low-grade UTUC lesions, which may be difficult to reach endoscopically. Durability of response appears to be encouraging, but longer-term data is clearly needed to understand if Jelmyto will decrease local recurrence rates compared to endoscopic ablative management alone. Potential disadvantages include increasing ureteral (and possibly intrarenal) stenosis, making future endoscopic surveillance challenging, as well as costly. For these reasons, it is very important to note that according to NCCN guidelines for low-grade UTUC lesions, mitomycin-containing reverse thermal gel is not a substitute for complete endoscopic ablation, whenever feasible [94].

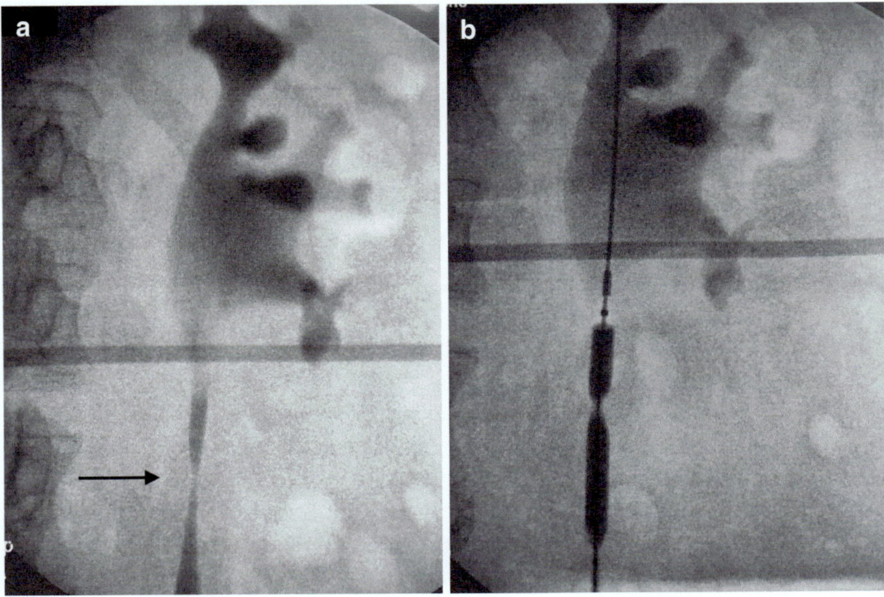

Fig. 6.13 (a) Retrograde pyelogram demonstrating a new proximal ureteral narrowing/stricture (arrow) in the same patient, 4 weeks after mitomycin-containing reverse thermal gel administration. (b) This sub-clinical ureteral stricture needed to be dilated with a balloon in order for subsequent ureteroscopic surveillance to be performed

BCG Treatment

Bacillus Calmette-Guérin (BCG) is an attenuated mycobacterium, which demonstrates an immunomodulatory effect treating urothelial cancer. For over four decades, BCG has been the standard adjuvant treatment for high-grade non-muscle-invasive bladder cancer (NMIBC) as well as the carcinoma in situ (CIS). BCG is used in the treatment of upper tract CIS as well as an adjuvant treatment of high-grade UTUC:

1. Treatment for CIS: The use of BCG to treat CIS of the upper tract has been described in a number of small retrospective series [146]. Typically, 6-weekly doses were instilled in most of the series. Kojima et al. used an 8-week course for CIS of upper tracts [149]. The change of urine cytology from positive to negative was defined as the response. The average response rate in these studies was greater than 60%. Further treatment was usually given if cytology remained positive. A subsequent recurrence rate of up to 55% is described. Hayashida et al. found a recurrence rate of 50% with mortality in all patients with recurrence [150].
2. Adjuvant treatment after the endoscopic treatment of UTUC: Various studies employing topical BCG in UTUC have defined efficacy, while small and often non-randomized retrospective analysis limits broad conclusions [146].
3. Combination of BCG and interferon-alpha topically, not unlike the in the bladder, appears to expand efficacy. In one small cohort of 11-patient series, there was a 73% initial complete response (CR), which increased to 82% after the second induction course [151].

Complications and Side Effects of BCG

The most common side effect of treatment of UTUC with BCG is fever. Twenty-five percent of patients were found to develop asymptomatic granulomatous involvement of the pelvis and of unclear clinical insignificance [152]. Hayashida et al. employed oral prophylactic isoniazid treatment halfway through BCG course to counter this risk [150].

Ureteral stenosis and hydronephrosis have been described after upper urinary tract application of BCG [152]. Granulomatous ureteric strictures have also been noted, precluding future endoscopic surveillance, ultimately requiring nephroureterectomy [152]. Rarely, fatal overwhelming sepsis can occur. Risk factors include colonization of the upper urinary tract secondary to chronic catheterization [132, 153].

Other Topical Agents

Thiotepa, an alkylating agent, has been employed topically in patients with urothelial malignancies. It has high hematopoietic toxicity as it has high systemic absorption due to small molecular weight and for those reasons is rarely administered today. The recurrence rate with thiotepa was reported as 60% in a five-patient series, compared to 12.5% for BCG [138].

The benefit of topical luminal therapy in UTUC is still incompletely understood for many reasons. Most published experience is that of retrospective series made up of a small number of patients with heterogeneic tumor characteristics including tumor grade, tumor multifocality, and completeness of endoscopic treatment prior to topical therapy. Most importantly is the lack of direct comparison to a well-matched control group undergoing effective and well-managed endoscopic treatment. In patient cohorts such as this, we know the local recurrence rate is variable but also relatively high ranging between 38 and 90% in series with long-term follow-up between 52 and 60 months [95–97, 154]. Given the potential liabilities of topical therapies, including multiple upper urinary tract manipulations, possibility of ureteral stricture or narrowing, potential for infection, and cost, this represents an area in a serious need of additional study.

Systemic Treatment for UTUC

UTUC is a relatively rare disease and represents 5–10% of all urothelial cancers with median age at presentation similar to bladder cancer. Radical nephroureterectomy is considered to be the standard of care for low- and high-risk disease. UTUC has recurrence rate reported in up to 50%, with both local disease in the lymph nodes, intraluminal including contralateral ureter, bladder, as well as metastatic disease. Patients with solitary kidney, underlying kidney insufficiency, bilateral disease, or not suitable for dialysis or transplant remains a challenge. Clinical trials of adjuvant immune and chemotherapies are few and mostly employed in advanced disease. Treatment in the UTUC is most often directly extrapolated from bladder cancer trials since there is paucity of data and subsequently guidelines. The trends in the last 20 years in the management of urothelial cancer include preoperative diagnostic endoscopies, improved surgical techniques including retroperitoneal lymph node dissection, and application of neo- and adjuvant chemotherapy that improved 2-year cancer-specific survival from 76% to 87% [155]. The upstaging from non-muscle-invasive to muscle-invasive cancer following the surgery happens in up to 30% of patients and is more frequent in UTUC than bladder cancer [156]. In the preoperative neoadjuvant settings, approximately 60% of patients are cisplatin eligible, and following nephroureterectomy due to decreased renal reserve and perioperative complications, only 15–30% is able to receive platinum-based adjuvant chemotherapy. There is a growing number of retrospective and prospective studies indicating that patients who received neoadjuvant chemotherapy had downstaging of the disease, pathologic CR, and better overall survival. MVAC (methotrexate, vinblastine, adriamycin, and cisplatin) or GC (gemcitabine, cisplatin), employed in a neoadjuvant setting for locally advanced high-grade bladder cancers (stage T2–T4a), has shown promising results in the neoadjuvant setting for UTUC, yielding ypT1 stage or less in 62% [157].

Evidence Suggesting a Role of Neoadjuvant Chemotherapy in UTUC

Significant pathologic downstaging was seen for patients who received neoadjuvant chemotherapy prior to nephroureterectomy (including a 25.4% reduction in the incidence of pT2 or higher disease and a 41.5% reduction in the incidence of pT3 or higher disease) [158]. In a series by Porten et al., neoadjuvant chemotherapy had 14% CR with significant downstaging and so emphasized the application in those with high-risk UTUC (clinical T4 disease or grossly involved lymph nodes) [159]. The 5-year rate of OS which was in those treated with neoadjuvant chemotherapy was statistically significant (80.2% vs. 57.6%, $p = 0.02$). Pathologic downstaging to pT1N0M0 in 75% and to pT0N0M0 in 38% with ddMVAC regimen of upper tract tumor was accomplished in 75% of patients with 2-year OS and DSS in 93% and 93% of patients. The response rate was better for patients in UTUC versus those with bladder cancer [160]. A multinational study underscored the safety and efficacy of neoadjuvant chemotherapy, with improved oncological outcomes in locally advanced regional node-positive UTUC [161]. EAU guidelines currently recommend perioperative chemotherapy for high-risk nonmetastatic UTUC, as there appears to be an overall and disease-free survival benefits for cisplatin-based chemotherapy [162].

Adjuvant Chemotherapy for UTUC

UTUC are chemo-sensitive similar to bladder urothelial malignancies. Retrospective studies have not shown any significant improvement in overall survival [163, 164]. A recent study has shown survival benefit of adjuvant chemotherapy versus observation after radical nephroureterectomy for pT3/T4 and/or lymph node-positive UTUC [165].

Adjuvant chemotherapy with either cisplatin or carboplatin for GFR < 50 ml/min in combination with gemcitabine day for upper tract urothelial carcinoma (POUT trial) for patient with pT2–pT4 pN0–N3 M0 and any T and N1–N3 M0 showed a significant advantage for disease-free survival with 3-year event-free survival 71% and 46%, respectively, in patient treated versus observation. There was an advantage of cisplatin versus carboplatin-based treatment, but there was definite benefit derived in patients with suboptimal renal function when carboplatin was substituted [166]. Based on the POUT study, adjuvant chemotherapy is the standard of care for patients who did not receive neoadjuvant chemotherapy and underwent nephroureterectomy.

Most chemotherapy regimens offered in the adjuvant setting are cisplatin based. A major limitation of this regimen is that not all patients are candidates for it because of comorbidities and impaired renal function after radical nephroureterectomy [86]. Chemotherapy-related toxicity, particularly nephrotoxicity due to platinum derivatives, may significantly reduce survival and quality of life in patients with postoperative renal dysfunction.

Adjuvant Check Point Inhibitors: Immunotherapy

Immune checkpoint inhibitors (CPI) are immune modulators, extending the life or T-cells and thus prolonging and enhancing the immune response to a malignancy. In recent trials for urothelial malignancies, checkpoint inhibitors have generated increased interest due to favorable objective response rate in comparison to standard chemotherapy [167, 168]. The FDA has approved the following five checkpoint inhibitors for the treatment of urothelial cancers in the first line for cisplatin-ineligible locally advanced or metastatic tumors: pembrolizumab, nivolumab, atezolizumab, durvalumab, and avelumab [169]. Only Pembrolizumab and atezolizumab have completed phase 3 trials in urothelial cancers and are approved as first line in cisplatin-ineligible tumors (KEYNOTE 045 trial and IMvigor211 trial, respectively [170–172]. Other agents have completed phase 2 trials with favorable response and adverse effect profile [173–176]. Within KEYNOTE and IMvigor trials, 27% of cases had UTUC, though no subgroup analysis was performed [170–172].

Patients with UTUC treated ureteroscopically tend to be those with low-grade disease. There are others who are either not candidates for NU or refuse extirpative surgery where systemic immunotherapy is being studied. Our preliminary experience defines increased survival, albeit not disease-free, in patients with high-grade UTUC treated endoscopically with concurrent adjuvant CPI. PDL1 tumor expression appears to correlate with response rates, with >10% expression being particularly favorable. Other potential indications for URS and adjuvant CPI include those patients with large-volume bilateral low-grade disease and those with Lynch syndrome, who are believed to be more susceptible to bilateral UTUC over time [129, 130].

Lynch Syndrome

Lynch syndrome or hereditary non-polyposis colorectal cancer (HNPCC) is an autosomal dominant multi-organ cancer syndrome with upper tract urothelial cancer ranking third after colorectal and endometrial cancer in patients diagnosed with a genetic mutation. Up to 21% of newly diagnosed patients with UTUC may have underlying HNPCC. Patients with hereditary UTUC were more likely to be females ($P = 0.047$), less likely smokers ($P = 0.012$), and no history of occupational carcinogens ($P = 0.037$) [177]. Identifying patients with Lynch syndrome not only allows to improve screening and early detection of other malignancies but also permits for effective and targeted treatment with immunotherapy in patients with UTUC thanks to increased neoantigen presentation with MSI-high tumors.

Solitary Kidney or Patients with Chronic Kidney Disease (CKD)

In patients with an anatomically solitary kidney, solitary functioning kidney, or suboptimal renal function, standard of care treatment with NU leads to dependence on hemodialysis. An estimated 7–10.9% of patients with localized upper tract urothelial cancer will not undergo definitive therapy with shorter overall survival in older age, male gender, and higher grade [178]. Approximately 40% of patients over age 70 will not meet criteria of adequate renal function to receive standard of care platinum-based chemotherapy either with ddMVAC or gemcitabine/cisplatin, and alternative regimen with carboplatin is not safe with GFR below 30 mL/min.

Patients such as these are a niche population that is not considered to be eligible for most clinical trials and are usually not identified in the guidelines. In this group of patients, a multidisciplinary approach with delineation of goals of treatment and good communication with the patient and family is needed. Combination chemotherapy in front-line treatment with gemcitabine, paclitaxel, and doxorubicin (GTA) with support of growth factors, showed response rate of 56.4% with median overall survival rate of 14.4 months and is considered a platinum-sparing alternative for patients with advanced urothelial cancer [179]. A clinical trial involving the combination of BCG and pembrolizumab in patients who are not a candidates for nephroureterectomy after endoscopic ablation of high-risk superficial upper urinary tract is ongoing (NCT03345134) (Table 6.6).

Toxicities associated with CPI are most often autoimmune in nature and require prompt treatment, most commonly with corticosteroids. Common adverse symptoms include fatigue (18.3%), pruritus (11%), and diarrhea (9.5%) and hypothyroidism [182]. Serious autoimmune effects include hypophysitis leading to Addisonian crisis, pneumonitis, colitis, myasthenia gravis, and nephritis. Steroid therapy is the mainstay of treatment for these complications [182]. Of note, combined CPI administrations appear to significantly increase the risk or autoimmune disorders.

Table 6.6 FDA-approved immunotherapeutic drugs for urothelial cancers

Agent	FDA approval	Mechanism of action	Brand	Landmark trial	Study population	Outcome
Atezolizumab	May 2016	PD L1/ IgG4	Tecentriq	IMvigor [180]	Metastatic urothelial cancers progressing after platinum-based chemotherapy	Overall survival: 11.1 months PFS: 2.1 months
Pembrolizumab	May 2017	PD L1/ IgG4	Keytruda	Keynote 052, [181] Keynote 045 [171]	Cisplatin-ineligible population and no prior chemotherapy	OS: 10.3 months PFS: 2.1 months
Nivolumab	Feb. 2017	PD L1/ IgG4	Opdivo	Checkmate 275 [173] and 032 [174]	Locally advanced or metastatic urothelial cancer which progressed after previous platinum-based CT	Confirmed objective response seen in 19.6%
Avelumab	May 2017	PD L1/ IgG4	Bavencio	Javelin [176]	Locally advanced or metastatic urothelial cancer which progressed after previous platinum-based CT	Complete or partial response was seen in 17%
Durvalumab	May 2017	PD L1/ IgG4 kappa	Imfinzi	Study 1108 [175]	Locally advanced or metastatic UC that progressed on, were eligible for, or refused CT	Objective response rate in 17.8%

Conclusion

Both topical and systemic chemotherapy and immunotherapy play a role in the treatment of UTUC. The true benefit of topical/luminal therapy is still not completely understood, especially against the experience of well-managed endoscopic treatment with strict surveillance. Systemic chemotherapy and immunotherapy may have a role in certain ureteroscopically treated UTUC patients. Such individuals include those with contraindications to NU and high-grade UTUC, those with bulky low-grade lesions difficult to clear endoscopically, and patients with mismatch repair-deficient tumors, as seen in Lynch syndrome.

Disclosures Financial Disclosure: Prof. Olivier Traxer is a consultant for Coloplast, Rocamed, Olympus, EMS, and Boston Scientific.

Funding Support: Dr. Etienne Xavier Keller is supported by a travel grant from the University Hospital Zurich and by a grant from the Kurt and Senta Herrmann Foundation. Dr. Vincent De Coninck is supported by a EUSP scholarship from the European Association of Urology and by a grant from the Belgische Vereniging voor Urologie (BVU).

References

Diagnosis of Upper Tract Urothelial Carcinoma

1. Chlapoutakis K, Theocharopoulos N, Yarmenitis S, Damilakis J. Performance of computed tomographic urography in diagnosis of upper urinary tract urothelial carcinoma, in patients presenting with hematuria: systematic review and meta-analysis. Eur J Radiol. 2010;73:334–8.
2. Albani JM, Ciaschini MW, Streem SB, Herts BR, Angermeier KW. The role of computerized tomographic urography in the initial evaluation of hematuria. J Urol. 2007;177:644–8.
3. Gray-Sears CL, Ward JF, Sears ST, Puckett MF, Kane CJ, Amling CL. Prospective comparison of computerized tomography and excretory urography in the initial evaluation of asymptomatic microhematuria. J Urol. 2002;168:2457–60.
4. Nawfel RD, Judy PF, Schleipman AR, Silverman SG. Patient radiation dose at CT urography and conventional urography. Radiology. 2004;232:126–32.
5. Van Der Molen AJ, Cowan NC, Mueller-Lisse UG, Nolte-Ernsting CCA, Takahashi S, Cohan RH. CT urography working Group of the European Society of urogenital radiology (ESUR): CT urography: definition, indications and techniques – a guideline for clinical practice. Eur Radiol. 2008;18:4–17.
6. Chen GL, El-Gabry EA, Bagley DH. Surveillance of upper urinary tract transitional cell carcinoma: the role of ureteroscopy, retrograde pyelography, cytology and urinalysis. J Urol. 2000;165:1901–4.
7. Takahashi N, Glockner JF, Hartman RP, King BF, Leibovich BC, Stanley DW, et al. Gadolinium enhanced magnetic resonance urography for upper urinary tract malignancy. J Urol. 2010;183:1330–6.
8. Tan WS, Sarpong R, Khetrapal P, Rodney S, Mostafid H, Cresswell J, et al. Can renal and bladder ultrasound replace CT urogram in patients investigated for microscopic hematuria? J Urol. 2018;200:973–80.
9. Miyake M, Owari T, Hori S, Nakai Y, Fujimoto K. Emerging biomarkers for the diagnosis and monitoring of urothelial carcinoma. Res Rep Urol. 2018;10:251–61.
10. Konety BR, Getzenberg RH. Urine based markers of urological malignancy. J Urol. 2001;165:600–11.
11. Zincke H, Aguillo JJ, Farrow GM, Utz DC, Khan AU. Significance of urinary cytology in the early detection of transitional cell cancer of the upper urinary tract. J Urol. 1976;116:781–3.
12. Renshaw AA. Comparison of ureteral washing and biopsy specimens in the community setting. Cancer Cytopathol. 2006;108:45–8.
13. Williams SK, Denton KJ, Minervini A, Oxley J, Khastigir J, Timoney AG, et al. Correlation of upper-tract cytology, retrograde pyelography, ureteroscopic appearance, and ureteroscopic biopsy with histologic examination of upper tract transitional cell carcinoma. J Endourol. 2008;22:71–6.
14. Sedlock DJ, MacLennan GT. Urine cytology in the evaluation of upper tract urothelial lesions. J Urol. 2004;172:2406.

15. Potretzke AM, Knight BA, Vetter JM, Anderson BG, Hardi AC, Bhayani SB, et al. Diagnostic utility of selective upper tract urinary cytology: a systematic review and meta-analysis of the literature. Urology. 2016;96:35–43.
16. Messer J, Shariat SF, Brien JC, Herman MP, Ng CK, Scherr DS, et al. Urinary cytology has a poor performance for predicting invasive or high-grade upper-tract urothelial carcinoma. BJU Int. 2011;108:701–5.
17. Gill WB, Lu CH, Bibbo M. Retrograde brush biopsy of the ureter and renal pelvis. Urol Clin North Am. 1979;6:573–86.
18. Blute RD Jr, Gittes RR, Gittes RF. Renal brush biopsy: survey of indications, techniques and results. J Urol. 1981;126:146.
19. Marin-Aguilera M, Mengual L, Ribal MJ, Musquera M, Ars E, Villavicencio H, et al. Utility of fluorescence in situ hybridization as a noninvasive technique in the diagnosis of upper urinary tract urothelial carcinoma. Eur Urol. 2007;51:409–15.
20. Gomella LG, Mann MJ, Cleary RC, Hubosky SG, Bagley DH, Thumar AB, et al. Fluorescence in situ hybridization (FISH) in the diagnosis of bladder and upper tract urothelial carcinoma: the largest single-institution experience to date. Can J Urol. 2017;24:8620–6.
21. Sassa N, Iwata H, Kato M, Murase Y, Seko S, Nishikimi T, Hattori R, et al. Diagnostic utility of UroVysion combined with conventional urinary cytology for urothelial carcinoma of the upper urinary tract. Am J Clin Pathol. 2019;151:469–78.
22. Chen AA, Grasso M. Is there a role for FISH in the management and surveillance of patients with upper tract transitional cell carcinoma? J Endourol. 2008;22:1371–4.
23. Konety B, Lotan Y. Urothelial bladder cancer: biomarkers for detection and screening. BJU Int. 2008;102:1234–41.
24. Xiong G, Liu J, Tang Q, Fan Y, Fang D, Yang K, et al. Prognostic and predictive value of epigenetic biomarkers and clinical factors in upper tract urothelial carcinoma. Epigenomics. 2015;7:733–44.
25. Guo RQ, Xiong GY, Yang KW, Zhang L, He SM, Gong YQ, et al. Detection of urothelial carcinoma, upper tract urothelial carcinoma, bladder carcinoma and urothelial carcinoma with gross hematuria using selected urine-DNA methylation biomarkers: a prospective, single center study. Urol Oncol. 2018;36:342e15–23.
26. Sfakianos JP, Cha EK, Iyer G, Scott SN, Zabor EC, Shah RH, et al. Genomic characterization of upper tract urothelial carcinoma. Eur Urol. 2015;68:970–7.
27. Hayashi Y, Fujita K, Matsuzaki M, Matsushita M, Kawamura N, Koh Y, et al. Diagnostic potential of TERT promoter and FGFR3 mutations in urinary cell-free DNA in upper tract urothelial carcinoma. Cancer Sci. 2019;110:1771–9.
28. Bier S, Hennenlotter J, Esser M, Mohrhardt S, Rausch S, Schwentner C et al. Performance of Urinary markers for detection of upper tract urothelial carcinoma: is upper tract urine more accurate than urine from the bladder? Dis Markers. 2018; 2018:5823870. Published 2018 Jan 30. https://doi.org/10.1155/2018/5823870
29. Lodde M, Mian C, Wiener H, Haitel A, Pycha A, Marberger M. Detection of upper urinary tract transitional cell carcinoma with ImmunoCyt: a preliminary report. Urology. 2001;58:362–6.
30. Johnson GB, Portella D, Grasso M. Advanced Ureteroscopy: wireless and Sheathless. J Endourol. 2006;20:552–5.
31. Kleinmann N, Healy KA, Hubosky SG, Margel D, Bibbo M, Bagley DH. Ureteroscopic biopsy of upper tract urothelial carcinoma: comparison of basket and forceps. J Endourol. 2013;27:1450–4.
32. Lama D, Safiullah S, Patel RM, Lee TK, Balani JP, Zhang L, et al. Multi-institutional evaluation of upper urinary tract biopsy using back loaded cup biopsy forceps, a nitinol basket, and standard cup biopsy forceps. Urology. 2018;117:89–94.
33. Breda A, Territo A, Sanguedolce F, Basile G, Subiela JD, Reyes HV, et al. Comparison of biopsy devices in upper tract urothelial carcinoma. World J Urol. 2019;39:1899–905.

34. Wason S, Seigne D, Schned R, Pais V. Ureteroscopic biopsy of upper tract urothelial carcinoma using a novel ureteroscopic biopsy forceps. Can J Urol. 2012;19(6):6560–5.
35. Holmquist M, Keebler C. A manual of cytotechnology. Chicago: American Society of Clinical Pathology; 1983. p. 335–6.
36. Keeley FX, Kulp DA, Bibbo M, McCue PA, Bagley DH. Diagnostic accuracy of ureteroscopic biopsy in upper tract transitional cell carcinoma. J Urol. 1997;157:33–7.
37. Sheridan TB, Walavalkar V, Yates JK, Owens CL, Fischer AH. Cytologic processing of ureteral microbiopsies is associated with higher sensitivity for detection of urothelial carcinoma compared with conventional biopsy processing. J Am Soc Cytopath. 2020;9:26–32.
38. Barkan GA, Tabatabai ZL, Kurtycz DF, Padmanabhan V, Souers RJ, Nayar R, et al. Practice patterns in urinary cytopathology prior to the Paris system for reporting urinary cytology. Arch Pathol Lab Med. 2020;144:172–6.
39. Mostofi FK, Sorbin LH, Torloni H. Histological typing of urinary bladder tumours, international classification of tumours, vol. 19. Geneva: World Health Organisation; 1973.
40. Pauwels RP, Schapers RF, Smeets AW, Debruyne FM, Geraedts JP. Grading in superficial bladder cancer. (1). Morphological criteria. Br J Urol. 1988;61:129–34.
41. Malmstrom PU, Busch C, Norlen BJ. Recurrence, progression and survival in bladder cancer. A retrospective analysis of 232 patients with greater than or equal to 5-year follow-up. Scand J Urol Nephrol. 1987;21:185–95.
42. Oosterhuis JWA, Schapers RFM, Janssen-Heijnen MLG, Pauwels RPE, Newling DW, Ten Kate FJW. Histological grading of papillary urothelial carcinoma of the bladder: prognostic value of the 1998 WHO/ISUP classification system and comparison with conventional grading systems. J Clin Pathol. 2002;55:900–5.
43. Epstein JI, Amin MB, Reuter VR, Mostofi FK. The World Health Organization/International Society of Urological Pathology consensus classification of urothelial (transitional cell) neoplasms of the urinary bladder. Bladder consensus conference committee. Am J Surg Pathol. 1998;22:1435–48.
44. Eble JN, Sauter G, Epstein JI, Sesterhenn IA. Pathology and genetics of tumours of the urinary system and male genital organs. World Health Organization classification of tumours. Lyon: IARC Press; 2004. p. 10.
45. Moch H, Humphrey PA, Ulbright TM, Reuter VE. WHO classification of tumours of the urinary system and male genital organs. Geneva: WHO Press; 2016.
46. Brown GA, Matin SF, Buzby JE, Dinney CPN, Grossman HB, Pettaway CA, et al. Ability of clinical grade to predict final pathologic stage in upper urinary tract transitional cell carcinoma: implications for therapy. Urology. 2007;70:252–6.
47. Rojas CP, Castle SM, Llanos CA, Santos Cortes JA, Bird V, Rodriguez S, et al. Low biopsy volume in ureteroscopy does not affect tumor biopsy grading in upper tract urothelial carcinoma. Urol Oncol. 2013;31:1696–700.
48. Clements T, Messer JC, Terrell JD, Herman MP, Ng CK, Scherr DS, et al. High-grade ureteroscopic biopsy is associated with advanced pathology of upper-tract urothelial carcinoma tumors at definitive surgical resection. J Endourol. 2012;26:398–402.
49. Margolin EJ, Matulay JT, Li G, Meng X, Chao B, Vijay V, et al. Discordance between ureteroscopic biopsy and final pathology for upper tract urothelial carcinoma. J Urol. 2018;199:1440–5.
50. Wang JK, Tollefson MK, Krambeck AE, Trost LW, Thompson RH. High rate of pathologic upgrading at nephroureterectomy for upper tract urothelial carcinoma. Urology. 2012;79:615–9.
51. Genega EM, Kapali M, Torres-Quinones M, Huang WC, Knauss JS, Wang LP, et al. Impact of the 1998 World Health Organization/International Society of Urological Pathology classification system for urothelial neoplasms of the kidney. Modern Pathol. 2005;18:11–8.
52. Guarnizo E, Pavlovich CP, Seiba M, Carlson DL, Vaughan ED, Sosa RE. Ureteroscopic biopsy of upper tract urothelial carcinoma: improved diagnostic accuracy and histopathological considerations using a multibiopsy approach. J Urol. 2000;163:52–5.
53. Vashistha V, Shabsigh A, Zynger DL. Utility and diagnostic accuracy of ureteroscopic biopsy in upper tract urothelial carcinoma. Arch Pathol Lab Med. 2013;137:400–7.

54. Jeon SS, Sung HH, Jeon HG, Han DH, Jeong BC, Seo SI, et al. Endoscopic management of upper tract urothelial carcinoma: improved prediction of invasive cancer using a ureteroscopic scoring model. Surg Oncol. 2017;26:252–6.
55. Scolieri MJ, Paik ML, Brown SL, Resnick MI. Limitations of computed tomography in the preoperative staging of upper tract urothelial carcinoma. Urology. 2000;56:930–4.
56. Buckley JA, Urban BA, Soyer P, Scherrer A, Fishman EK. Transitional cell carcinoma of the renal pelvis: a retrospective look at CT staging with pathologic correlation. Radiology. 1996;201:194–8.
57. Ng CK, Shariat SF, Lucas SM, Bagrodia A, Lotan Y, Scherr DS, et al. Does the presence of hydronephrosis on preoperative axial CT imaging predict worse outcomes for patients undergoing nephroureterectomy for upper-tract urothelial carcinoma? Urol Oncol. 2008;29:27–32.
58. Brien JC, Shariat SF, Herman MP, Ng CK, Scherr DS, Scoll B, et al. Preoperative hydronephrosis, ureteroscopic biopsy grade and urinary cytology can improve prediction of advanced upper tract urothelial carcinoma. J Urol. 2010;184:69–73.
59. Favaretto RL, Shariat SF, Savage C, Godoy G, Chade DC, Kaag M, et al. Combining imaging and ureteroscopy variables in a preoperative multivariable model for prediction of muscle-invasive and non-organ confined disease in patients with upper tract urothelial carcinoma. BJU Int. 2012;109:77–82.
60. Farnum JA, Vikram R, Rao A, Bedi D, Dinney CP, Matin SF. Accuracy of high-frequency endoluminal ultrasonography for clinical staging of upper tract urothelial carcinoma. J Endourol. 2018;32:806–11.
61. Matin SF, Kamat AM, Grossman HB. High-frequency endoluminal ultrasonography as an aid to the staging of upper tract urothelial carcinoma. J Ultrasound Med. 2010;29:1277–84.
62. Bus MT, de Bruin DM, Faber DJ, Kamphuis GM, Zondervan PJ, Laguna-Pes MP, et al. Optical coherence tomography as a tool for in vivo staging and grading of upper urinary tract urothelial carcinoma: a study of diagnostic accuracy. J Urol. 2016;196:1749–55.

Enhanced Endoscopic Imaging Techniques for Upper Tract Urothelial Carcinoma

63. Smith AK, Stephenson AJ, Lane BR, Larson BT, Thomas AA, Gong MC, et al. Inadequacy of biopsy for diagnosis of upper tract urothelial carcinoma: implications for conservative management. Urology. 2011;78(1):82–6.
64. Tavora F, Fajardo DA, Lee TK, Lotan T, Miller JS, Miyamoto H, et al. Small endoscopic biopsies of the ureter and renal pelvis: pathologic pitfalls. Am J Surg Pathol. 2009;33(10):1540–6.
65. Rouprêt M, Babjuk M, Burger M, Capoun O, Cohen D, Comperat M, et al. European Association of Urology guidelines on upper urinary tract urothelial carcinoma: 2020 update. Eur Urol. 2021;79:62–79.
66. Altobelli E, Zlatev DV, Liao JC. Role of narrow band imaging in Management of Urothelial Carcinoma. Curr Urol Rep. 2015;16(8):58.
67. Traxer O, Geavlete B, de Medina SGD, Sibony M, Al-Qahtani SM. Narrow-band imaging digital flexible ureteroscopy in detection of upper urinary tract transitional-cell carcinoma: initial experience. J Endourol. 2011;25(1):19–23.
68. Keller EX, Doizi S, Villa L, Traxer O. Which flexible ureteroscope is the best for upper tract urothelial carcinoma treatment? World J Urol. 2019;37:2325–33.
69. Kamphuis GM, de Bruin DM, de Reijke TM, de la Rosette J. íSPIES–a novel approach to advanced endoscopic imaging. J Endourol. 2014;28(8):894–5.
70. Kamphuis GM, de Bruin DM, Brandt MJ, Knoll T, Conort P, Lapini A, et al. Comparing image perception of bladder tumors in four different Storz professional image enhancement system modalities using the íSPIES app. J Endourol. 2016;30(5):602–8.

71. Bus MTJ, de Bruin DM, Faber DJ, Kamphuis GM, Zondervan PJ, Laguna Pes MP, et al. Optical diagnostics for upper urinary tract urothelial cancer: technology, thresholds, and clinical applications. J Endourol. 2015;29(2):113–23.
72. Baard J, Freund JE, de la Rosette JJMCH, Laguna MP. New technologies for upper tract urothelial carcinoma management. Curr Opin Urol. 2017;27(2):170–5.
73. Jocham D, Stepp H, Waidelich R. Photodynamic diagnosis in urology: state-of-the-art. Eur Urol. 2008;53:1138–48.
74. Kata SG, Aboumarzouk OM, Zreik A, Somani B, Ahmad S, Nabi G, et al. Photodynamic diagnostic ureterorenoscopy: a valuable tool in the detection of upper urinary tract tumour. Photodiagn Photodyn Ther. 2016;13:255–60.
75. Ahmad S, Aboumarzouk O, Somani B, Nabi G, Kata SG. Oral 5-aminolevulinic acid in simultaneous photodynamic diagnosis of upper and lower urinary tract transitional cell carcinoma – a prospective audit. BJU Int. 2012;110(11 Pt B):E596–600.
76. Osman E, Alnaib Z, Kumar N. Photodynamic diagnosis in upper urinary tract urothelial carcinoma: a systematic review. Arab J Urol. 2017;15(2):100–9.
77. Aboumarzouk OM, Mains E, Moseley H, Kata SG. Diagnosis of upper urinary tract tumours: is photodynamic diagnosis assisted ureterorenoscopy required as an addition to modern imaging and ureterorenoscopy? Photodiagn Photodyn Ther. 2013;10(2):127–33.
78. Baard J, de Bruin DM, Zondervan PJ, Kamphuis G, de la Rosette J, Laguna MP. Diagnostic dilemmas in patients with upper tract urothelial carcinoma. Nat Rev Urol. 2017;14(3):181–91.
79. Chen SP, Liao JC. Confocal laser endomicroscopy of bladder and upper tract urothelial carcinoma: a new era of optical diagnosis? Curr Urol Rep. 2014;15(9):437.
80. Bui D, Mach KE, Zlatev DV, Rouse RV, Leppert JT, Liao JC. A pilot study of in vivo confocal laser endomicroscopy of upper tract urothelial carcinoma. J Endourol. 2015;29(12):1418–23.
81. Villa L, Cloutier J, Cotè J-F, Salonia A, Montorsi F, Traxer O. Confocal laser endomicroscopy in the management of endoscopically treated upper urinary tract transitional cell carcinoma: preliminary data. J Endourol. 2016;30(2):237–42.
82. Breda A, Territo A, Guttilla A, Sanguedolce F, Manfredi M, Quaresima L, et al. Correlation between confocal laser endomicroscopy (Cellvizio®) and histological grading of upper tract urothelial carcinoma: a step forward for a better selection of patients suitable for conservative management. Eur Urol Focus. 2018;4:954–9.

Ureteroscopic Treatment of Upper Tract Urothelial Carcinoma

83. Go AS, Chertow GM, Fan D, McCulloch CE, Hsu CY. Chronic kidney disease and the risks of death, cardiovascular events, and hospitalization. NEJM. 2004;351:1296–305.
84. Huang WC, Levey AS, Serio AM, Snyder M, Vickers AJ, Raj GV, et al. Chronic kidney disease after nephrectomy in patients with renal cortical tumours: a retrospective cohort study. Lancet Oncol. 2006;7:735–40.
85. Lane BR, Campbell SC, Demirjian S, Fergany A. Surgically induced chronic kidney disease may be associated with a lower risk of progression and mortality than medical chronic kidney disease. J Urol. 2013;189:1649–55.
86. Kaag MG, O'Malley RL, O'Malley PO, Godoy G, Chen M, Smaldone MC, et al. Changes in renal function following nephroureterectomy may affect the use of perioperative chemotherapy. Eur Urol. 2010;58:581–7.
87. Bagley DH, Grasso M. Ureteroscopic laser treatment of upper urinary tract neoplasms. World J Urol. 2010;28:143–9.
88. Grasso M, Bagley D. Small diameter, actively deflectable, flexible ureteropyeloscopy. J Urol. 1998;160:1648–53.
89. Yakoubi R, Colin P, Seisen T, Léon P, Nison L, Bozzini G, et al. Radical nephroureterectomy versus endoscopic procedures for the treatment of localized upper tract urothelial carcinoma: a meta-analysis and a systematic review of current evidence from comparative studies. Eur J Surg Oncol. 2014;40:1629–34.

90. Seisen T, Peyronnet B, Dominguez-Escrig JL, Bruins HM, Yuan CY, Babjuk M, et al. Oncologic outcomes of kidney-sparing surgery versus radical Nephroureterectomy for upper tract urothelial carcinoma: a systematic review by the EAU non-muscle invasive bladder cancer guidelines panel. Eur Urol. 2016;70:1052–68.
91. Chen GL, Bagley DH. Ureteroscopic management of upper tract transitional cell carcinoma in patients with normal contralateral kidneys. J Urol. 2000;164:1173–6.
92. Elliott DS, Segura JW, Lightner D, Patterson DE, Blute ML. Is nephroureterectomy necessary in all cases of upper tract transitional cell carcinoma? Long-term results of conservative endourologic management of upper tract transitional cell carcinoma in individuals with a normal contralateral kidney. Urology. 2001;58:174–8.
93. Rouprêt M, Babjuk M, Burger M, Capoun O, Cohen D, Compérat EM, et al. European association of urology guidelines on upper urinary tract urothelial carcinoma: 2020 update. Eur Urol. 2020;79:62–79.
94. National Comprehensive Cancer Network. (2020). Bladder cancer (version 6.2020). Retrieved from: https://www.nccn.org/professionals/physician_gls/pdf/bladder.pdf.
95. Cutress ML, Stewart GD, Wells-Cole S, Phipps S, Thomas BG, Tolley DA. Long-term endoscopic management of upper tract urothelial carcinoma: 20-year single-centre experience. BJU Int. 2012;110:1608–17.
96. Grasso M, Fishman AI, Cohen J, Alexander B. Ureteroscopic and extirpative treatment of upper urinary tract urothelial carcinoma: a 15-year comprehensive review of 160 consecutive patients. BJU Int. 2012;110:1618–26.
97. Pak R, Moskowitz E, Bagley DH. What is the cost of maintaining a kidney in upper tract transitional cell carcinoma? J Endourol. 2009;23:341–6.
98. Scotland KB, Kleinmann N, Cason D, Hubbard L, Tanimoto R, Healy KA, et al. Ureteroscopic management of large≥ 2 cm upper tract urothelial carcinoma: a comprehensive 23-year experience. Urology. 2018;121:66–73.
99. Cohen JH, Cohen SD, Grasso M. Flexible ureteroscopy: wireless and sheathless. In: Monga M, editor. Ureteroscopy: indications, instrumentation and technique. New York: Humana Press; 2013. p. 291–302.
100. Malloy TR. Laser treatment of ureter and upper collecting system. In: Smith JA, editor. Lasers in urologic surgery. Chicago: YearBook Medical Publishers; 1985. p. 82–93.
101. Blute ML, Segura JW, Patterson DE, Benson RC Jr, Zincke H. Impact of endourology on diagnosis and management of upper urinary tract urothelial cancer. J Urol. 1989;141:1298–301.
102. Schmeller NT, Hofstetter AG. Laser treatment of ureteral tumors. J Urol. 1989;141:840–3.
103. Erhard MJ, Bagley DH. Urologic applications of the holmium laser: preliminary experience. J Endourol. 1995;9:383–6.
104. Razvi HA, Chun SS, Denstedt JD, Sales JL. Soft-tissue applications of the holmium: YAG laser in urology. J Endourol. 1995;9:387–90.
105. Hubosky SG, Bagley DH. Ureteroscopic diagnosis and treatment of upper urinary tract neoplasms. In: Smith A, Preminger G, Kavoussi L, Badlani G, editors. Smith's textbook of endourology. Oxford: Wiley-Blackwell; 2019. p. 568–83.
106. Defidio L, De Dominicis M, Di Gianfrancesco L, Fuchs G. First collaborative experience with thulium laser ablation of localized upper urinary tract urothelial tumors using retrograde intra-renal surgery. Arch Ital Urol Androl. 2011;83:147–53.
107. Breda A, Territo A, Sanguedolce F. Combination of holmium and thulium laser ablation in upper tract urothelial carcinoma. World J Urol. 2020;38:2661–2.
108. Villa L, Cloutier J, Letendre J, Ploumidis A, Salonia A, Cornu JN, Montorsi F, Traxer O. Early repeated ureteroscopy within 6-8 weeks after a primary endoscopic treatment in patients with upper tract urothelial cell carcinoma: preliminary findings. World J Urol. 2016;34:1201–6.
109. Huang A, Low RK, deVere White R. Nephrostomy tract tumor seeding following percutaneous manipulation of a ureteral carcinoma. J Urol. 1995;153:1041–2.
110. Stewart GD, Tolley DA. What are the oncological risks of minimal access surgery for the treatment of urinary tract cancer? Eur Urol. 2004;46(4):415–20.

111. Cutress ML, Stewart GD, Zakikhani P, Phipps S, Thomas BG, Tolley DA. Ureteroscopic and percutaneous management of upper tract urothelial carcinoma (UTUC): systematic review. BJU Int. 2012;110(5):614–28.
112. Irwin BH, Berger AK, Brandina R, Stein R, Desai MM. Complex percutaneous resections for upper-tract urothelial carcinoma. J Endourol. 2010;24(3):367–70.
113. Cheng L, Neumann RM, Nehra A, Spotts BE, Weaver AL, Bostwick DG. Cancer heterogeneity and its biological implications in the grading of urothelial carcinoma. Cancer. 2000;88:1663–70.
114. Skolarikos A, Griffiths TRL, Powell PH, Thomas DJ, Neal DE, Kelly JD. Cytologic analysis of ureteral washings is informative in patients with grade 2 upper tract TCC considering endoscopic treatment. Urology. 2003;61:1146–50.
115. Weizer AZ, Faerber GJ, Wolf S. Progression of disease despite good endoscopic local control of upper tract urothelial carcinoma. Urology. 2007;70:469–72.
116. Cosentino M, Palou J, Gaya JM, Breda A, Rodriguez-Faba O, Villavicencio-Mavrich H. Upper urinary tract urothelial carcinoma: location as a predictive factor for concomitant bladder carcinoma. World J Urol. 2013;31:141–5.
117. Sowter SJ, Ilie CP, Efthimiou I. Endourologic management of patients with upper tract transitional cell carcinoma: long term follow up in a single center. J Endourol. 2007;21:1005–9.
118. Cornu TN, Roupret M, Carpentier X, Geavlete B, Diez de Medina SG, Cussenot O, et al. Oncologic control obtained after exclusive flexible ureteroscopic management of upper urinary tract urothelial cell carcinoma. World J Urol. 2010;28:151–6.
119. Kang CH, Yu TJ, Hsieh HH, Yang JW, Shu K, Huang CC. The development of bladder tumors and contralateral upper urinary tract tumors after primary transitional cell carcinoma of the upper urinary tract. Cancer. 2003;98:1620–6.
120. Raman JD, Ng CK, Boorjian SA, Vaughan ED, Sosa RE, Scherr DS. Bladder cancer after managing upper urinary tract transitional cell carcinoma: predictive factors and pathology. BJUI. 2005;96:1031–5.
121. Matsui Y, Utsunomiya N, Ichioka K, Ueda N, Yoshimura K, Terai A, et al. Risk factors for subsequent development of bladder cancer after primary transitional cell carcinoma of the upper urinary tract. Urology. 2005;65:279–83.
122. Liu Y, Lu J, Hong K, Huang Y, Ma L. Independent prognostic factors for initial intravesical recurrence after laparoscopic nephroureterectomy for upper urinary tract urothelial carcinoma. Urol Oncol. 2014;32:146–52.
123. O'Brien T, Ray E, Singh R, Coker B, Beard R, British Association of Urological Surgeons Section of Oncology. Prevention of bladder tumours after nephroureterectomy for primary upper urinary tract urothelial carcinoma: a prospective, multicentre, randomised clinical trial of a single postoperative intravesical dose of mitomycin C (the ODMIT-C Trial). Eur Urol. 2011;60:703–10.
124. Kulp DA, Bagley DH. Does flexible ureteropyeloscopy promote local recurrence of transitional cell carcinoma? J Endourol. 1994;8:111–3.
125. Hendin BN, Streem SB, Levin HS, Klein EA, Novick AC. Impact of diagnostic ureteroscopy on long-term survival in patients with upper tract transitional cell carincoma. J Urol. 1999;161:783–5.
126. Linehan J, Schoenberg M, Seltzer E, Thacker K, Smith AB. Complications associated with ureteroscopic management of upper tract urothelial carcinoma. Urology. 2021;147:87–95.
127. Grasso M. Ureteropyeloscopic treatment of ureteral and intrarenal calculi. Urol Clin North Am. 2000;27:623–31.
128. Johnson DB, Pearle MS. Complications of ureteroscopy. Urol Clin North Am. 2004;31:157–71.
129. Hubosky SG, Boman BM, Charles S, Bibbo M, Bagley DH. Ureteroscopic management of upper tract urothelial carcinoma (UTUC) in patients with Lynch syndrome (hereditary non-polyposis colorectal cancer syndrome). BJU Int. 2013;112:813–9.
130. Crockett DG, Wagner DG, Holmang S, Johansson SL, Lynch HT. Upper urinary tract carcinoma in Lynch syndrome cases. J Urol. 2011;185:1627–30.
131. Mork M, Hubosky SG, Roupret M, Margulis V, Raman J, Lotan Y, et al. Lynch syndrome: a primer for urologists and panel recommendations. J Urol. 2015;194:21–9.

Adjuvant Treatment for Upper Tract Urothelial Carcinoma: Topical and Systemic

132. Thalmann GN, Markwalder R, Walter B, Studer UE. Long-term experience with bacillus Calmette-Guerin therapy of upper urinary tract transitional cell carcinoma in patients not eligible for surgery. J Urol. 2002;168:1381–5.
133. Katz MH, Lee MW, Gupta M. Setting a new standard for topical therapy of upper-tract transitional-cell carcinoma: BCG and interferon-α2B. J Endourol. 2007;21:374–7.
134. Irie A, Iwamura M, Kadowaki K, Ohkawa A, Uchida T, Baba S. Intravesical instillation of bacille Calmette-Guérin for carcinoma in situ of the urothelium involving the upper urinary tract using vesicoureteral reflux created by a double-pigtail catheter. Urology. 2002;59:53–7.
135. Patel A, Fuchs GJ. New techniques for the administration of topical adjuvant therapy after endoscopic ablation of upper urinary tract transitional cell carcinoma. J Urol. 1998;159:71–5.
136. Liu Z, Ng J, Yuwono A, Lu Y, Tan YK. Which is best method for instillation of topical therapy to the upper urinary tract? An in vivo porcine study to evaluate three delivery methods. Int Braz J Urol. 2017;43:1084–91.
137. Pollard ME, Levinson AW, Shapiro EY, Cha DY, Small AC, Mohamed NE, et al. Comparison of 3 upper tract anticarcinogenic agent delivery techniques in an ex vivo porcine model. Urology. 2013;82:1451.e1–6.
138. Martínez-Piñeiro JA, García Matres MJ, Martínez-Piñeiro L. Endourological treatment of upper tract urothelial carcinomas: analysis of a series of 59 tumors. J Urol. 1996;156:377–85.
139. Keeley FX, Bagley DH. Adjuvant mitomycin C following endoscopic treatment of upper tract transitional cell carcinoma. J Urol. 1997;158:2074–7.
140. Aboumarzouk OM, Somani B, Ahmed S, Nabi G, Townell N, Kata SG. Mitomycin C instillation following ureteroscopic laser ablation of upper urinary tract carcinoma. Urol Ann. 2013;5:184–9.
141. Metcalfe M, Wagenheim G, Xiao L, Papadopoulos J, Navai N, Davis JW, et al. Induction and maintenance adjuvant mitomycin C topical therapy for upper tract urothelial carcinoma: tolerability and intermediate term outcomes. J Endourol. 2017;31:946–53.
142. Gallioli A, Boissier R, Territo A, Vila-Reyes H, Sanguedolce F, Gaya JM, et al. Adjuvant single-dose upper urinary tract instillation of mitomycin C after therapeutic ureteroscopy for upper tract urothelial carcinoma: a single-centre prospective non-randomized trial. J Endourol. 2020;34:573–80.
143. Balasubramanian A, Metcalfe MJ, Wagenheim G, Xiao L, Papadopoulos J, Navai N, et al. Salvage topical therapy for upper tract urothelial carcinoma. World J Urol. 2018;36:2027–34.
144. Eastham JA, Huffman JL. Technique of mitomycin C instillation in the treatment of upper urinary tract urothelial tumors. J Urol. 1993;150:324–5.
145. Goel MC, Mahendra V, Roberts JG. Percutaneous management of renal pelvic urothelial tumors: long-term follow-up. J Urol. 2003;169:925–9.
146. Hoffman-Censits J. Systemic chemotherapy for upper tract urothelial cancer. In: Grasso M, Bagley DH, editors. Upper urinary tract urothelial carcinoma, vol. 2015. Heidelberg: Springer; 2015. p. 75–81.
147. Donin NM, Duarte S, Lenis AT, Caliliw R, Torres C, Smithson A, et al. Sustained-release formulation of mitomycin C to the upper urinary tract using a thermosensitive polymer: a preclinical study. Urology. 2017;99:270–7.
148. Kleinmann N, Matin SF, Pierorazio PM, Gore JL, Shabsigh A, Hu B, et al. Primary chemoablation of low-grade upper tract urothelial carcinoma using UGN-101, a mitomycin-containing reverse thermal gel (OLYMPUS): an open-label, single-arm, phase 3 trial. Lancet Oncol. 2020;21:776–85.
149. Kojima Y, Tozawa K, Kawai N, Sasaki S, Hayashi Y, Kohri K. Long-term outcome of upper urinary tract carcinoma in situ: effectiveness of nephroureterectomy versus bacillus Calmette-Guérin therapy. Int J Urol. 2006;13:340–4.

150. Hayashida Y, Nomata K, Noguchi M, Eguchi J, Koga S, Yamashita S, et al. Long-term effects of bacille Calmette-Guérin perfusion therapy for treatment of transitional cell carcinoma in situ of upper urinary tract. Urology. 2004;63:1084–8.

151. Giannarini G, Kessler TM, Birkhäuser FD, Thalmann GN, Studer UE. Antegrade perfusion with bacillus Calmette- Guérin in patients with non-muscle-invasive urothelial carcinoma of the upper urinary tract: who may benefit? Eur Urol. 2011;60:955–60.

152. Bellman GC, Sweetser P, Smith AD. Complications of intracavitary bacillus Calmette-Guerin after percutaneous resection of upper tract transitional cell carcinoma. J Urol. 1994;151:13–5.

153. Schnapp DS, Weiss GH, Smith AD. Fever following intracavitary bacillus Calmette-Guerin therapy for upper tract transitional cell carcinoma. J Urol. 1996;156:386–8.

154. Elliott DS, Blute ML, Patterson DE, Bergstralh EJ, Segura JW. Long-term follow up of endoscopically treated upper urinary tract transitional cell carcinoma. Urology. 1996;47:819–25.

155. Wong NC, Assel M, Tracey A, Alvim R, Almassi N, Singla N et al. Trends in management and outcomes in patients with upper tract urothelial carcinoma following radical nephroureterectomy at Memorial Sloan Kettering Cancer Center. J Clin Oncol. 2020; 38: (suppl 6; abstr 469).

156. Nagumo Y, Kojima T, Kojo K, Kimura T, Kandori S, Kawai K et al. Discrepancy between clinical stage and pathological stage based on the tumor location of urothelial carcinoma: a hospital-based cancer registry in Japan. J Clin Oncol. 2020; 38: (suppl 6; abstr 579).

157. Margulis V, Puligandla M, Trabulsi EJ, Plimack ER, Kessler ER, Matin SF, et al. Phase II trial of neoadjuvant systemic chemotherapy followed by extirpative surgery in patients with high grade upper tract urothelial carcinoma. J Urol. 2020;203:690–8.

158. Matin SF, Margulis V, Kamat A, Wood CG, Grossman HB, Brown GA, et al. Incidence of downstaging and complete remission after neoadjuvant chemotherapy for high-risk upper tract transitional cell carcinoma. Cancer. 2010;116:3127–34.

159. Porten S, Siefker-Radtke AO, Xiao L, Margulis V, Kamat AM, Wood CG, et al. Neoadjuvant chemotherapy improves survival of patients with upper tract urothelial carcinoma. Cancer. 2014;120:1794–9.

160. Siefker-Radtke AO, Kamat, AM, Corn PG, Matin SF, Grossman HB, et al. Neoadjuvant chemotherapy with DD- MVAC and bevacizumab in high-risk urothelial cancer: Results from phase II at the M.D. Anderson Cancer Center. J Clin Oncol. 2012; 30: (suppl abstr 4523).

161. Hosogoe S, Hatakeyama S, Kusaka A, Hamano I, Iwamura H, Fujita N, et al. Platinum-based neoadjuvant chemotherapy improves oncological outcomes in patients with locally advanced upper tract urothelial carcinoma. Eur Urol Focus. 2018;4:946–53.

162. Roupret M, Babjuk M, Burger M, Capoun O, Cohen D, Comperat EM, et al. European Association of Urology guidelines on upper tract urothelial carcinoma: 2020 update. Eur Urol. 2021;79:62–79.

163. Soga N, Arima K, Sugimura Y. Adjuvant methotrexate, vinblastine, adriamycin, and cisplatin chemotherapy has potential to prevent recurrence of bladder tumors after surgical removal of upper urinary tract transitional cell carcinoma. Int J Urol. 2008;15:800–3.

164. Vassilakopoulou M, de la Motte RT, Colin P, Ouzzane A, Khayat D, Dimopoulos MA, et al. French collaborative National Database on UUT-UCC. Outcomes after adjuvant chemo- therapy in the treatment of high-risk urothelial carcinoma of the upper urinary tract (UUT-UC): results from a large multicenter collaborative study. Cancer. 2011;117:5500–8.

165. Seisen T, Jindal T, Karabon P, Sood A, Bellmunt J, Roupret M, et al. Efficacy of systemic chemotherapy plus radical nephroureterectomy for metastatic upper tract urothelial carcinoma. Eur Urol. 2017;71:714–8.

166. Birtle A, Johnson M, Chester J, Jones R, Dolling D, Bryan RT, et al. Adjuvant chemotherapy in upper tract urothelial carcinoma (the POUT trial): a phase 3, open-label, randomised controlled trial. Lancet. 2020;395:1268–77.

167. Weng YM, Peng M, Hu MX, Yao Y, Song QB. Clinical and molecular characteristics associated with the efficacy of PD-1/ PD-L1 inhibitors for solid tumors: a meta-analysis. Onco Targets Ther. 2018;11:7529–42.

168. Stenehjem DD, Tran D, Nkrumah MA, Gupta S. PD1/PDL1 inhibitors for the treatment of advanced urothelial bladder cancer. Onco Targets Ther. 2018;11:5973–89.
169. Baldini C, Champiat S, Vuagnat P, Massard C. Durvalumab for the management of urothelial carcinoma: a short review on the emerging data and therapeutic potential. Onco Targets Ther. 2019;12:2505–12.
170. Rosenberg JE, Hoffman-Censits J, Powles T, van der Heijden MS, Balar AV, Necchi A, et al. Atezolizumab in patients with locally advanced and metastatic urothelial carcinoma who have progressed following treatment with platinum-based chemotherapy: a single-arm, multicentre, phase 2 trial. Lancet. 2016;387:1909–20.
171. Fradet Y, Bellmunt J, Vaughn DJ, Lee JL, Fong L, Vogelzang NJ, et al. Randomized phase III KEYNOTE-045 trial of pembrolizumab versus paclitaxel, docetaxel, or vinflunine in recurrent advanced urothelial cancer: results of >2 years of follow-up. Ann Oncol. 2019;30:970–6.
172. Powles T, Duran I, van der Heijden MS, Loriot Y, Vogelzang NJ, De Giorgi U, et al. Atezolizumab versus chemotherapy in patients with platinum-treated locally advanced or metastatic urothelial carcinoma (IMvigor211): a multicentre, open-label, phase 3 randomised controlled trial. Lancet. 2018;24:748–57.
173. Sharma P, Retz M, Siefker-Radtke A, Baron A, Necchi A, Bedke J, et al. Nivolumab in metastatic urothelial carcinoma after platinum therapy (CheckMate 275): a multicentre, single-arm, phase 2 trial. Lancet Oncol. 2017;18:312–22.
174. Sharma P, Callahan MK, Bono P, Kim J, Spiliopoulou P, Calvo E, et al. Nivolumab monotherapy in recurrent metastatic urothelial carcinoma (CheckMate 032): a multicentre, open-label, two-stage, multi-arm, phase 1/2 trial. Lancet Oncol. 2016;17:1590–8.
175. Powles T, O'Donnell PH, Massard C, Arkenau HT, Friedlander TW, Hoimes CJ, et al. Efficacy and safety of durvalumab in locally advanced or metastatic urothelial carcinoma: updated results from a phase 1/2 open-label study. JAMA Oncol. 2017;3(9):e172411.
176. Patel MR, Ellerton J, Infante JR, Agrawal M, Gordon M, Aljumaily R, et al. Avelumab in metastatic urothelial carcinoma after platinum failure (JAVELIN solid tumor): pooled results from two expansion cohorts of an open-label, phase 1 trial. Lancet Oncol. 2018;19:51–64.
177. Audenet F, Colin P, Yates DR, Ouzzane A, Pignot G, Long JA, et al. A proportion of hereditary upper urinary tract urothelial carcinomas are misclassified as sporadic according to a multi-institutional database analysis: proposal of patient- specific risk identification tool. BJU Int. 2012;110:e583–9.
178. Syed JS, Nguyen KA, Suarez-Sariemento A, Leung C, Casilla-Lennon M, Raman JD, et al. Outcomes of upper tract urothelial cancer managed non-surgically. Can J Urol. 2019;26:9699–707.
179. Siefker-Radtke AO, Campbell MT, Munsell MF, Harris DR, Carolla RL, Pagliaro LC. Frontline treatment with gemcitabine, paclitaxel and doxorubicin for patients with unresectable or metastatic urothelial cancer and poor renal function: final results from a phase II study. Urology. 2016;89:83–9.
180. Balar AV, Galsky MD, Rosenberg JE, Powles T, Petrylak DP, Bellmunt J, et al. Atezolizumab as first-line treatment in cisplatin-ineligible patients with locally advanced and metastatic urothelial carcinoma: a single-arm, multicentre, phase 2 trial. Lancet. 2017;389:67–76.
181. Balar AV, Castellano D, O'Donnell PH, Grivas P, Vuky J, Powles T, et al. First-line pembrolizumab in cisplatin-ineligible patients with locally advanced and unresectable or metastatic urothelial cancer (KEYNOTE-052): a multicentre, single-arm, phase 2 study. Lancet Oncol. 2017;18:1483–92.
182. Haanen J, Carbonnel F, Robert C, Kerr KM, Peters S, Larkin J, et al. Management of toxicities from immunotherapy: ESMO clinical practice guidelines for diagnosis, treatment and follow-up. Ann Oncol. 2018; 29 (Supplement_4):iv264–iv266. 71. Gayed BA, Thoreson GR, Margulis V. The role of systemic chemotherapy in management of upper tract urothelial cancer. Curr Urol Rep 2013;14:94–101.

Chapter 7
Ureteroscopic Management of Upper Urinary Tract Obstruction

Scott G. Hubosky and Demetrius H. Bagley

Introduction

When faced with upper urinary tract obstruction, the ultimate treatment goal should be to obtain durable, tubeless, efficient drainage with the least amount of imposed procedural morbidity for the patient whenever possible. Treatment must be tailored to the individual situation, given the many etiologies for upper tract obstruction and the various options for intervention. Two common forms of upper tract obstruction include ureteropelvic junction (UPJ) obstructions and ureteral strictures, both of which can be congenital or acquired. The broad treatment categories for upper tract obstruction include formal surgical reconstruction, which can be performed open or laparoscopically, with or without robotic assistance, and endourological incision of the obstruction. Given the higher long-term patency rates of pyeloplasty [1, 2], minimally invasive advantages of laparoscopy, and widespread dissemination of robotics, endopyelotomy rates have significantly declined. Nevertheless, endopyelotomy and endoureterotomy are still indicated in select cases.

S. G. Hubosky (✉)
Department of Urology, Sidney Kimmel Medical College at Thomas Jefferson University Hospital, Philadelphia, PA, USA
e-mail: Scott.Hubosky@jefferson.edu

D. H. Bagley
Department of Urology and Radiology, Sidney Kimmel Medical College at Thomas Jefferson University Hospital, Philadelphia, PA, USA
e-mail: Demetrius.BagleyJr@jefferson.edu

© Springer Nature Switzerland AG 2022
S. G. Hubosky et al. (eds.), *Advanced Ureteroscopy*,
https://doi.org/10.1007/978-3-030-82351-1_7

Ureteropelvic Junction (UPJ) Obstruction

Etiology

UPJ obstructions can be congenital or acquired. Congenital UPJ obstructions often manifest in the pediatric population either on prenatal ultrasound screening as hydronephrosis or with postnatal symptoms such as flank or abdominal pain, renal colic, fever, or a combination of these. Not uncommonly, patients with congenital UPJ obstructions present with symptoms in young adulthood or later. Congenital UPJ obstructions are usually classified into one of three main categories, which are not necessary mutually exclusive. These are intrinsic obstruction, extrinsic obstruction from lower pole crossing vessels, and high insertion morphology.

The exact etiology of UPJ obstructions is still not entirely clear, as multiple embryological and histopathological studies over the years have demonstrated conflicting findings [3, 4]. Cases of intrinsic obstruction demonstrate focal luminal narrowing at the UPJ in the absence of any factor contributing to extrinsic compression (Fig. 7.1). Accessory crossing blood vessels are often found anterior to the UPJ and have actually been noted in almost 20% of patients with normal, patent UPJs [5]. Although seemingly dependent on patient age, the presence of crossing vessels in obstructed UPJs has been reported at 50% [6] and, in some cases, is responsible for extrinsic compression (Fig. 7.2). Debate exists as if the crossing vessels are the actual cause of obstruction or if they simply simultaneously coexist in some cases of intrinsic obstruction. Nevertheless,

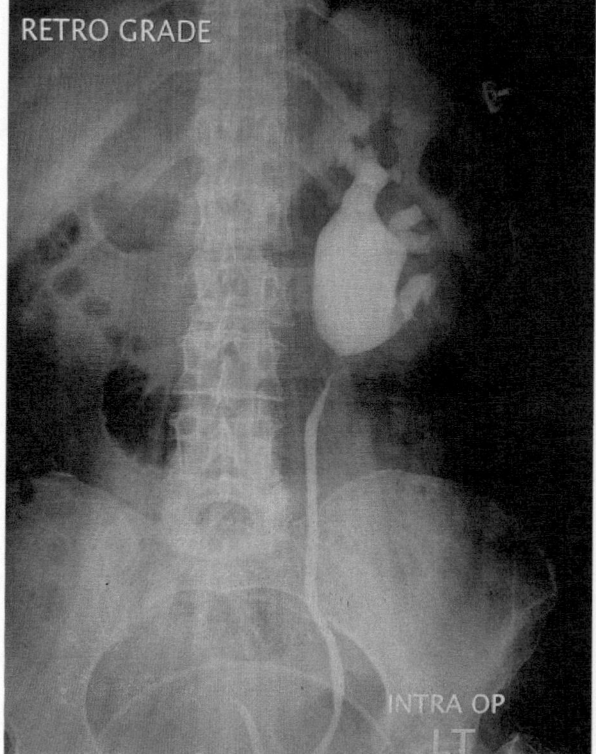

Fig. 7.1 Retrograde pyelogram demonstrating focal stenosis of the left ureteropelvic junction (UPJ). Additional imaging during workup showed no evidence of extrinsic obstruction

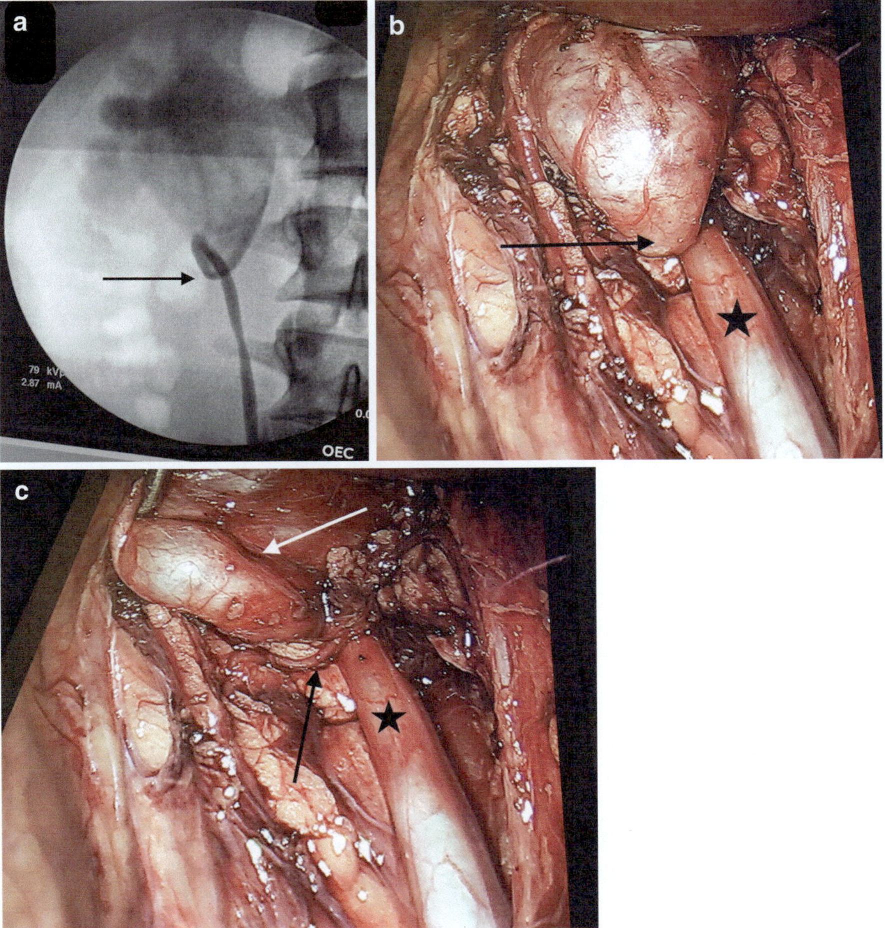

Fig. 7.2 (**a**) Retrograde pyelogram of a patient with right-sided ureteropelvic junction obstruction secondary to an anterior crossing vessel. Arrow marks the apex of the redundant anterior renal pelvis, "draped over" anterior crossing vessels. (**b**) Same patient during laparoscopic pyeloplasty. Star marks the right ureter, and arrow marks the redundant renal pelvis, which overlies the crossing vessels, not seen in this view. (**c**) Right renal pelvis is retracted cranially and laterally (white arrow), exposing anterior crossing vessel (black arrow) and ureter (black star)

multiple groups over time have shown the presence of crossing vessels to be negatively correlated with durable patency following endopyelotomy [7–9]. Additionally, these crossing vessels can be violated during ureteroscopic endopyelotomy and be a source of significant hemorrhage [10]. High insertion morphology is less commonly seen but has a distinctive appearance on retrograde pyelogram (Fig. 7.3).

Secondary UPJ obstructions are acquired. These can arise from frequent stone passage and/or treatments but most commonly result from previously unsuccessful primary treatments of a UPJ obstruction. Defining failure of a primary procedure used to treat UPJ obstruction has historically not been uniform, making results among different studies difficult to objectively judge. Nevertheless, success is usually defined by a radiographic study to determine upper tract patency and improvement in symptoms, although the use of standardized questionnaires is uncommon.

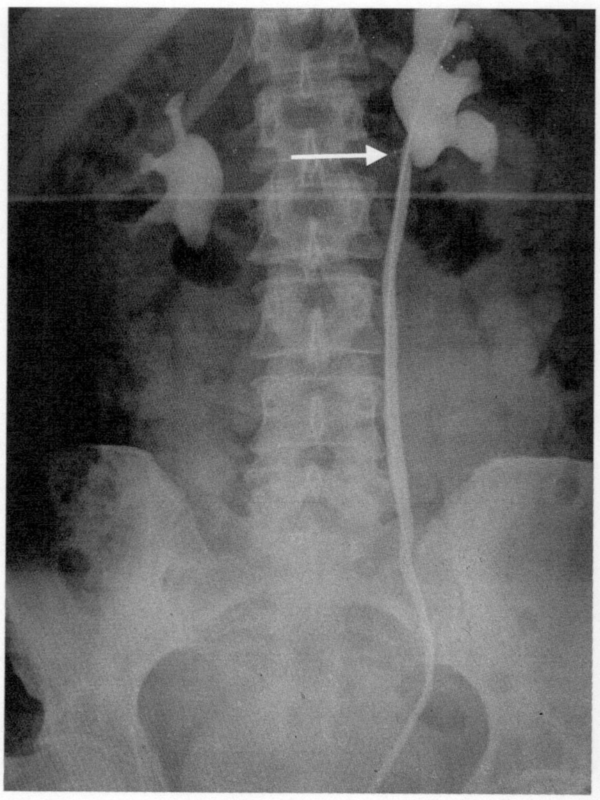

Fig. 7.3 High insertion morphology can be seen on the left retrograde pyelogram. Arrow shows the origin of the left ureteropelvic junction is not in the most dependent position to allow for maximized drainage

A third and quite practical criterion to determine success is the absence of further needed intervention [11], which is inconsistently reported.

Endopyelotomy

The foundation for current endoscopic management of UPJ obstructions and ureteral strictures was provided by David M. Davis. In his description of the intubated ureterotomy during the 1940s, he demonstrated in a canine model that a stented incision of the UPJ epithelialized in 1 week and that almost complete smooth muscle regeneration occurred circumferentially in 6 weeks [12]. It is this healing by secondary intention of the ureter over a stent that makes endoscopic incision an effective treatment option.

The first endopyelotomy was performed in 1983 by way of a percutaneous antegrade approach using cold-knife incision of the UPJ [13]. This technique was attractive as a less invasive alternative to open pyeloplasty and was further advanced by Arthur Smith and colleagues, who in 1997 reported an 85% success rate with at least 6 months of follow-up, in a series of 401 antegrade endopyelotomies [14]. A combined antegrade and retrograde approach was described by Bagley et al. in order to regain patency to obliterated UPJ obstructions [15]. A purely retrograde ureteroscopic approach to endopyelotomy was described in 1986 by Inglis and Tolley, using a diathermy hook and semi-rigid ureteroscopy [16]. Since then, retrograde ureteroscopic endopyelotomy has evolved to include the routine use of flexible ureteroscopy so the incision can be performed under direct vision. Incisions can be made with a cold knife or electrocautery using a hook, but the holmium (Ho) laser has become more popular, given its versatility in lithotripsy and widespread availability.

In 1993, Schuessler et al. described the first case series of laparoscopic dismembered pyeloplasty resulting in resolution of obstruction in five patients with an average of 12-month follow-up [17]. This technique quickly gained popularity due not only to its minimally invasive nature compared to open pyeloplasty but also for its versatility [18]. Purely laparoscopic pyeloplasty could be tailored to the specific pathology around the UPJ. Anderson-Hynes dismembered pyeloplasty could be performed for crossing vessel etiologies. In the absence of crossing vessels, Heineke-Mikulicz type repairs could be performed for short stenotic segments, and a Foley V-Y plasty repair could be applied to high insertion-type morphologies. With time and experience, the durable patency rate of laparoscopic pyeloplasty was shown in multiple studies to be superior to endopyelotomy for treatment of primary UPJ obstructions (Table 7.1). Yanke et al. reported 76% patency rate for laparoscopic pyeloplasty at 7 years of follow-up compared to 50% patency for those patients undergoing retrograde ureteroscopic endopyelotomy [1]. Dimarco et al. showed 75% patency rate for open pyeloplasty at 10 years versus 41% for antegrade endopyelotomy [2]. The refinement and widespread availability of robotic assistance have diminished the learning curve of laparoscopic pyeloplasty, and as a result, endopyelotomy has assumed a secondary role in the treatment of UPJ obstructions.

Table 7.1 Postoperative patency rates of pyeloplasty versus endopyelotomy

	Number	Median months follow-up (range)	Patency at 1 year	Patency at 3 years	Patency at 7 years
TJU series [1]	–	–	–	–	–
Retrograde Endopyelotomy	128	20 (1–165)	82%	62%	50%
Laparoscopic Pyeloplasty	116	20 (1–87)	93%	86%	76%
Mayo series [2]	–	–	**Patency at 1 year**	**Patency at 5 years**	**Patency at 10 years**
Antegrade Endopyelotomy	182	37 (1–1674)	63%	55%	41%
Pyeloplasty	174	47 (1–240)	85%	80%	75%

Patient Selection

Laparoscopic pyeloplasty with or without robotic assistance should always be primarily considered as the gold standard treatment for patients with UPJ obstruction given its minimally invasive nature, high long-term success rate, and versatility. It is clearly the superior choice in relatively young patients and those with preoperatively detected crossing vessels. If calculi are present, they can also be removed with this approach in the majority of cases. If significant cortical deterioration and truly minimal split function is present, the patient will likely be best served with simple nephrectomy if a normal contralateral kidney is present.

Nevertheless, endopyelotomy still maintains a role in those patients who are not ideal candidates for pyeloplasty. This includes patients with significant medical comorbidities or previous abdominal or retroperitoneal surgery in which laparoscopic or open pyeloplasty would be prohibitively risky. Furthermore, the surgeon must evaluate the body habitus of the patient and expected approach to the UPJ. Patients with minimal collecting system dilation or kidney malrotation may offer significant technical challenge if pyeloplasty is selected. In cases such as these, endopyelotomy can offer an ideal alternative (Fig. 7.4). Once pyeloplasty has been deferred in favor of endopyelotomy, additional factors must be considered, which will affect treatment success. The European Association of Urology (EAU) guidelines suggest, based mostly on single-institutional retrospective studies, that ideal endopyelotomy candidates have short (< 2-cm-long) stenotic segments without any component of extrinsic obstruction [19]. In accordance with other published series, the presence of massive hydronephrosis or split renal function less than 20% will render lower success rates for endopyelotomy [14].

Surgical Planning

Attention should be paid to the presence of crossing vessels at the UPJ since significant intraoperative hemorrhage can result if they are incised and transfusion rates during endopyelotomy can range from 1% to 16% [20]. Computerized tomography (CT) is useful for preoperative workup to rule out the presence of significantly sized crossing vessels. Intraoperative endoluminal ultrasound (ELUS) has been shown to be more sensitive for the detection of crossing vessels relative to helical CT angiography by multiple groups [10, 21]. Empiric incision at the lateral position relative to the UPJ during endopyelotomy has been suggested [22] since this area has been considered relatively devoid of significant vascular structures according to cadaveric studies [23]. Experience using ELUS however has shown, in both patients with UPJ obstructions and those with normal anatomy around the UPJ, that primarily

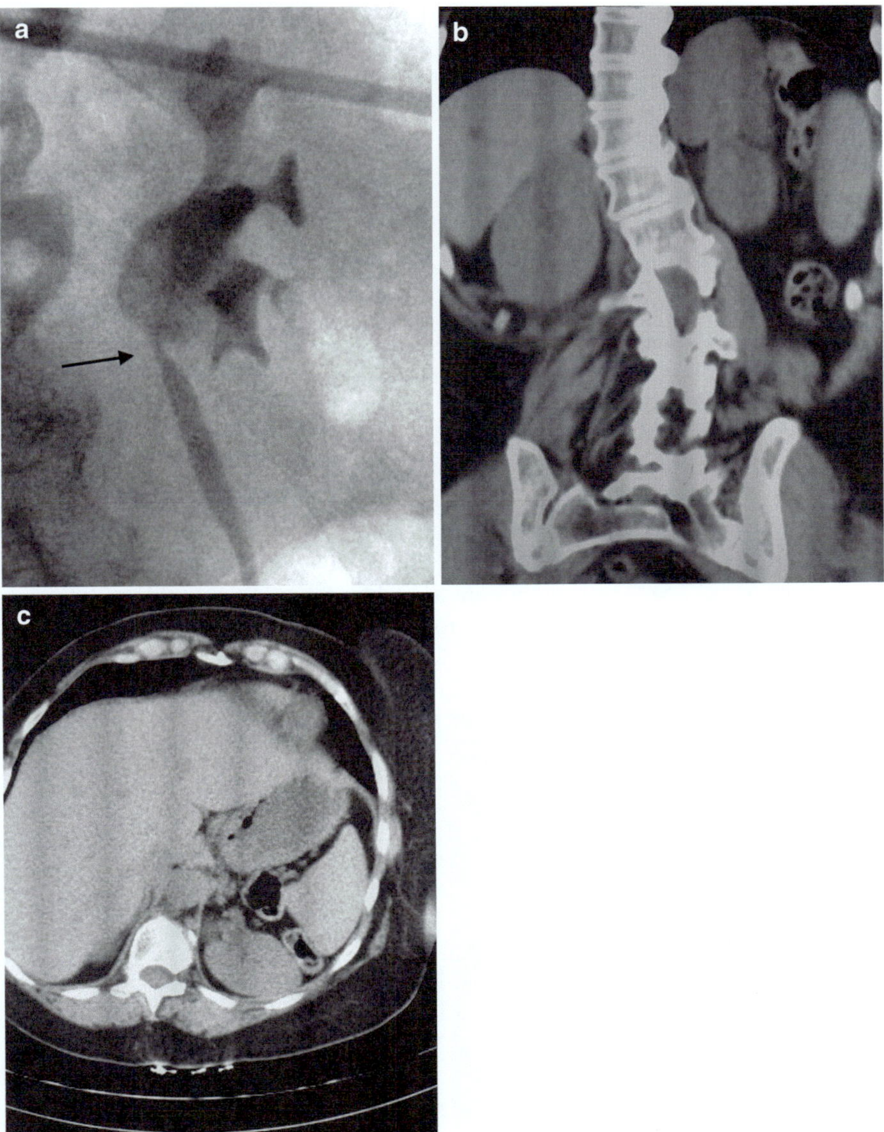

Fig. 7.4 Characteristics of the ideal candidate for ureteroscopic endopyelotomy are shown. (**a**) Retrograde pyelogram shows a short stenotic segment (black arrow) with mild to moderate hydronephrosis. (**b**) Coronal CT scan view and (**c**) axial views of the same patient show minimal hydronephrosis. A minimally dilated system, obese body habitus, and spinal curvature make this patient a technical challenge for pyeloplasty

anterior or posterior crossing vessels can have a lateral component in 18.8% and 28%, respectively [5, 24]. Therefore, we suggest the use of intraoperative ELUS during retrograde ureteroscopic endopyelotomy, if available. It should be acknowledged that cost can be a limiting factor, since ELUS units have capital acquisition costs of approximately $75,000.00.

Surgical Technique

Cystoscopy with retrograde pyelogram (RGP) is the initial step of the procedure and serves to define the exact location and length of the obstructed segment as well as the degree of hydronephrosis. Retrograde placement of a safety wire is highly recommended in these cases. Flexible ureteroscopy is then performed in order to visually inspect the entire upper urinary tract for any additional pathology such as tumor or calculus. Retrograde pyelogram can be repeated by injecting contrast through the ureteroscope in order to further study the area of interest. Next, ELUS is then performed. ELUS probes are catheter-based and are placed over a guidewire under fluoroscopy (Fig. 7.5). These probes are available in round-tip or side-saddle configurations and range in size from 5.0 to 8.5F diameter. The frequency of these

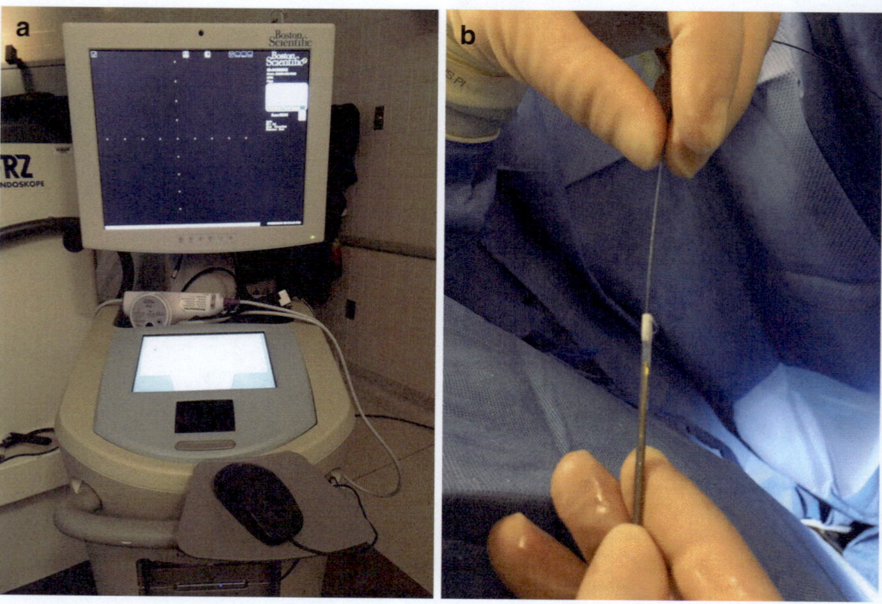

Fig. 7.5 Endoluminal ultrasound (ELUS) is a portable unit (**a**) and is manufactured by Boston Scientific as well as Olympus. The pictured probe (**b**) is a round-tip design, measuring 8.5 French, and provides resolution up 2.0 cm from the center of ureteral lumen

Fig. 7.6 View of the right ureter, as seen with endoluminal ultrasound. Long black arrow marks the ureteral wall. Short black arrow demonstrates a blood vessel parallel to the ureter. White star marks the shadow produced by the guidewire

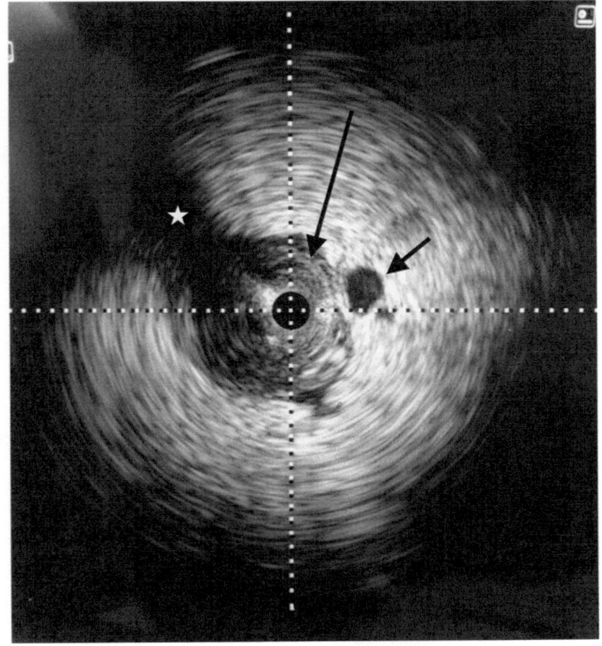

probes ranges from 12.5 to 20 MHz which provides resolution up to 1.5–2.0 cm of distance from the center of the ureteral lumen, allowing for adequate observation of any pathology in close proximity to the ureter [25]. ELUS should be performed immediately following a RGP with the fluoroscopic C-arm in a locked position. The ELUS probe is placed over a wire and up to the renal pelvis, initially. Next, in order to properly set the orientation, the position of the safety wire relative to the ELUS probe must be noted and maintained, usually at either the 3 or 9 o'clock position. The safety wire can be appreciated on ELUS since it provides a shadow (Fig. 7.6). The ELUS probe is then slowly withdrawn across the UPJ while maintaining orientation to the safety wire and correlating with the location of obstruction on the original RGP, using bony landmarks as provided by fluoroscopy. Deference to the posterior-lateral position should be made, but it is important to rule out the presence of any crossing vessels prior to performing laser incision. Once the decision has been made in terms of location of the incision, the flexible ureteroscope is then replaced, and the ureteropelvic junction is again inspected. A laser fiber is then placed through the ureteroscope, and the incision is made with holmium laser at settings of 1.2 J and 15 Hz, moving superiorly to inferiorly across the obstructed area. More than one pass may be required, and the incision should be taken down until peri-ureteral adipose tissue is seen (Figs. 7.7 and 7.8). Once this has been achieved, a balloon dilator measuring 6 or 7 mm is placed and inflated in order to further dilate the area. A stent is then placed for at least 6 weeks. Patients can typically be discharged the same day.

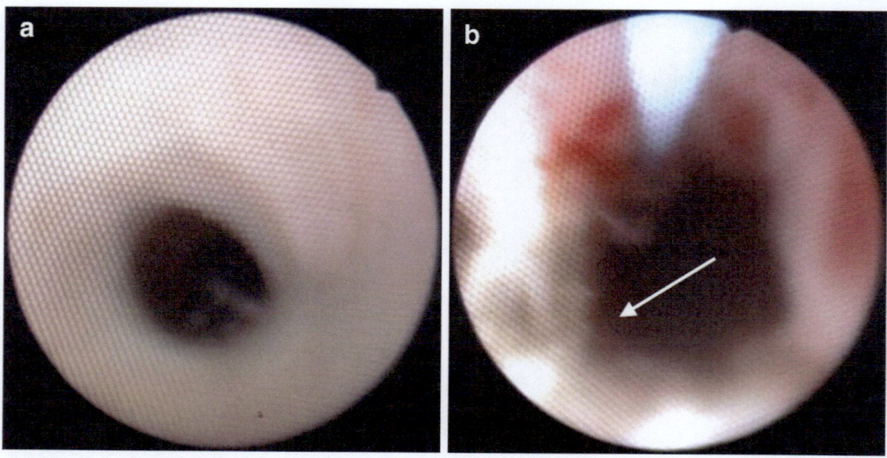

Fig. 7.7 (**a**) Ureteroscopic view of ischemic stenosis at the right ureteropelvic junction (UPJ). (**b**) Right UPJ after laser incision in the posterior-lateral position. Note the incision has been taken down to peri-ureteral adipose (white arrow)

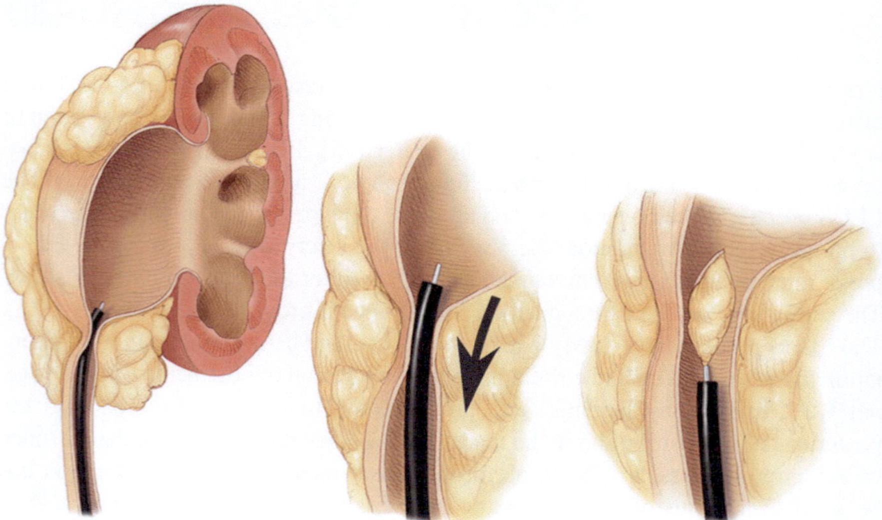

Fig. 7.8 Schematic shows the approach to retrograde ureteroscopic endopyelotomy for UPJ obstruction. The flexible ureteroscope is advanced above the UPJ under direct vision. The incision is carried down moving from a superior position to an inferior one until peri-ureteral adipose tissue is reached. Of note, it may take multiple passes for this outcome to be achieved. It is important to carry the incision in the exact same location, always moving from a superior to inferior position. (With permissions from "© M. Grasso, D. H. Bagley / KARL STORZ SE & Co. KG, Germany")

Outcomes

Multiple published single-center experiences provide outcome data for ureteroscopic endopyelotomy with a great deal of heterogeneity in terms of patient population, method of incision, definitions of success, and length of follow-up. A recent systematic review of the contemporary literature on retrograde ureteroscopic endopyelotomy found a pooled success rate of 79% for primary UPJ obstruction and 71% for secondary UPJ obstructions with mean follow-up of 29 months [26]. Generally, when reported, cases of intrinsic obstruction had higher success rates compared to those with crossing vessels, and if the procedure failed, it would usually occur within 2 years' time or sooner.

In terms of secondary UPJ obstruction, multiple retrospective series made up of small numbers of patients describe patency rates between 70% and 83% with follow-up between 15 and 47 months [27–29]. Interestingly, in a non-randomized retrospective study, Vannahme et al. found better patency rates in patients with secondary UPJ obstruction treated with salvage laparoscopic pyeloplasty compared to those treated with endopyelotomy, 87.5% versus 44%, respectively [11]. This was regardless of the primary procedure used to treat the original UPJ obstruction. Importantly, they noted that some of the patients, who had initially failed primary pyeloplasty, still were found to have anterior crossing vessels present during salvage pyeloplasty. This highlights the need for extensive preoperative workup of referred patients with secondary UPJ obstruction following pyeloplasty and the importance of not assuming that transposition of crossing vessels had been routinely performed.

Ureteral Stricture

Etiology

Similar to UPJ obstructions, ureteral strictures can be congenital, but acquired strictures are much more common. Acquired ureteral strictures are further categorized into malignant or benign etiologies. Upper tract urothelial carcinoma (UTUC) is primary malignancy of the ureter and is not uncommonly seen by endourologists. Most times, UTUC of ureteral origin will manifest with an obvious luminal component such as a papillary tumor but rarely will present as a tight, indurated, luminal narrowing, possibly resulting in hydronephrosis. A high index of suspicion for UTUC should exist in elderly patients when no other obvious etiology for ureteral stricture formation is present, especially when history of tobacco use or personal history of urothelial carcinoma of the bladder is present. These strictures should be thoroughly biopsied and closely followed even if initial biopsies are unrevealing.

Secondary malignancies can cause ureteral obstruction either from direct metastatic involvement or extrinsic compression either directly or from adjacent lymphadenopathy. Malignant ureteral stricture disease should be treated with either surgical removal, if indicated, or conservatively with either stent or percutaneous drainage, depending on the individual aspects of the case including cancer prognosis, renal function, and comorbidities.

Benign ureteral strictures have many etiologies but can also be further classified as ischemic or non-ischemic. Ischemic strictures commonly follow pelvic radiation for malignancy or surgery requiring dissection near the ureter [30]; both instances can negatively affect blood supply in the vicinity of the ureter. Other characteristics of ureteral strictures, which will affect treatment choice, include stricture length and location along the ureter. The sacroiliac (SI) joint serves as a well-known and convenient anatomic landmark, easily noted on fluoroscopy, to define sections of the ureter [31]. By convention, the area above the SI joint defines the proximal ureter, while the ureter below the SI joint is designated as distal. The length of the ureter, which lies along the SI joint, is the mid-ureter.

Patient Selection

As mentioned above, malignant ureteral strictures are not well suited to endoureterotomy. In UTUC, if curative intent is the goal and malignant stricture is present, segmental ureterectomy or radical nephroureterectomy needs to be considered and can be performed with open, laparoscopic, or robotic approaches. Secondary malignancies causing ureteral stricture or obstruction may benefit from the same approach or, depending on the unique situation, may benefit from drainage either with an indwelling stent or percutaneous drain.

According to multiple contemporary reviews of endoureterotomy series [30, 32, 33], the best surgical candidates are those with benign, non-ischemic, short (< 2 cm) segments, in the distal or proximal ureter with relatively robust split renal function (> 20%). In patients with diminished split renal function, endoureterotomy may be attempted in lieu of a major reconstructive procedure, but ultimately, nephrectomy is likely the best option, especially if there is persistent infection or pain from obstruction. For patients with benign ureteral strictures longer than 2 cm and robust split renal function, a formal reconstruction should be considered, and the approach will depend on the location of the obstruction. Open [34–36], laparoscopic [37], and robotic approaches [38] offer great versatility when formal reconstruction is needed. The recent incorporation of buccal mucosal grafts allows for the minimally invasive treatment of proximal and mid-ureteral strictures up to 5 cm in length [39]. Nevertheless, the appeal of endoureterotomy lies in its minimally invasive approach and low morbidity, especially in those patients in whom abdominal surgery would present a high risk.

Surgical Technique

Cystoscopy with retrograde pyelogram is performed with fluoroscopy in order to define stricture characteristics (length and location), as well as degree of obstruction and ureteral dilation/tortuosity. Retrograde access is then obtained using a PTFE or hydrophilic tip wire as necessary. Direct inspection of the ureter is then made with either flexible or semi-rigid ureteroscopy, as needed. Repeat retrograde pyelogram can then be performed directly through the ureteroscope, if needed to further clarify stricture characteristics. The ureteroscope is then advanced beyond the stricture until the normal ureteral lumen is encountered. This might require a stiff wire through the channel of the ureteroscope or calibration with a ureteral dilator. At times, balloon dilation is necessary in order to facilitate ureteroscope advancement. Once the entire length of stricture has been inspected, then endoscopic incision can be made. Options for this step include cold-knife or electrocautery incision, although holmium (Ho) laser is the preferred contemporary modality at most institutions. Ho laser settings for incision are 1.2 J and 15 Hz. In order to avoid violation of adjacent blood vessels, the direction of the proposed incision will depend on the location of the stricture along the length of the ureter. For proximal ureteral strictures, the incision is made laterally, while for distal ureteral strictures, the incision will be made relatively medially. For incisions that lie over the iliac artery, the incision should be made anteriorly. The incision should be made deep enough to see peri-ureteral adipose tissue. Dilation should then be performed over the incised area with a 6- or 7-mm balloon. Either a relatively large diameter stent or alternatively two parallel stents should then be placed for at least 6 weeks.

Outcomes

Reported success rates for endoureterotomy in well-selected patients range from 60% to 86% with follow-up ranging between 12 and 60 months, depending on the series [30, 33]. Higher patency rates are noted in non-ischemic strictures of relatively shorter length [40]. Significant complications are relatively rare. Patients should be carefully followed up for either clinical or radiographic evidence of recurrent obstruction.

Conclusion

Although less frequently indicated today for upper urinary tract obstruction, retrograde ureteroscopic endopyelotomy and endoureterotomy remain well-studied, safe, and effective treatment options. This is particularly true for patients who are not ideal candidates for laparoscopic or open reconstructive procedures. Since long-term patency rates are superior in formal reconstructions, these procedures should be considered the gold standard, especially since the majority of them can be performed laparoscopically with or without robotic assistance.

References

1. Yanke BV, Lallas CD, Pagnani C, McGinnis DE, Bagley DH. The minimally invasive treatment of ureteropelvic junction obstruction: a review of our experience during the last decade. J Urol. 2008;180:1397–402.
2. Dimarco DS, Gettman MT, McGee SM, Chow GK, Leroy AJ, Slezak J, et al. Long-term success of antegrade endopyelotomy compared with pyeloplasty at a single institution. J Endourol. 2006;20:707–12.
3. Williams B, Tareen B, Resnick MI. Pathophysiology and treatment of ureteropelvic junction obstruction. Curr Urol Rep. 2007;8:111–7.
4. Cancian M, Pareek G, Caldamone A, Aguiar L, Wang H, Amin A. Histopathology in ureteropelvic junction obstruction with and without crossing vessels. Urology. 2017;107:209–13.
5. Zeltser IS, Liu JB, Bagley DH. The incidence of crossing vessels in patients with normal ureteropelvic junction examined with endoluminal ultrasound. J Urol. 2004;172:2304–7.
6. Rooks VJ, Lebowitz RL. Extrinsic ureteropelvic junction obstruction from a crossing renal vessel: demography and imaging. Pediatr Radiol. 2001;31:120–4.
7. Van Cangh PJ, Nesa S, Galeon M, Tombal B, Wese FX, Dardenne AN, et al. Vessels around the ureteropelvic junction: significance and imaging by conventional radiology. J Endourol. 1996;10:111–9.
8. Conlin MJ, Bagley DH. Ureteroscopic endopyelotomy at a single setting. J Urol. 1998;159:727–31.
9. Giddens JL, Grasso M. Retrograde ureteroscopic endopyelotomy using the holmium: YAG laser. J Urol. 2000;164:1509–12.
10. Hendrikx AJ, Nadorp S, De Beer N, Van Beekum JB, Gravas S. The use of endoluminal ultrasonography for preventing significant bleeding during endopyelotomy: evaluation of helical computed tomography vs endoluminal ultrasonography for detecting crossing vessels. BJU. 2006;97:786–90.
11. Vannahme M, Mathur S, Davenport K, Timoney AG, Keeley FX. The management of secondary pelvi-ureteric junction obstruction – a comparison of pyeloplasty and endopyelotomy. BJU. 2014;113:108–12.
12. Davis DM, Strong GH, Drake WM. Intubated ureterotomy: experimental work and clinical results. J Urol. 1948;59:851–62.
13. Wickham JE, Kellet MJ. Percutaneous pyelolysis. Eur Urol. 1983;9:122–4.
14. Gupta M, Tuncay OL, Smith AD. Open surgical exploration after failed endopyelotomy: a 12-year perspective. J Urol. 1997;157:1613–9.
15. Bagley DH, Huffman J, Lyon E, McNamara T. Endoscopic ureteropyelostomy: opening the obliterated ureteropelvic junction with nephroscopy and flexible ureteroscopy. J Urol. 1985;133:462–4.
16. Inglis JA, Tolley DA. Ureteroscopic pyelolysis for pelviureteric junction obstruction. BJU. 1986;58:250–2.
17. Schuessler WW, Grune MT, Tecuanhuey LV, Preminger GM. Laparoscopic dismembered pyeloplasty. J Urol. 1993;150:1795–9.
18. Jarrett TW, Chan DY, Charambura TC, Fugita O, Kavoussi LR. Laparoscopic pyeloplasty: the first 100 cases. J Urol. 2002;167:1253–6.

19. Herrmann TRW, Liatsikos EN, Nagele U, Traxer O, Merseburger AS. EAU guidelines on laser technologies. Eur Urol. 2012;61:783–95.
20. Van Cangh PJ, Nesa S, Galeon M, Tombal B, Wese FX, Dardenne AN, et al. Vessels around the ureteropelvic junction: significance and imaging by conventional radiology. J Endourol. 1996;10(2):111–9.
21. Keeley FX, Moussa SA, Miller J, Tolley DA. Prospective study of endoluminal ultrasound versus computerized tomography angiography for detecting crossing vessels at that ureteropelvic junction. J Urol. 1999;162:1938–41.
22. Nakada SY, Wolf JS, Brink JA, Quillen SP, Nadler RB, Gaines MV, et al. Retrospective analysis of the effect of crossing vessels on successful retrograde endopyelotomy outcomes using spiral computerized tomography angiography. J Urol. 1998;159:62–5.
23. Sampaio FJ. Vascular anatomy at the ureteropelvic junction. Urol Clin North Am. 1998;25:251–8.
24. Tawfiek ER, Liu JB, Bagley DH. Ureteroscopic treatment of ureteropelvic junction obstruction. J Urol. 1998;160:1643–7.
25. Bagley DH, Liu JB. Endoureteral sonography to define the anatomy of the obstructed ureteropelvic junction. Urol Clin North Am. 1998;25:271–9.
26. Elmussareh M, Traxer O, Somani BK, Biyani CS. Laser endopyelotomy in the management of pelviureteric junction obstruction in adults: a systematic review of the literature. Urology. 2017;107:11–22.
27. Geavlete P, Georgescu D, Mirciulescu V, Nita G. Ureteroscopic laser approach in recurrent ureteropelvic junction stenosis. Eur Urol. 2007;51:1542–8.
28. Park J, Kim WS, Hong B, Park T, Park HK. Long-term outcome of secondary endopyelotomy after failed primary intervention for ureteropelvic junction obstruction. Int J Urol. 2008;15:490–4.
29. Acher PL, Nair R, Abburaju JS, Dickinson IK, Vohra A, Sriprasad S. Ureteroscopic holmium laser endopyelotomy for ureteropelvic junction stenosis after pyeloplasty. J Endourol. 2009;23:899–902.
30. Hafez KS, Wolf S. Update of minimally invasive management of ureteral strictures. J Endourol. 2003;17:453–64.
31. Faerber G, Lebastchi AH, Jen RP. Ureteral anatomy. In: Smith AD, Preminger GM, Kavoussi LR, Badlani GH, editors. Smith's textbook of endourology. Oxford: Wiley-Blackwell; 2019. p. 455–64.
32. Lucas JW, Ghiraldi E, Ellis J, Friedlander JI. Endoscopic management of ureteral strictures: an update. Curr Urol Rep. 2018;19:24. https://doi.org/10.1007/s11934-018-0773-4.
33. Emiliani E, Breda A. Laser endoureterotomy and endopyelotomy: an update. World J Urol. 2015;33:583–7.
34. Wenske S, Olsson CA, Benson MC. Outcomes of distal ureteral reconstruction through reimplantation with psoas hitch, Boari flap, or ureteroneocystostomy for benign or malignant ureteral obstruction or injury. Urology. 2013;82:231–6.
35. Roth JD, Monn MF, Szymanski KM, Bihrle R, Mellon MJ. Ureteral reconstruction with ileum: long-term follow-up of renal function. Urology. 2017;104:225–9.
36. Wotkowicz C, Libertino JA. Renal autotransplantation. BJUI. 2004;93:253–7.
37. Simmons MN, Gill IS, Fergany AF, Kaouk JH, Desai MM. Laparoscopic ureteral reconstruction for benign stricture disease. Urology. 2007;69:280–4.
38. Schiavina R, Zaramella S, Chessa F, Pultrone CV, Borghesi M, Minervini A, et al. Laparoscopic and robotic ureteral stenosis repair: a multi-institutional experience with a long-term follow-up. J Robotic Surg. 2016;10:323–30.
39. Lee Z, Waldorf BT, Cho EY, Liu JC, Metro MJ, Eun DD. Robotic ureteroplasty with buccal mucosa graft for the management of complex ureteral strictures. J Urol. 2017;198:1430–5.
40. Gnessin E, Yossepowitch O, Holland R, Livne PM, Lifshitz DA. Holmium laser endoureterotomy for benign ureteral stricture: a single center experience. J Urol. 2009;182:2775–9.

Chapter 8
Ureteroscopic Treatment of Chronic Unilateral Hematuria

Abhay A. Singh, Scott G. Hubosky, Ryuta Tanimoto, and Demetrius H. Bagley

Introduction

Flexible ureteroscopy provides diagnostic information and allows for control of upper urinary tract hemorrhage from both benign and malignant etiologies. Chronic unilateral hematuria (CUH) refers to gross hematuria that lateralizes to an upper tract source and is diagnosed by bloody efflux from a ureteral orifice on cystoscopy without an obvious radiographic etiology or oncologic origin. Over the years, CUH has also been referred to in the literature as benign essential hematuria, lateralizing essential hematuria, benign lateralizing hematuria, unilateral primary hematuria, unilateral essential hematuria, and idiopathic renal bleeding. The etiology of CUH can be defined with ureteroscopic assessment and broadly be categorized as a discrete lesion (s), diffuse lesions, or no identifiable lesion. Our experience reflects that the vast majority of cases can be diagnosed and managed with ureteroscopic laser ablation or diathermy fulguration.

A. A. Singh · S. G. Hubosky (✉)
Department of Urology, Sidney Kimmel Medical College at Thomas Jefferson University Hospital, Philadelphia, PA, USA
e-mail: Abhay.singh@jefferson.edu; Scott.Hubosky@jefferson.edu

D. H. Bagley
Department of Urology and Radiology, Sidney Kimmel Medical College at Thomas Jefferson University Hospital, Philadelphia, PA, USA
e-mail: Demetrius.BagleyJr@jefferson.edu

R. Tanimoto
Department of Urology, Graduate School of Medicine, Dentistry & Pharmaceutical Sciences, Okayama University, Okayama, Japan

© Springer Nature Switzerland AG 2022
S. G. Hubosky et al. (eds.), *Advanced Ureteroscopy*,
https://doi.org/10.1007/978-3-030-82351-1_8

Etiology

As is the standard of care for patients with gross hematuria, work-up begins with cross-sectional imaging and cystoscopy. Whenever clinically possible, CT urogram should be obtained. MR urogram can be substituted in patients with suboptimal renal function. If neither of the above is acceptable, a renal ultrasound may be obtained with subsequent retrograde pyelography. The diagnosis of CUH is predicated on a radiological exam that does not find an overt upper urinary tract etiology for the hematuria in combination with a cystoscopic examination, which demonstrates gross hematuria emanating from one or both ureteral orifice(s). At this juncture, flexible ureteroscopy is indicated to help with diagnosis and treatment.

The potential etiologies of CUH include peripapillary varices, often referred to as minute venous ruptures (MVRs), renal hemangioma, upper tract urothelial cancer or stones not detected by standard imaging, exercise-induced hematuria, fibroepithelial polyps, arteriovenous fistula, and papillary necrosis. As mentioned before, classification can split into discrete lesions, diffuse lesions, and no identifiable lesions. A recent review of the world literature on ureteroscopic evaluation of CUH reported 73% of 288 reported cases were secondary to a discrete lesion, while no lesion or etiology was identifiable in 16% [1].

While all are rare, the most common discrete lesions in the kidneys are minute venous ruptures and renal hemangiomas. In the ureter, fibroepithelial polyps and hemangiomas can be present. When a discrete lesion is identified, a biopsy should certainly be obtained if there is concern for malignancy. The most frequently encountered etiology of CUH, as documented by Araki et al. in the largest single-center experience compromising 22 years, was that of minute venous rupture (MVR), "a venous bleeding without clear abnormality" [2]. MVR is characterized by small lesions in the collecting system that result from fragile vasculature in the renal papilla or fornix [3]. In our experience, this is akin to peripapillary varices (Fig. 8.1). These entities are small, but sometimes, prominent blood vessels, which are found around the circumference of the papilla and ooze blood of a seemingly venous source. They can also arise from the papillary tips. A high index of suspicion should exist in patients presenting with CUH and very robust-appearing renal papilla on retrograde pyelogram (Fig. 8.2). A recent report of 75 patients with CUH noted that bleeding is more often seen in the upper or lower pole positions, specifically involving compound papillae in the majority of cases [4].

Hemangiomas of the urinary tract are rare and most occur in the kidney followed by the bladder and then ureter [5]. The lesions can vary in size from nearly invisible to several centimeters. They are usually solitary and found at the tips or bases of the papilla, in the mucosa, or subepithelial tissue [6]. Under direct vision with ureteroscopy, hemangiomas appear as a red- or blue-colored mulberry-like lesion or spherical mass with a vascular rich surface over the papilla [7] (Fig. 8.3). Another benign and even more rare neoplastic vascular lesion is anastomosing hemangioma. It can

Fig. 8.1 Fiberoptic flexible ureteroscopic view of peripapillary varices (black arrows) around the circumference of a renal papilla

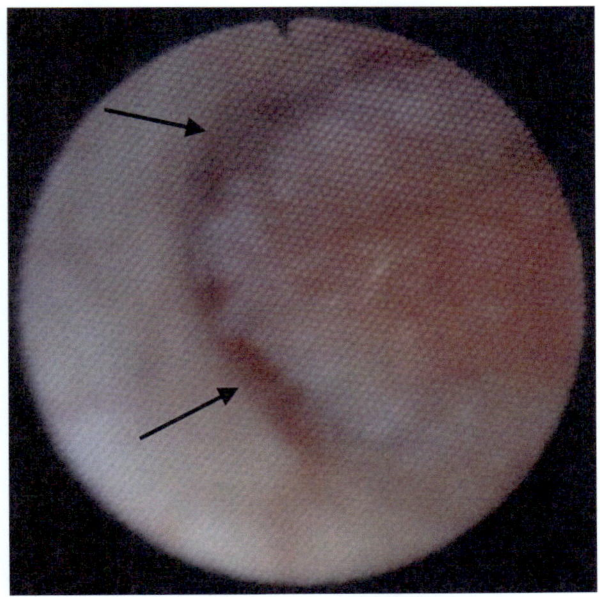

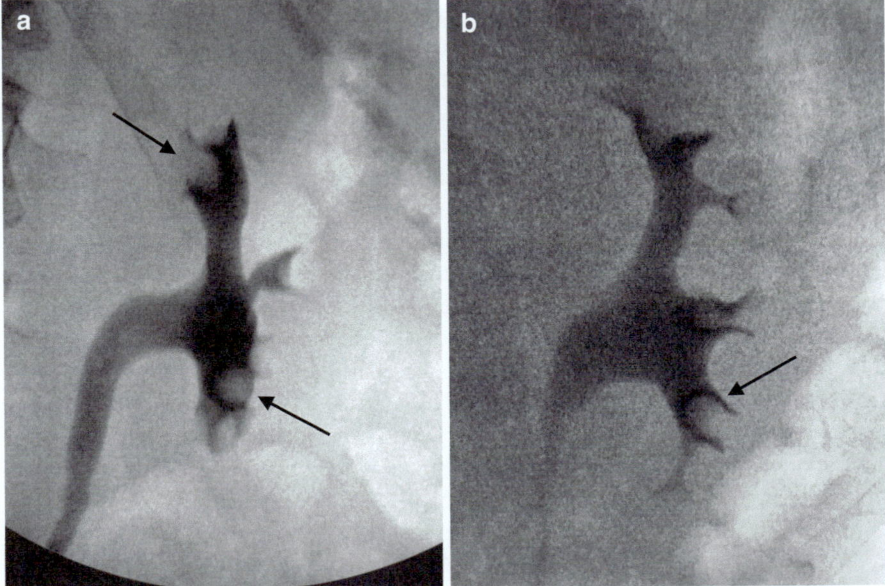

Fig. 8.2 (**a**, **b**) Retrograde pyelograms of patients with benign essential hematuria and very prominent renal papilla appearing as filling defects (black arrows). Peripapillary varices often are seen endoscopically around the circumference of prominent papilla

A. A. Singh et al.

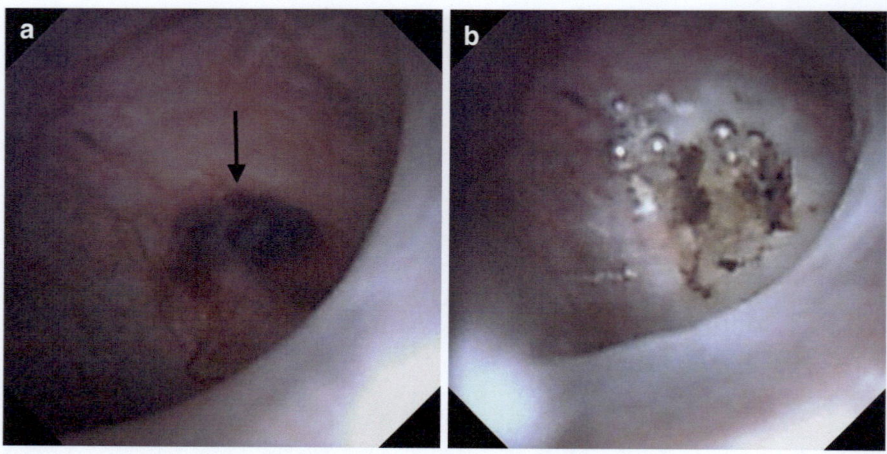

Fig. 8.3 (**a**) Digital ureteroscopic view of a renal hemangioma (black arrow) toward the periphery of a renal calyx. (**b**) Cauterization of hemangioma in same case

be found in various organs but was first described in the kidney where it is usually found in association with end- stage renal disease [8]. Histologically it resembles angiosarcoma.

Renal papillary necrosis (RPN) can manifest as gross or microhematuria and sometimes with obstruction if the papilla sloughs off the urothelial surface. Ischemic necrosis at the papilla is the end result of many potential etiologies such as diabetes and sickle cell disease or can be drug induced [9, 10]. RPN is most commonly associated with overuse of non-steroidal anti-inflammatory drugs (NSAIDS) and is due to inhibition of cyclooxygenase, which results in decreased prostaglandin production. As a result, vascular perfusion is decreased, leading to vasoconstriction and local ischemia [11]. The ureteroscopic appearance of papillary necrosis has recently been reported. On flexible ureteroscopy, the necrotic papillae have a white or grey color and appear cottony and friable. They can be freely floating in the collecting system or attached to the urothelial surface by a small pedicle [12]. Bleeding can be diffuse but usually limited to the calyx in which the papilla has sloughed.

There have been several case reports of diffuse lesions, but interestingly the prevalence of these has decreased dramatically with time such that there have not been any reported cases since 1999. This is presumably a reflection of the improvements in imaging and endoscopic technology such that once poorly defined collecting systems diagnosed as having nonspecific pyelitis can now be more accurately studied.

Potential sources of undefined lesions include exercise-induced hematuria. While gross hematuria is more common in contact sports, it can also occur secondary to physiologic changes during exercise. Endurance sports especially can lead to shunting of blood away from the kidneys with resulting hypoxic nephron damage and increased glomerular permeability along with vasoconstriction of efferent glomerular arterioles resulting in excretion of red cells [13].

Diagnosis

The first description of endoscopy to aid in the diagnosis of CUH was from 1981, when Gittes described the placement of an angled rigid nephroscope through a small pyelotomy in patients undergoing open exploration [14]. The endoscopic visualization of discrete bleeding sites then guided definitive treatment, usually in the form of partial nephrectomy. With the evolution of improved instrumentation, the diagnosis and often treatment of CUH now rest on flexible ureteroscopy, independently and simultaneously reported in 1990 by both Bagley [15] and Kumon [16]. Their fundamental operative principles still are the essence of contemporary practice.

The ureter and collecting system require thorough visual examination in an atraumatic fashion. This is facilitated by practicing a "no-touch technique," which will increase the specificity of the procedure. Some authors prefer to utilize a narrow (<7Fr) semi-rigid ureteroscope, which is used to intubate the ureteral orifice under direct vision [17, 18]. The distal ureter is evaluated before introducing a guide wire. Once the ureteroscope travels past the iliac vessels, a guidewire can be deployed through the scope with care taken to only place the wire into the explored section of the ureter (to avoid iatrogenic trauma by the wire) after which the semi-rigid scope is exchanged for a flexible ureteroscope over the wire, under fluoroscopic guidance. The flexible ureteroscope is then advanced to examine the remainder of the ureter and the entire renal pelvis.

Another technique simply employs flexible ureteroscopy exclusively. This is possible due to improved durometer or shaft stiffness, particularly at the most distal portion of the flexible ureteroscope. The flexible instrument is passed into the ureteral orifice and up the ureter without the aid of a preceding semi-rigid scope or a wire. In some cases, buckling of the distal portion of the flexible ureteroscope will require a guidewire to facilitate access.

The diagnostic yield of ureteroscopy is felt to increase when active bleeding is present. Therefore, Mugiya and colleagues recommended patients be physically active and not to take bed rest prior to endoscopic evaluation [19]. While performing ureteroscopy it is important to ensure the irrigation pressure is not too great. This is important for two reasons. Higher pressure may obscure minute venous bleeding, and also higher-pressure irrigation may itself traumatize the collecting system. Araki et al. reported the use of a monitored irrigation pressure system to maintain pressure at 40 mmHg, which facilitated increased diagnostic yield of MVR and fewer unidentified lesions [2]. Irrigation by hand using syringes and tubing is perfectly acceptable, provided the surgical assistant appreciates the importance of utilizing gentle pressure and stays attentive during the case. If during ureteroscopic evaluation, there is no obvious source of hemorrhage, it is recommended to consider stopping irrigation [6] or creating a slight negative pressure by syringe aspiration through the working channel of the ureteroscope, in order to unmask subtle discrete bleeding points [4].

The careful and selective use of sterile water for irrigant rather than saline may also increase the diagnostic yield of ureteroscopy. Sterile water offers optical advantages as it lyses red blood cells, which in turn improve visibility and light transmission. Cybulski et al. showed that there is minimal fluid absorption during ureteroscopy, estimated to be 54 ml, for cases up to 83 minutes [20]. Even with pressures up to 200 mmHg and in the event of ureteral perforations, it appears the fluid absorbed is a fraction of the volume typically associated with a risk of TUR syndrome [21]. The volume of fluid absorbed during URS is far less than that expected during a TURP (150–3600 mL) or a PCNL (50–2200 mL) [20]. In a contemporary study of the safety of sterile water as an irrigant during ureteroscopy, Pirani et al. prospectively randomized 139 patients to water versus saline irrigation during ureteroscopy for laser lithotripsy. For cases taking up to 63 minutes at maximum and utilizing up to 1450 mL of irrigation, they found no difference in the safety profile of water while noting a significant visual advantage compared to saline, based on both objective turbidity clarity and subjective surgeon visualization scores [22]. Therefore, careful and conservative use of sterile water in ureteroscopic cases in which luminal bleeding is anticipated can provide a clear technical advantage without detriment to the patient.

Treatment

The majority of lesions responsible for CUH, namely, MVRs and hemangiomas, can be treated via ureteroscopy with fulguration or laser ablation. Fulguration is usually performed with a 2- or 3-French ureteroscopic electrode set at 10 watts in coagulation mode (Figs. 8.4 and 8.5). Using the minimal amount of power possible will optimize hemostasis, since higher levels will induce the electrode tip to stick to the cauterized tissue surface, which will re-bleed when the electrode is pulled back. Options for laser treatment include holmium:YAG and neodymium:YAG lasers. Holmium:YAG penetrates tissue <0.5 mm whereas neodymium has an affinity for hemoglobin and can penetrate tissue to a depth of 5 mm. Brito addressed lesions with a 200-μm holmium:YAG laser with settings of 1.0 J and 8 Hz [6]. ND:YAG is used at powers of 15–30 W [3, 23].

Hemangiomas can spontaneously regress as a result of fibrosclerosis, so observation is a potential option in the minimally symptomatic patient [5]. As mentioned above, ureteroscopy is a logical first-line intervention since it offers diagnosis and potential treatment with fulguration and is appropriate for most encountered lesions. For the rare lesion too large for endoscopic treatment, selective embolization can be performed, when the diagnosis of benign hemangioma is confirmed [24, 25]. Formal surgical excision can be considered if there is any doubt that malignancy might coexist. This translates to partial or complete nephrectomy for renal lesions [26, 27] or segmental ureterectomy in the ureter [28].

Ureteroscopic treatment is associated with high rates of success for discrete lesions. A 2017 review of prior CUH literature found a 95% success rate [1]. There

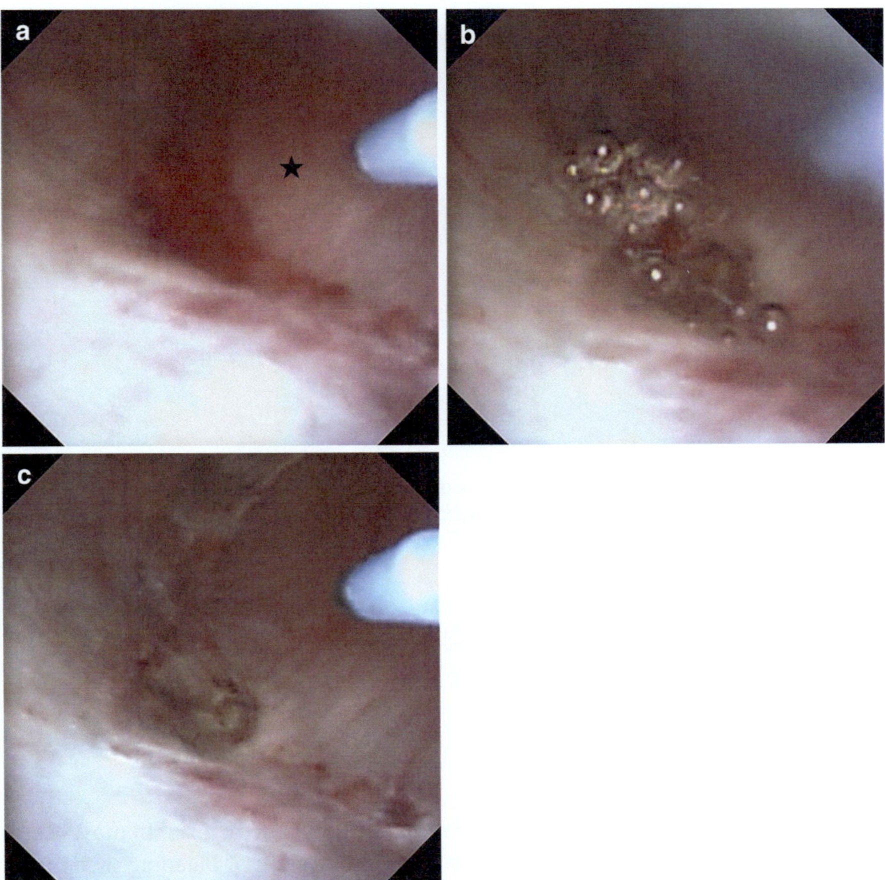

Fig. 8.4 (**a**) Digital ureteroscopic image of hemorrhage from peripapillary varices around the partial circumference of a renal papilla (black star marks papilla). A 2-French electrode is seen extending from the 3 o'clock position of the ureteroscope. (**b**) Hemorrhagic area immediately after cauterization. (**c**) Peripapillary hemorrhage now well hemostatic following cauterization

is not a standardized algorithm for follow-up after ureteroscopic treatment of CUH. Brito and coworkers performed urinalysis at 1, 3, 6, and 12 months and then annually [7]. Anecdotally, we have observed that certain patient behaviors in this population of benign bleeders can trigger recurrence of gross hematuria such as heavy lifting, high-impact exercise, or uncontrolled hypertension. Lifestyle modification can decrease bleeding recurrence.

If a lesion is not amenable to endoscopic treatment secondary to size or a diffuse process, then consideration can be made for topical or oral treatments. Silver nitrate has been used in the collecting system (10 mL of 0.25–1%) but has become a rare treatment in part related to potential, serious side effects to include sepsis, ureteral stricture, and interstitial nephritis [2]. Oral treatment with aminocaproic acid can be

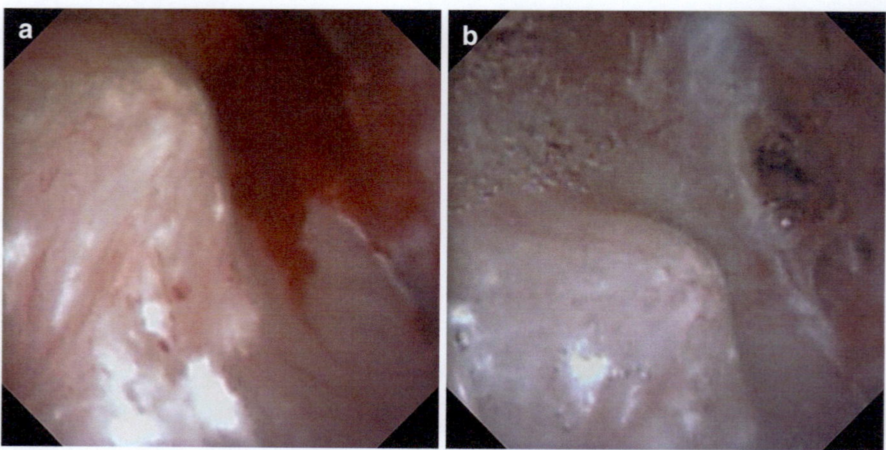

Fig. 8.5 (**a**) Hemorrhage is noted on the right-sided periphery of this renal calyx with papilla present in the center of the calyx. (**b**) Peripheral bleeder is effectively hemostatic after ureteroscopic cauterization

successful but also has a potential adverse safety profile to include microangiopathic thrombosis and clot obstruction [29, 30].

Conclusion

Ureteroscopy is necessary to diagnosis chronic unilateral hematuria. In most cases, ureteroscopy will result in effective treatment and cessation of bleeding with precision coagulation as provided by cautery or laser. Meticulous no-touch ureteroscopic technique with relatively low irrigation pressures and careful use of sterile water as an irrigant can maximize successful outcomes.

References

1. Tanimoto R, Kumon H, Bagley DH. Development of endoscopic diagnosis and treatment for chronic unilateral hematuria: 35 years experience. J Endourol. 2017;31:S76–80.
2. Araki M, Uehara S, Sasaki K, Monden K, Tsugawa M, Watanabe T, et al. Ureteroscopic management of chronic unilateral hematuria: a single-center experience over 22 years. PLoS One. 2012;7:e36729.
3. Rowbotham C, Anson KM. Benign lateralizing haematuria: the impact of upper tract endoscopy. BJU Int. 2001;88:841–9.
4. Waseda Y, Takazawa R, Kobayashi M, Tsujii T. Chronic unilateral hematuria: compound papillae are likely to bleed. J Endourol. 2021; Ahead of print: https://doi.org/10.1089/end.2020.0783.

5. Jahn H, Nissen HM. Haemangioma of the urinary tract: review of the literature. Br J Urol. 1991;68:113–7.

6. Hagen A. Renal angioma. Four cases of angioma of the renal pelvis. Acta Chir Scand. 1963;126:657–67.

7. Brito AH, Mazzucchi E, Vicentini FC, Danilovic A, Chedid Neto EA, Srougi M. Management of chronic unilateral hematuria by ureterorenoscopy. J Endourol. 2009;23:1273–6.

8. Lappa E, Drakos E. Anastomosing hemangioma: short review of a benign mimicker of angiosarcoma. Arch Pathol Lab Med. 2020;144:240–4.

9. Bach PH, Nguyen TK. Renal papillary necrosis--40 years on. Toxicol Pathol. 1998;26:73–91.

10. Henderickx M, Brits T, De Baets K, Seghers M, Maes P, Trouet D, et al. Renal papillary necrosis in patients with sickle cell disease: how to recognize this 'forgotten' diagnosis. J Pediatr Urol. 2017;13:250–6.

11. Brix AE. Renal papillary necrosis. Toxicol Pathol. 2002;30:672–4.

12. Panach-Navarrete J, Medina-Gonzalez M, Alarcon-Molero L, Sanchez-Cano E, Pastor-Hernandez F, Martinez-Jabaloyas JM. Renal papillary necrosis, an endoscopic vision. Scand J Urol. 2019;53:361–3.

13. Akiboye RD, Sharma DM. Haematuria in sport: a review. Eur Urol Focus. 2019;5:912–6.

14. Gittes RF, Varady S. Nephroscopy in chronic unilateral hematuria. J Urol. 1981;126:297–300.

15. Bagley DH, Allen J. Flexible ureteropyeloscopy in the diagnosis of benign essential hematuria. J Urol. 1990;143:549–53.

16. Kumon H, Tsugawa M, Matsumura Y, Ohmori H. Endoscopic diagnosis and treatment of chronic unilateral hematuria of uncertain etiology. J Urol. 1990;143:554–8.

17. Abdel-Razzak OM, Ehya H, Cubler-Goodman A, Bagley DH. Ureteroscopic biopsy in the upper urinary tract. Urology. 1994;44:451–7.

18. Tawfiek E, Bibbo M, Bagley DH. Ureteroscopic biopsy: technique and specimen preparation. Urology. 1997;50:117–9.

19. Mugiya S, Ozono S, Nagata M, Takayama T, Furuse H, Ushiyama T. Ureteroscopic evaluation and laser treatment of chronic unilateral hematuria. J Urol. 2007;178:517–20.

20. Cybulski P, Honey RJ, Pace K. Fluid absorption during ureterorenoscopy. J Endourol. 2004;18:739–42.

21. Hahn RG. Fluid absorption in endoscopic surgery. Br J Anaesth. 2006;96:8–20.

22. Pirani F, Makhani SS, Kim FY, Lay AH, Cimmino CB, Hartsell L, et al. Prospeective randomized trial comparing the safety and clarity of water versus saline irrigant in ureteroscopy. Eur Urol Focus. 2020;S2405-4569(20):30066.

23. Tawfiek ER, Bagley DH. Ureteroscopic evaluation and treatment of chronic unilateral hematuria. J Urol. 1998;160:700–2.

24. Lang EK, Atug F, Thomas R. Selective embolization of capillary hemangioma of the renal papilla. J Urol. 2007;177:1146.

25. Laucirica O, Izquierdo F, Marti J, Laguna P, Palou J, Vicente J. Renal hemangiomas: a clinical case and review of the literature. Actas Urol Esp. 1992;16:366–70.

26. Ceccarelli G, Codacci Pisanelli M, Patriti A, Biancafarina A. Renal cavernous hemangioma: robot-assisted partial nephrectomy with selective warm ischemia. Case report and review of the literature. G Chir. 2015;36:197–200.

27. Zhao X, Zhang J, Zhong Z, Koh CJ, Xie HW, Hardy BE. Large renal cavernous hemangioma with renal vein thrombosis: case report and review of literature. Urology. 2009;73:443 e1–3.

28. Tak GR, Agrawal S, Desai MR, Ganpule AP, Singh AG, Sabnis RB. Hemangioma of ureter: a diagnostic dilemma-managed surgically using robotic platform. J Endourol Case Rep. 2020;6:128–31.

29. Nash DA Jr, Henry AR. Unilateral essential hematuria. Therapy with epsilon aminocaproic acid. Urology. 1984;23:297–8.

30. Stefanini M, English HA, Taylor AE. Safe and effective, prolonged administration of epsilon aminocaproic acid in bleeding from the urinary tract. J Urol. 1990;143:559–61.

Chapter 9
Antegrade Ureteroscopy

Anthony T. Tokarski and Demetrius H. Bagley

Introduction

Antegrade ureteroscopy is usually not the first choice as an approach to a ureteral lesion but is extremely useful in certain circumstances. When the distal ureter is completely obstructed or severely compromised or altered, the antegrade approach may be the only choice. The need for percutaneous renal access is necessary for this approach. The indications, instruments, and techniques for antegrade ureteroscopy are considered.

Indications

There is a wide range of indications for antegrade ureteroscopy, some nearly mandatory and others more elective. For example, severe distal ureteral damage or obliteration with a more proximal target lesion renders the antegrade approach preferable. Similarly, bladder diversion or ureteral reimplantation can make retrograde ureteroscopy problematic and favor antegrade access. One of the more common indications is residual calculi after percutaneous nephrolithotomy. The decision for the direction of ureteroscopy is then based on the stone burden, location, collecting system morphology, as well as patient factors related to positioning. These and other considerations are discussed in detail.

A. T. Tokarski (✉)
Department of Urology, Sidney Kimmel Medical College at Thomas Jefferson University Hospital, Philadelphia, PA, USA
e-mail: Anthony.Tokarski@jefferson.edu

D. H. Bagley
Department of Urology and Radiology, Sidney Kimmel Medical College at Thomas Jefferson University Hospital, Philadelphia, PA, USA
e-mail: Demetrius.BagleyJr@jefferson.edu

© Springer Nature Switzerland AG 2022
S. G. Hubosky et al. (eds.), *Advanced Ureteroscopy*,
https://doi.org/10.1007/978-3-030-82351-1_9

Complete Ureteral Obstruction

Severe scarring can result in complete ureteral obstruction or obliteration of a ureteral segment. This has been reported after disruption of a surgical repair; severe inflammation from an impacted ureteral stone or with repetitive shockwave lithotripsy; proximal drainage with a dry, inflamed ureteral segment; and other rare episodes. Initial retrograde ureteroscopy may find the lesion and in some very short segments allow for recanalization. The situation may require an antegrade approach combined with retrograde ureteroscopy for recanalization. This technique was first described by Bagley et al., in two patients with a complete ureteropelvic junction obstruction [1]. Since that time, while scant data have been published, some authors have published larger case series showing the efficacy and safety of this procedure. Conlin and colleagues reported on a series of eight patients who underwent combined antegrade and retrograde ureteroscopy for the treatment of a complete ureteral obstruction secondary to iatrogenic or traumatic injury [2]. Many variations of this technique have been developed, including the rendezvous procedure, which involves the antegrade insertion of guidewires across the obliterated ureteral segment [3–5]. Similar to the approach used for posterior urethral strictures, the cut-to-the-light technique can be used for ureteral strictures and requires both antegrade and retrograde ureteroscopy [6–9].

From a technical standpoint, cut-to-the-light procedures, or endoscopic ureteroureterostomy or recanalizations of obliterated ureteral segments, should begin with simultaneous antegrade and retrograde pyelograms. Preferably these are performed with contrast placed through the endoscopes simultaneously with fluoroscopy available (Fig. 9.1). This defines the exact length and location of the obliterated segment, which will determine the likelihood of treatment success. Patients should be counseled appropriately in order to set realistic expectations. Obliterated segments >2 cm are usually not amenable to endoscopic recanalization (Fig. 9.2).

Once the obliterated segment has been defined, and it has been determined that the patient is a candidate for recanalization, simultaneous antegrade and retrograde ureteroscopy should be performed by two experienced ureteroscopists, with two separate endoscopic monitors and multi-planar fluoroscopy available. When the obliterated segment is sufficiently short, it is possible to see the illumination of one ureteroscope's light when the other has its light source disconnected (Fig. 9.3a). Therefore, a fiberoptic ureteroscope is necessary for this step, since digital ureteroscopes cannot separate image from light source. The "dark ureteroscope" is then used to perform laser incision "towards the light" of the second ureteroscope until the actual endoscope is seen in the ureteral lumen (Fig. 9.3b). Holmium laser set at 1.2 Joules and 15 Hertz serves well for this technique. Next, a wire should be placed under direct vision across the defect, followed by balloon dilation of the strictured segment and ultimately stent placement (Fig. 9.4) The durable ureteral patency rate in the published literature for this approach is between 44 and 75% (Table 9.1), and close follow-up is needed. If recurrent stricture is encountered, more definitive treatment with open, laparoscopic, or robotic surgery might be indicated versus

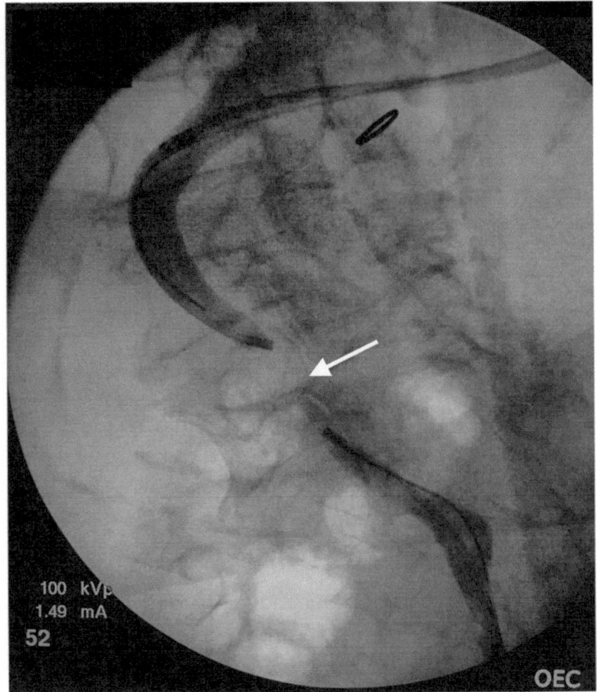

Fig. 9.1 Simultaneous antegrade and retrograde ureteroscopy allow for simultaneous contrast studies from above and below, which precisely define the length of the obliterated ureteral segment (arrow)

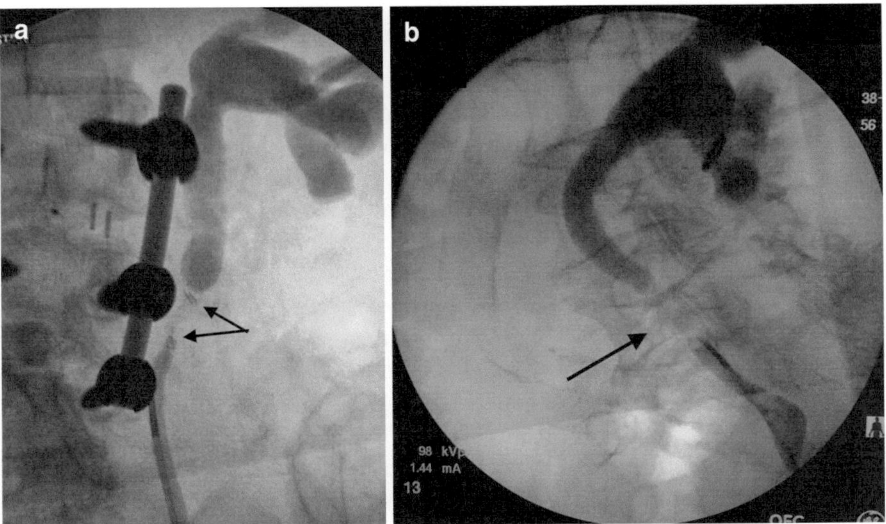

Fig. 9.2 (**a**) Simultaneous left antegrade nephrostogram and retrograde pyelogram show a long obliterated segment of the proximal ureter secondary to iatrogenic clipping and ligation of the ureter during spinal fusion surgery. Black arrows demonstrate the clips, responsible for the defect. (**b**) Another simultaneous antegrade and retrograde study defines a long segment of ureteral obliteration, not amenable to ureteroscopic recanalization

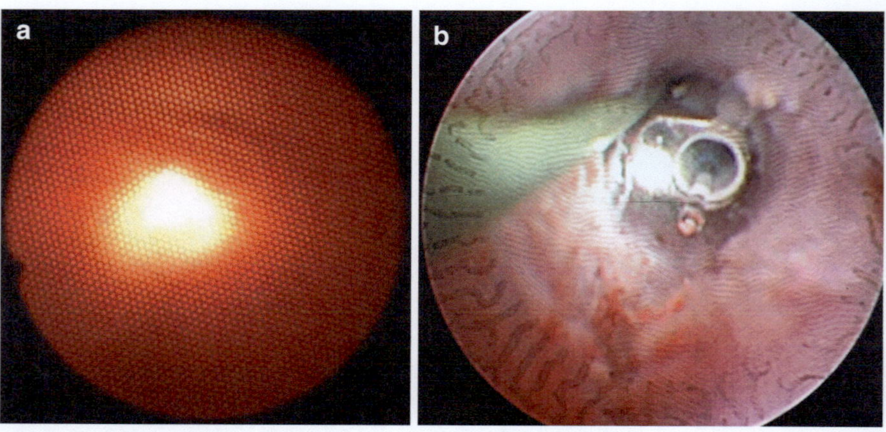

Fig. 9.3 (**a**) Ureteroscopic view of "cut-to-the-light" procedure during endoscopic ureteroureterostomy. The ureteroscopist doing the "cutting" must turn off their light source in order to see the light from the opposing ureteroscope. (**b**) After successful recanalization, the opposing ureteroscope tip can be clearly seen in the ureteral lumen

repetitive stent changes, depending on the treatment goal. At the very least, successful endoscopic ureteroureterostomy results in trading a long-term nephrostomy for internal ureteral stent drainage.

Difficulty Accessing the Ureteral Orifice

Patient anatomy, surgical or pathologic, can make accessing the ureteral orifice in a retrograde fashion difficult and can necessitate antegrade ureteroscopy. Urinary diversions (ileal conduit, orthotopic neobladder, pouch diversions) involve an ureteroenteric anastomosis, which may be difficult to identify with retrograde endoscopy. Further complicating matters is the development of a ureteroenteric anastomotic stricture which have an incidence of 2.6–13% following radical cystectomy with diversion [10] and can make retrograde access not feasible. In addition, metabolic derangements associated with intestinal absorption as well as bacterial colonization can predispose these patients to stone formation. Several authors have described safe and effective techniques of antegrade ureteroscopy to treat a variety of conditions. In a small consecutive series, Stuurman et al. were able to render 82.3% of patients stone-free in one procedure using an antegrade approach with minimal complications using the aid of a 28–30 Fr renal access sheath [11]. Other authors have also achieved good results in the prone position [12].

Pediatric patients with vesicoureteral reflex often require surgical correction, which will distort the anatomy of the ureteral orifice, particularly patients undergoing a Cohen cross-trigonal reimplant. Retrograde access has been reported in these

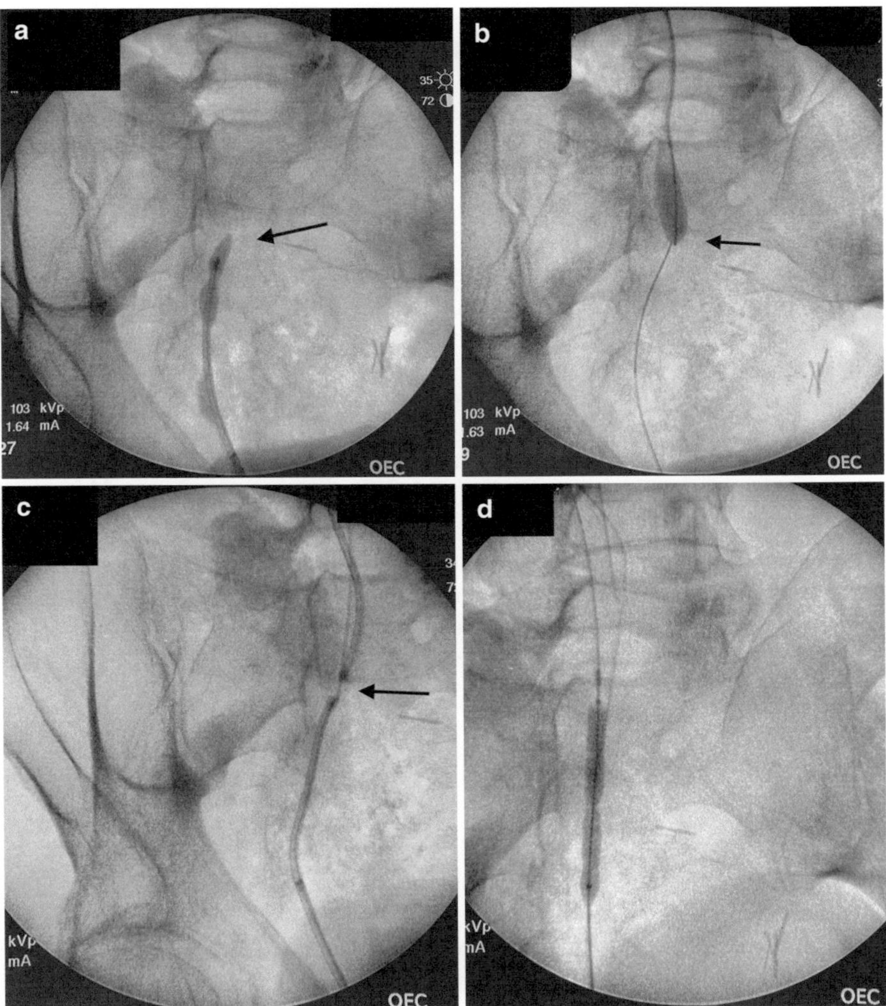

Fig. 9.4 (**a**) Right retrograde pyelogram demonstrates complete ureteral obstruction at upper aspect of distal ureter (arrow). (**b**) Right antegrade ureterogram confirms complete ureteral obstruction (black arrow). (**c**) Simultaneous antegrade and retrograde ureteroscopic evaluation clearly defines the relatively short length of ureteral obstruction (arrow). (**d**) Successful endoscopic ureteroureterostomy with subsequent balloon dilation showing wasting of strictured segment. Immediate stent placement followed full inflation with the balloon dilator

Table 9.1 Durable patency rates after cut-to-the-light and rendezvous procedures

Authors (year)	Number of patients	Durable patency rate
Conlin [2] (1996)	8	75%
Keoghane [3] (2019)	18	44%
Pastore [4] (2014)	18	67%
Watson [5] (2002)	15	47%
Lingeman [7] (1995)	9	44%
Lopatkin [40] (2000)	21	67%

patients but can prove difficult because of the angle required to place a guidewire across the ureteral orifice. Percutaneous antegrade ureteroscopy through a ureteral access sheath has been described as an effective option when the ureter cannot be accessed via a retrograde approach [13]. Antegrade ureteroscopy has also been employed when patients failed to pass stone fragments through the intramural potion of the reimplanted ureter after shockwave lithotripsy [14].

Accessing a transplant ureter in a retrograde fashion can be difficult as the ureteral orifice is not always readily identified and placement of the ureteroneocystostomy is not standardized. When a preexisting percutaneous tract was placed, Hyams et al. were able to successfully treat small ureteral or renal stone burdens with antegrade ureteroscopy in a non-dilated tract [15]. Larger series have found antegrade ureteroscopy to have a superior stone-free rate compared to shockwave lithotripsy [16]. Other authors have demonstrated the safety and efficacy of dilating a percutaneous tract to 14–15 Fr to facilitate antegrade ureteroscopy with a high stone-free rate [17]. With advances in flexible ureteroscopic techniques, antegrade approaches to dealing with pathology in renal transplants remains a useful tool for urologists [18].

Several other clinical scenarios exist that make identifying the ureteral office challenging. These include severe benign prostatic hyperplasia, cystoceles, ureteroceles, and invasive gynecologic malignancies. Antegrade ureteroscopy can provide a means of treating upper tract pathology that would otherwise not be feasible through a retrograde approach.

Proximal Ureteral Stones

Antegrade ureteroscopy is most commonly used as an adjuvant procedure, in conjunction with primary PCNL (percutaneous nephrolithotomy), to retrieve fragments of stone, which have passed into the proximal ureter. Although a rigid or flexible nephroscope may be used, a smaller-diameter flexible ureteroscope may be required depending on the size of the ureter. Large, impacted proximal ureteral stones can be difficult to treat completely with retrograde ureteroscopy, particularly when there is ureteral stricture or narrowing distal to the impacted stone. Ureteral inflammation can cause protrusion of the mucosa, surrounding the stone making it difficult to fragment and cause bleeding that can obscure visibility. Furthermore, stones large enough to cause significant hydronephrosis may retropulse into a dilated and capacious renal pelvis making fragmenting and extraction challenging. These factors can be mitigated by antegrade approaches to stone treatment. Historically, antegrade ureteroscopy for large proximal ureteral stones had been attempted as an alternative to open surgery [19], and early studies showed its safety and effectiveness in achieving stone clearance [20]. As equipment and techniques have evolved, this approach has become a more viable option for primary treatment and is included as a recommended approach in contemporary guidelines [21]. One randomized, controlled trial found that antegrade ureteroscopy with a semi-rigid ureteroscope had a higher stone-free rate when compared to retrograde ureteroscopy [22]. More recent series have demonstrated the safety and efficacy of achieving stone-free status with flexible antegrade ureteroscopy dilating the tract up to 30 Fr or as small as 15 Fr [23, 24].

Other Considerations

There are several other scenarios where antegrade ureteroscopy can be helpful in treating upper tract pathology. During percutaneous nephrolithotomy (PCNL), fragments may be displaced into the ureter, or patients may present with concomitant ureteral stones. Antegrade ureteroscopy allows for effective treatment without the time-consuming measure of repositioning the patient into dorsal lithotomy. The antegrade approach has also been proven useful in treating upper tract urothelial carcinoma, particularly in those patients with high-volume disease, technically challenging location such as dependent lower poles, and after urinary diversion [25, 26]. This technique has also been described in the treatment of large-volume fibroepithelial polyps of the renal pelvis and ureter [27].

Positioning

As with all urologic procedures, proper patient positioning is crucial when preparing for antegrade ureteroscopy (see Chap. 5). There are certain considerations that must be taken when preparing the patient for this procedure. When positioning the patient, the goal should be to have adequate access to the antegrade tract as well as the urethra. Neither prone nor dorsal lithotomy will provide access to both sites, and a hybrid of the two positions is the preferred method. Variations of these have been described. Many of these positions were originally conceived for access during PCNL and were later adapted for antegrade ureteroscopy. Valdivia et al. described positioning the patient supine, with the legs flexed in supports and the ipsilateral leg higher than contralateral leg with the goal of facilitating the use of a rigid ureteroscope. This position was further modified to provide better retrograde access. The patient is placed in the lithotomy position with a 3-liter bag of saline or other roll to raise the flank. The ipsilateral leg is extended, and the contralateral leg is flexed and abducted [28]. Grasso et al. described a modified flank roll position wherein the patient is placed in lithotomy and the flank is tilted 45° to allow access to a previously placed nephrostomy tube [29]. As with all procedures, care should be taken to pad all pressure points, taking into account not only the standard considerations for patients in lithotomy but also pressure points generated by better exposure of the flank.

In order to maintain a sterile field, the patient will need to be prepped and draped to include both the flank and urethra. A povidone-iodine-based solution can be used both on the flank that contains a pre-placed nephrostomy tube and the genitalia. Positioning of the fluoroscope is another important consideration. The surgical team must have access to the ipsilateral flank. This requires that the fluoroscope be placed on the contralateral side.

Endoscopic Access

While the percutaneous access point is governed in part by the location of the pathology being treated by antegrade ureteroscopy and patient anatomy, several principles can be adhered to in order to optimize procedural success. Accessing the renal pelvis and ureter through a dependent lower-pole calyx may create an angle that causes the ureteroscope to buckle and limit defection of the scope, impeding navigation (Fig. 9.5). A middle-pole or even an upper-pole calyceal access point may facilitate a straighter angle to approach the ureter. Ureteral access sheaths can be placed through the percutaneous tract not only to aid in the case of stone fragment or neoplasm removal but also add a layer of protection for the ureteroscope [30]. When ureteroscope mobility is limited at the level of the skin or fascia, dilating balloons can aid in enlarging the tract and allow the ureteroscope to move more freely, in addition to facilitating introduction of a sheath. The degrees of deflection and angles needed during antegrade ureteroscopy can put the endoscope at risk of being damaged, due to torque on the shaft, leading some authors to recommend the use of single-use ureteroscopes when available [13] (Fig. 9.6). The flexible endoscope being placed antegrade through a nephrostomy tract into the kidney and ureter should always be protected by a sheath or by placing it over a guidewire, preferably a double floppy-tipped stiff wire. A flexible ureteroscope is also at considerable risk when in place and manipulated within the ureter. The surgeon must always be cognizant of the appropriate endoscope for each procedure. For percutaneous ureteroscopy, often the proximal ureter is adequately dilated enough to accept a flexible nephroscope, which is much stronger and more durable than the smaller-diameter ureteroscope. Single-use instruments also have value here.

Post Treatment

Drainage

The principles of drainage for antegrade ureteroscopy are similar to those used in the decision-making process for retrograde ureteroscopy and PCNL. The surgeon must decide whether to leave a nephrostomy tube, a ureteral stent, both, or none. Currently, there is no universally agreed upon method of post-procedural drainage. Several authors have described the safety of forgoing nephrostomy tube drainage

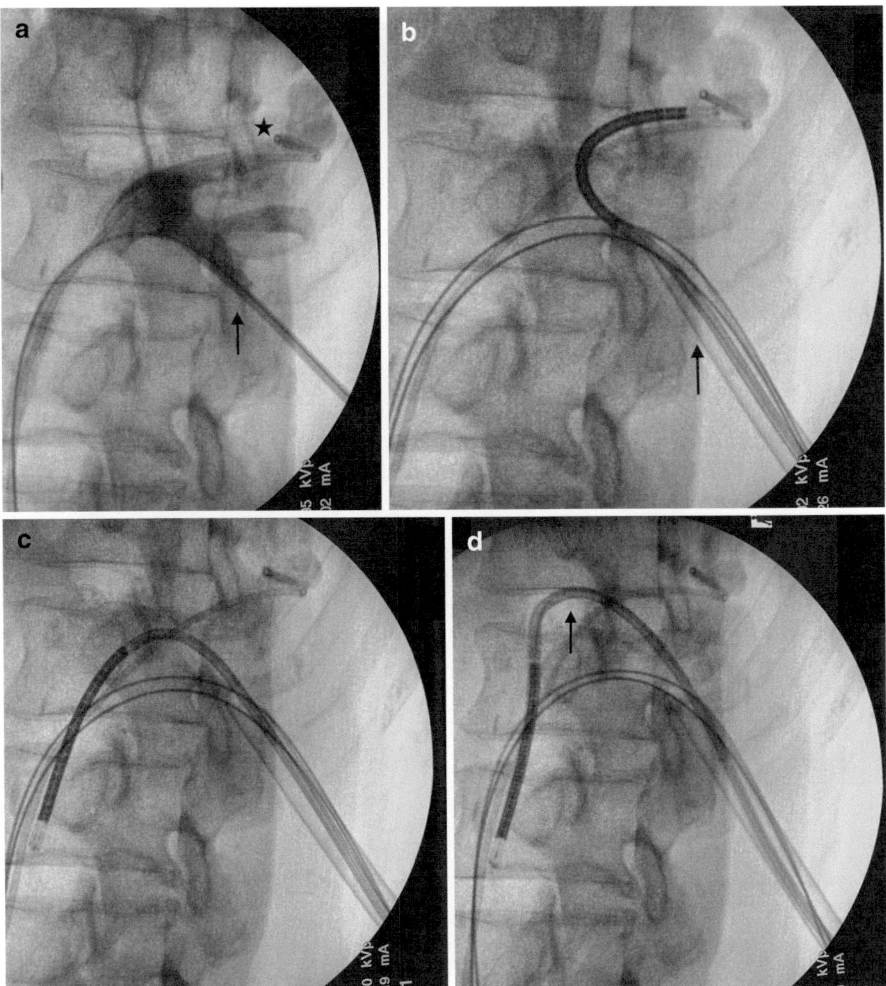

Fig. 9.5 (**a**) Left antegrade nephrostogram with lower-pole percutaneous access (black arrow). Note the proximal curl of an encrusted ureteral stent (black star). (**b**) Lower-pole percutaneous access allows antegrade ureteroscopic treatment of upper-pole stone burden. Black arrow marks renal access sheath. (**c**) Same lower-pole access allows limited antegrade ureteroscopic treatment of stent encrustations in the proximal ureter. (**d**) Dependent lower-pole access may limit antegrade ureteroscopic advancement down the ureter. Black arrow shows buckling of ureteroscopic shaft against the inside of the renal pelvis upon advancement down the proximal ureter

after percutaneous renal surgery [31–34]. Commonly, nephrostomy tubes are left in place when there is concern for a large amount of bleeding, purulence in the collecting system requiring reliable drainage, or extensive injury to the collecting system. Some of these complicating factors may be mitigated when performing true antegrade ureteroscopy through a non-dilated tract or a tract dilated to 15 French rather

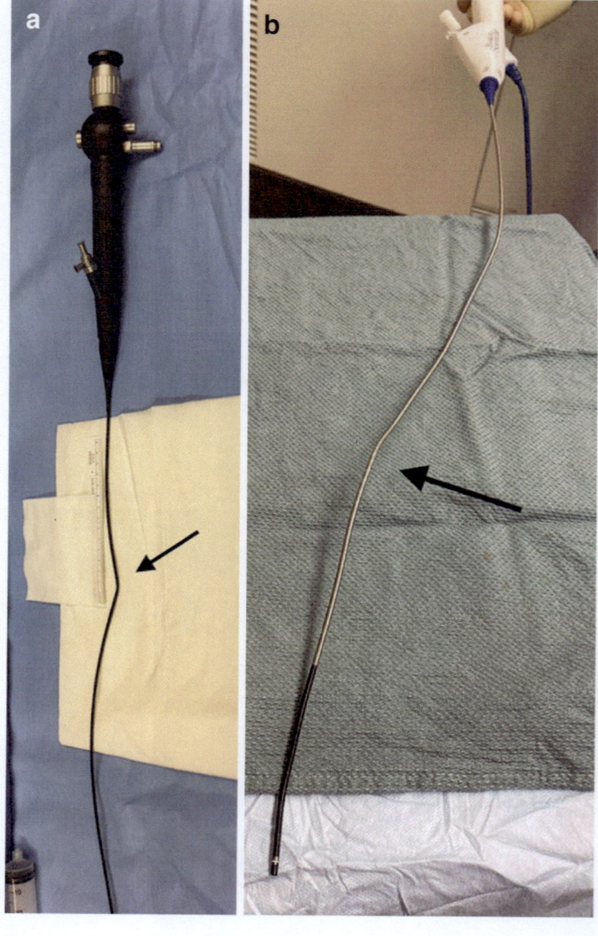

Fig. 9.6 (a) Reusable flexible ureteroscope with crushed shaft (arrow) secondary to torque applied by the surgeon for endoscope rotation during antegrade ureteroscopy. (**b**) Same phenomena is seen with single-use instruments (arrow) but with less economic impact due to avoidance of repair costs

than the larger tracts required for PCNL. In the absence of strong evidence to guide practices, the decision on whether to place a nephrostomy tube or ureteral stent is ultimately at the discretion of the surgeon based on intraoperative factors and anticipation of requiring further intervention. We have found it useful to place relatively wide-diameter stents or two stents side by side in cases involving recanalization of obliterated ureteral segments.

Antibiotics

Current AUA best practice statements advise that less than 24 hours of perioperative antibiotics be used a prophylaxis for PCNL and one dose of perioperative antibiotics is sufficient for ureteroscopy [35]. Multiple authors have shown there to be no benefit from the standpoint of postoperative infection by extending antibiotic prophylaxis beyond 24 hours for either PCNL or ureteroscopy [36–39]. Surgeons should identify those patients they deem at higher risk of postoperative sepsis and tailor their antibiotic prophylaxis accordingly.

Conclusion

Antegrade ureteroscopy is a useful part of the endourological armamentarium to treat upper urinary tract conditions, either as a primary, adjuvant, or combined approach. It is helpful when the ureter is not accessible in the customary retrograde fashion or when both simultaneous retrograde and antegrade approaches are needed, as seen in patients with relatively short, complete ureteral obliterations. Special considerations must be given to the equipment and personnel needed to achieve treatment success.

References

1. Bagley DH, Huffman J, Lyon E, McNamara T. Endoscopic ureteropyelostomy: opening the obliterated ureteropelvic junction with nephroscopy and flexible ureteropyeloscopy. J Urol. 1985;133:462–4.
2. Conlin MJ, Gomella LG, Bagley DH. Endoscopic ureteroureterostomy for obliterated ureteral segments. J Urol. 1996;156:1394–9.
3. Keoghane SR, Deverill SJ, Woodhouse J, Shennoy V, Johnston T, Osborn P. Combined antegrade and retrograde access to difficult ureters: revisiting the rendezvous technique. Urolithiasis. 2019;47:383–90.
4. Pastore AL, Palleschi G, Silvestri L, Leto A, Autieri D, Ripoli A, et al. Endoscopic rendezvous procedure for ureteral iatrogenic detachment: report of a case series with long-term outcomes. J Endourol. 2014;29:415–20.
5. Watson JM, Dawkins GPC, Whitfield HN, Philp T, Kellett MJ. The rendezvous procedure to cross complicated ureteric strictures. BJU Int. 2002;89:317–9.
6. Goda K, Kawabata G, Yasufuku T, Hara I, Fujisawa M, Kamidono S, et al. Cut-to-the-light technique and potassium titanyl phosphate laser ureterotomy for complete ureteral obstruction. Int J Urol. 2004;11:427–8.
7. Lingeman JE, Wong MY, Newmark JR. Endoscopic management of total ureteral occlusion and ureterovaginal fistula. J Endourol. 1995;9:391–6.
8. Niesel T, Moore RG, Alfert HJ, Kavoussi LR. Alternative endoscopic management in the treatment of urethral strictures. J Endourol. 1995;9:31–9.
9. Zhang M, Fathollahi A, Hillesohn J, Eshghi M. Endoscopic management of distal ureteral strictures. In: Smith AD, Preminger GM, Kavoussi LR, Badlani GH, editors. Smith's textbook of endourology. 4th ed. Oxford: Wiley Blackwell; 2019. p. 620.
10. Ericson KJ, Thomas LJ, Zhang JH, Knorr JM, Khanna A, Crane A, et al. Uretero-enteric anastomotic stricture following radical cystectomy: a comparison of open, robotic extracorporeal, and robotic intracorporeal approaches. Urology. 2020;144:130–5.

11. Stuurman RE, Al-Qahtani SM, Cornu J-N, Traxer O. Antegrade percutaneous flexible endoscopic approach for the management of urinary diversion-associated complications. J Endourol. 2013;27:1330–4.
12. Zhong W, Yang B, He F, Wang L, Swami S, Zeng G. Surgical management of urolithiasis in patients after urinary diversion. PLoS One. 2014;9:e111371.
13. Inoue T, Yamamichi F, Endo T, Kaku Y, Horikoshi M, Hara S, et al. Successful percutaneous flexible ureteroscopy for treatment of distal ureteral stones under modified Valdivia position after Cohen reimplantation. IJU Case Rep. 2019;2:245–8.
14. Krambeck AE, Gettman MT, BaniHani AH, Husmann DA, Kramer SA, Segura JW. Management of nephrolithiasis after Cohen cross-trigonal and Glenn-Anderson advancement ureteroneocystostomy. J Urol. 2007;177:174–8.
15. Hyams E, Marien T, Bruhn A, Quirouet A, Andonian S, Shah O, et al. Ureteroscopy for transplant lithiasis. J Endourol. 2011;26:819–22.
16. Emiliani E, Subiela JD, Regis F, Angerri O, Palou J. Over 30-yr experience on the management of graft stones after renal transplantation. Eur Urol Focus. 2018;4:169–74.
17. Rifaioglu MM, Berger AD, Pengune W, Stoller ML. Percutaneous management of stones in transplanted kidneys. Urology. 2008;72:508–12.
18. Harraz AM, Kamal AI, Shokeir AA. Urolithiasis in renal transplant donors and recipients: an update. Int J Surg. 2016;36:693–7.
19. Gumpinger R, Miller K, Fuchs G, Eisenberger F. Antegrade ureteroscopy for stone removal. Eur Urol. 1985;11:199–202.
20. Maheshwari PN, Oswal AT, Andankar M, Nanjappa KM, Bansal M. Is antegrade ureteroscopy better than retrograde ureteroscopy for impacted large upper ureteral calculi? J Endourol. 1999;13:441–4.
21. Türk C, Petřík A, Sarica K, Seitz C, Skolarikos A, Straub M, et al. EAU guidelines on interventional treatment for urolithiasis. Eur Urol. 2016;69:475–82.
22. Sun X, Xia S, Lu J, Liu H, Han B, Li W. Treatment of large impacted proximal ureteral stones: randomized comparison of percutaneous antegrade ureterolithotripsy versus retrograde ureterolithotripsy. J Endourol. 2008;22:913–8.
23. Elgebaly O, Abdeldayem H, Idris F, Elrifai A, Fahmy A. Antegrade mini-percutaneous flexible ureteroscopy versus retrograde ureteroscopy for treating impacted proximal ureteric stones of 1-2 cm: a prospective randomised study. Arab J Urol. 2020;18:176–80.
24. Sfoungaristos S, Mykoniatis I, Isid A, Gofrit ON, Rosenberg S, Hidas G, et al. Retrograde versus Antegrade Approach for the Management of Large Proximal Ureteral Stones. BioMed Res Int [Internet]. 2016 [cited 2020 Dec 5]; 2016. Available from: https://www.ncbi.nlm.nih.gov/pmc/articles/PMC5059524/
25. Petros FG, Li R, Matin SF. Endoscopic approaches to upper tract urothelial carcinoma. Urol Clin North Am. 2018;45:267–86.
26. Park BH, Jeon SS. Endoscopic management of upper urinary tract urothelial carcinoma. Korean J Urol. 2013;54:426–32.
27. Lam JS, Bingham JB, Gupta M. Endoscopic treatment of fibroepithelial polyps of the renal pelvis and ureter. Urology. 2003;62:810–3.
28. Ibarluzea G, Scoffone CM, Cracco CM, Poggio M, Porpiglia F, Terrone C, et al. Supine Valdivia and modified lithotomy position for simultaneous anterograde and retrograde endourological access. BJU Int. 2007;100:233–6.
29. Grasso M, Nord R, Bagley DH. Prone Split leg and flank roll positioning: simultaneous antegrade and retrograde access to the upper urinary tract. J Endourol. 1993;7:307–10.
30. Winter M, Lynch C, Appu S, Kourambas J. Access sheath-aided percutaneous antegrade ureteroscopy; a novel approach to the ureter. BJU Int. 2011;108:620–2.
31. Ichaoui H, Samet A, Ben Hadjalouane H, Hermi A, Hedhli H, Bakir MA, et al. Percutaneous Nephrolithotomy (PCNL): Standard Technique Versus Tubeless - 125 Procedures. Cureus [Internet]. [cited 2020 Dec 6];11(3). Available from: https://www.ncbi.nlm.nih.gov/pmc/articles/PMC6516629/

32. Yoon GH, Bellman GC. Tubeless percutaneous nephrolithotomy: a new standard in percutaneous renal surgery. J Endourol. 2008;9:1865–7; discussion 1869.
33. Desai MR, Kukreja RA, Desai MM, Mhaskar SS, Wani KA, Patel SH, et al. A prospective randomized comparison of type of nephrostomy drainage following percutaneous nephrostolithotomy: large bore versus small bore versus tubeless. J Urol. 2004;172:565–7.
34. Zhao PT, Hoenig DM, Smith AD, Okeke Z. A randomized controlled comparison of nephrostomy drainage vs ureteral stent following percutaneous nephrolithotomy using the Wisconsin StoneQOL. J Endourol. 2016;30:1275–84.
35. Lightner DJ, Wymer K, Sanchez J, Kavoussi L. Best practice statement on urologic procedures and antimicrobial prophylaxis. J Urol. 2020;203:351–6.
36. Chew BH, Miller NL, Abbott JE, Lange D, Humphreys MR, Pais VM, et al. A randomized controlled trial of preoperative prophylactic antibiotics prior to percutaneous nephrolithotomy in a low infectious risk population: a report from the EDGE consortium. J Urol. 2018;200:801–8.
37. Greene DJ, Gill BC, Hinck B, Nyame YA, Almassi N, Krishnamurthi V, et al. American urological association antibiotic best practice statement and ureteroscopy: does antibiotic stewardship help? J Endourol. 2018;32:283–8.
38. Chew BH, Flannigan R, Kurtz M, Gershman B, Arsovska O, Paterson RF, et al. A single dose of intraoperative antibiotics is sufficient to prevent urinary tract infection during ureteroscopy. J Endourol. 2016;30:63–8.
39. Deshmukh S, Sternberg K, Hernandez N, Eisner BH. Compliance with American Urological Association guidelines for post-percutaneous nephrolithotomy antibiotics does not appear to increase rates of infection. J Urol. 2015;194:992–6.
40. Lopatkin NA, Martov AG, Gushchin BL. An endourologic approach to complete ureteropelvic junction and ureteral strictures. J Endourol. 2000;14:721–6.

Chapter 10
Complications of Ureteroscopy

Scott G. Hubosky and Brian P. Calio

Introduction

The practice of ureteroscopy has significantly evolved over the last 35 years [1]. Advancements in instrument design and miniaturization along with the development of laser technology and other endourological instrumentation have led to widespread utilization of ureteroscopy for treatment of upper urinary tract stones, neoplasms, and strictures. With the increased practice of ureteroscopy has come a host of variable complications, which have been described both in the literature and anecdotally. These complications are generally characterized as minor or major. While minor complications are often transient and well managed with stent placement, major complications can have serious implications for the patient. Despite strong educational efforts, devastating ureteroscopic complications are still reported in the contemporary literature [2] and via anonymous, passive Internet surveillance systems, such as the MAUDE (Manufacturer and User Facility Device Experience) database [3]. Although seemingly rare, major complications of ureteroscopy are likely underreported, and awareness of them is paramount in order to limit their incidence.

S. G. Hubosky (✉) · B. P. Calio
Department of Urology, Sidney Kimmel Medical College at Thomas Jefferson University Hospital, Philadelphia, PA, USA
e-mail: Scott.Hubosky@jefferson.edu; Brian.calio@jefferson.edu

© Springer Nature Switzerland AG 2022
S. G. Hubosky et al. (eds.), *Advanced Ureteroscopy*,
https://doi.org/10.1007/978-3-030-82351-1_10

Classification Systems for Complications of Ureteroscopy/ Ureteral Injury

Formal classification systems for ureteral injury exist to provide uniformity in the reporting of complications. The first such classification scheme was put forth in the trauma surgery literature and is known as the "American Association for the Surgery of Trauma Organ Injury Severity Scale for the Ureter" [4] (Table 10.1). This system broadly categorizes the extent of ureteral injury in order to direct the practitioner to whether stenting or formal surgical repair is indicated. It applies to blunt or penetrating trauma and iatrogenic injuries of the ureter. There is limited practical value for endourologists with this scheme.

The Clavien-Dindo classification system introduced in 2004 stratified complications into grades based on the level of intervention required for treatment and is presented in Table 10.2 [5]. This system includes not just surgical interventions for a given complication but also considers pharmacological treatment and the need for intensive care unit (ICU) monitoring, allowing it to account for post-ureteroscopic sepsis. Thus far, this system is the most comprehensive and the most commonly applied in the contemporary literature.

In 2012 the post-ureteroscopic lesion scale (PULS) was introduced as an injury scale geared specifically toward complications encountered during ureteroscopy [6]. This scale stratifies injuries to the ureter in a way that provides the urologist a systematic approach to determine when post-ureteroscopic stent placement is indicated. Although high inter-rater reliability has been demonstrated using this system, it has not yet been validated for standardization of stent placement following ureteroscopy [7].

Formal classification systems are necessary to consistently report ureteroscopic complications across studies and to best judge the safety of new procedures. If, however, the goal of classifying complications is for the surgeon to anticipate, recognize, and avoid them, then the classification system must be practical and easily remembered. Such classification schemes have been put forth by authors of review papers on ureteroscopic complications [2, 8], and they broadly organize ureteroscopic complications as intraoperative, postoperative early, or postoperative late.

Table 10.1 American Association for the Surgery of Trauma (AAST) ureter organ injury scale [4]

Grade[a]	Injury type	Description of injury	ICD-9	AIS-85	AIS-90
I	Hematoma	Contusion of hematoma without devascularization	867.2/867.3	2	2
II	Laceration	<50% transection	867.2/867.3	2	2
III	Laceration	>50% transection	867.2/867.3	3	3
IV	Laceration	Complete transection with 2-cm devascularization	867.2/867.3	3	3
V	Laceration	Avulsion with >2 cm of devascularization	867.2/867.3	3	3

[a]Advance one grade if multiple lesions exist

Table 10.2 Modified Clavien classification of surgical complications [5]

Grade	Definition
Grade I	Any deviation from the normal postoperative course without the need for pharmacological treatment or surgical, endoscopic, and radiological interventions Allowed therapeutic regimens are drugs as antiemetics, antipyretics, analgetics, diuretics, electrolytes, and physiotherapy. This grade also includes wound infections opened at the bedside
Grade II	Requiring pharmacological treatment with drugs other than such allowed for grade 1 complications. Blood transfusions and total parenteral nutrition are also included
Grade III	Requiring surgical, endoscopic, or radiological intervention
Grade IIIa	Intervention not under general anesthesia
Grade IIIb	Intervention under general anesthesia
Grade IV	Life-threatening complication (including CNS complications)[a] requiring IC/ICU management
Grade IVa	Single organ dysfunction (including dialysis)
Grade IVb	Multiorgan dysfunction
Grade V	Death of a patient
Suffix "d"	If the patient suffers from a complication at the time of discharge, the suffix "d" (for disability) is added to the respective grade of complication. This label indicates the need for a follow-up to fully evaluate the complication

CNS central nervous system, *IC* intermediate care, *ICU* intensive care unit
[a]Brain hemorrhage, ischemic stroke, and subarachnoidal bleeding, but excluding transient ischemic attacks

Each of these three categories is further subdivided into major or minor sequelae. The major category includes any complication that results in the need for additional, otherwise unexpected, major operative intervention or results in patient mortality or severe morbidity such as in postsurgical sepsis. Minor complications are typically self-limiting and, although potentially morbid, usually are well treated with temporary postoperative stent placement.

Intraoperative Complications (Major)

Ureteral Avulsion

Ureteral avulsion, defined as discontinuation of the full thickness of the ureter, is one of the most devastating complications involving either flexible or semi-rigid ureteroscopy. In almost all cases, repair requires open or laparoscopic intervention, and in certain cases, nephrectomy may be required [9]. Historically, before ureteroscopy became almost universally available, ureteral avulsion had been a complication of so-called blind basketing of ureteral stones. With the advent of digital and fiberoptic ureteroscopy, the practice of blind basketing is obsolete and no longer advocated and has been replaced by stone manipulation under direct ureteroscopic visualization. As such, the incidence of ureteral avulsion has decreased significantly, to the point that the complication has become extremely rare. Estimates from several reviews place the incidence of ureteral avulsion between 0% and 0.5% of all ureteroscopic cases. In a literature search of the MEDLINE database on stone basketing between 1970 and 2005, ureteral avulsion occurred in 0.3% of cases [10]. Similar results were reported in a large study performed by the Clinical Research Office of the Endourological Society (CROES) encompassing 9681 patients who underwent ureteroscopy in 2012, in which ureteral avulsion had a prevalence of 0.1% [11], and a recent review by Grasso reported 0% incidence of avulsion in 1059 cases [12].

Although quite rare, contemporary reports of ureteral avulsion still occur, even when basket extraction is performed under direct ureteroscopic visualization, usually when fundamental ureteroscopic principles are not followed. In some cases the avulsed, inverted ureter can be seen on cystoscopy floating within the lumen of the bladder (Fig. 10.1). In other cases, the surgeon stops short of complete inversion, even though the ureter has been completely avulsed and the basket remains in the patient with the stone still engaged (Fig. 10.2).

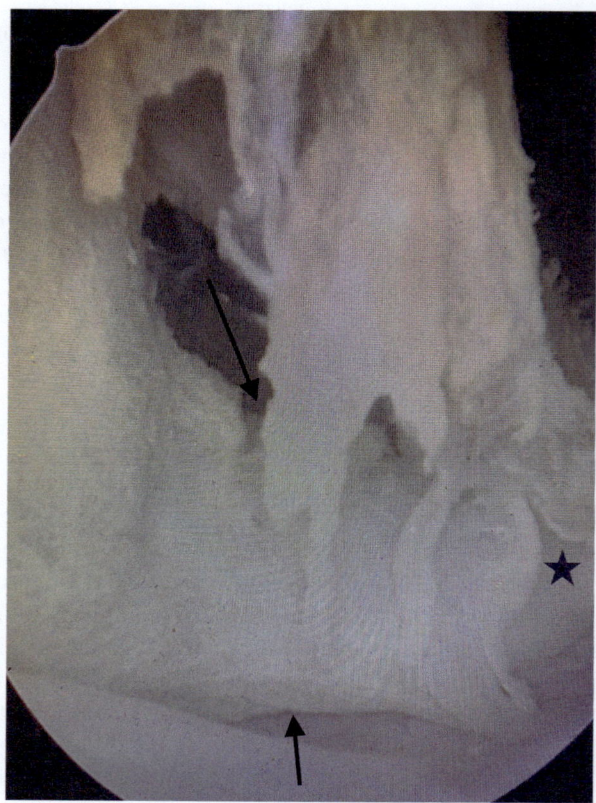

Fig. 10.1 Close-up cystoscopic view of a completely avulsed, inverted, and devitalized left ureter within the bladder lumen. Black arrows mark the ureteral wall edges. A black star marks the position of the former left ureteral orifice. This patient was transferred after failed basket extraction of a ureteral calculus. Ultimately a renal autotransplant was required

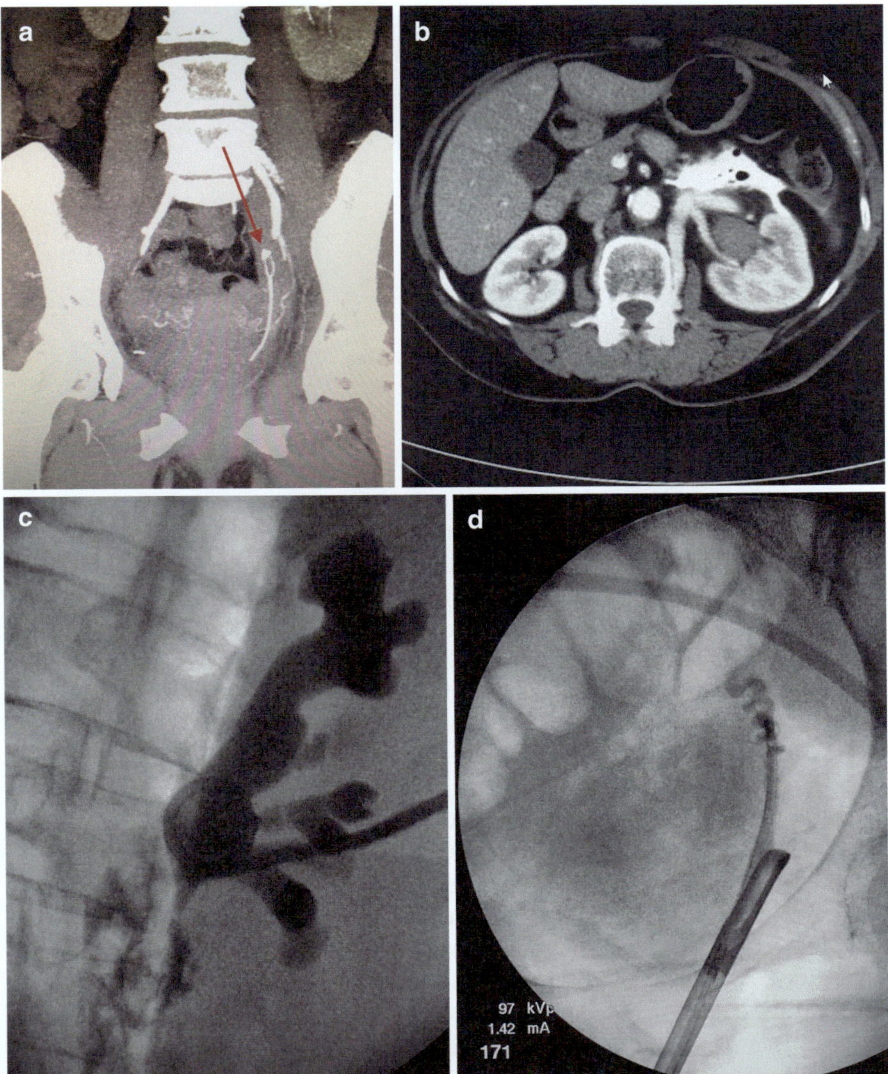

Fig. 10.2 A patient transferred with suspected ureteral avulsion secondary to basket extraction of an 8-mm calculus. (**a**) Coronal view CT scan shows retained calculus in stone basket wires along the expected course of the left ureter (red arrow). (**b**) Axial view of a CT scan from same patient demonstrates contrast extravasation from the left proximal ureter. (**c**) Left antegrade nephrostogram through percutaneous nephrostomy shows contrast extravasation with no continuity to the ureter. (**d**) Retrograde ureteroscopic evaluation along retained stone basket shows blind-ending ureter confirmed with retrograde pyelogram showing bunching of avulsed ureter like an accordion. (**e**) Avulsed ureter with retained basket noted during subsequent renal autotransplant (blue vessel loop marks common iliac artery). (**f**) Devitalized left ureter and stone basket removed

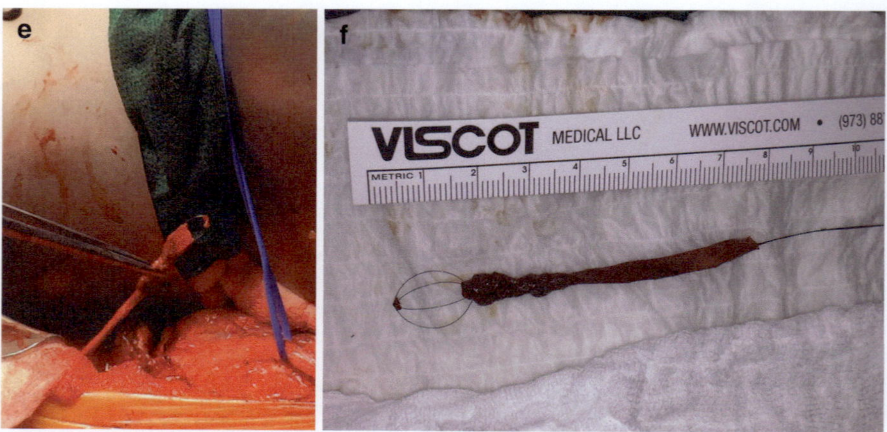

Fig. 10.2 (continued)

Ureteral avulsion can be avoided by maintaining proper technique and patience while removing ureteral stones with a basket or other grasping devices. Retrieving stones intact also increases the risk of avulsion, particularly in the case of large calculi. Whole-stone extraction should only be attempted in cases of very small stones and not when the maximal stone diameter is greater than the diameter of the narrowest portion of the ureter, in the surgeon's judgment. Intracorporeal lithotripsy prior to stone extraction is a safer alternative that minimizes the risk of avulsion in most cases. Visualization of the entire length of ureteral mucosa with the ureteroscope during extraction is a fundamental safety principle. The stone should be held several millimeters from the tip of the ureteroscope (Fig. 10.3), and the ureteral mucosa should be seen moving away from the surgeon while the stone is being withdrawn. Keeping the stone in clear view may require deflection or rotation of the ureteroscope as the surgeon navigates down the ureteral lumen. Nitinol baskets or three-pronged graspers are the safest instruments for ureteroscopic stone removal since they can resume their original shape for stone release. Baskets with stainless steel wires should be avoided for ureteroscopic stone removal since they do not reliably return to their original shape and make stone release potentially difficult.

In addition to basket extraction of calculi, other less often encountered etiologies of ureteral avulsion exist, as reported by Tanimoto et al. in a review of the MAUDE database [3]. These cases seem to all involve ureteroscopic entrapment in the upper urinary tract, and independent reports have also been recently published, bringing these rare complications to our attention. Etiologies for ureteroscopic entrapment include locked deflection of flexible ureteroscopes [13, 14], bunching of the distal bending rubber [15], resultant stone fragment impaction along the ureteroscope shaft during laser lithotripsy [3, 16, 17], and scabbard avulsions [18]. Due to the rarity of these complications, no standard protocol to mitigate them exists, although anecdotally, careful retrograde manipulations with coaxial dilators have been reported to help [13, 15], as have gentle rotational maneuvers with muscle relaxants

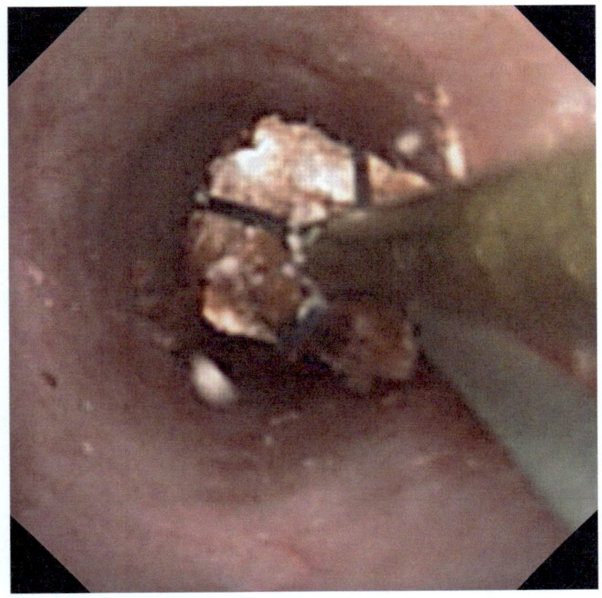

Fig. 10.3 Safe stone removal entails direct visualization of the calculus and the ureteral mucosa at all times. Note the presence of a safety wire at the 4 o'clock position

and bladder emptying [17]. In other cases, controlled open surgery was required to remove the entrapped ureteroscope and avoid avulsion [14–16].

Awareness of these rare complications is the best defense against them. Locked deflection occurs secondary to suboptimal surgical technique in which stress is placed on the deflection cables of the flexible ureteroscope causing the inner bend radius cable to kink (Fig. 10.4), resulting in the inability of the ureteroscope to revert back to a straight configuration. This instrument stress can ensue from pulling a fully deflected ureteroscope through an intrarenal stricture such as a stenotic infundibulum (Fig. 10.5) or by the use of extreme secondary deflection as is sometimes necessary to reach very dependent lower pole positions (Fig. 10.6). Constant awareness of the position of the ureteroscope within the confines of the given collecting system will help avoid situations resulting in locked deflection. Rippling or bunching of the distal bending rubber of a flexible ureteroscope is difficult to predict but enforces the fact that every flexible ureteroscope, including the distal bending rubber, should be examined by operating room personnel prior to placement. Additionally, medical device safety notices provided by manufacturers recommend refraining from ureteroscope placement if significant resistance is met during insertion [15], reinforcing the need for sound surgical judgment in every case. Ureteroscope entrapment secondary to intraluminal stone fragment impaction is best avoided by regular fluoroscopic evaluation along the ureter in cases involving treatment of relatively large stone burdens to allow for intermittent basket extraction or early intraoperative stent placement. Ureteral access sheaths may also be beneficial in these cases. Index of suspicion should be higher for this complication in cases with large stone burdens.

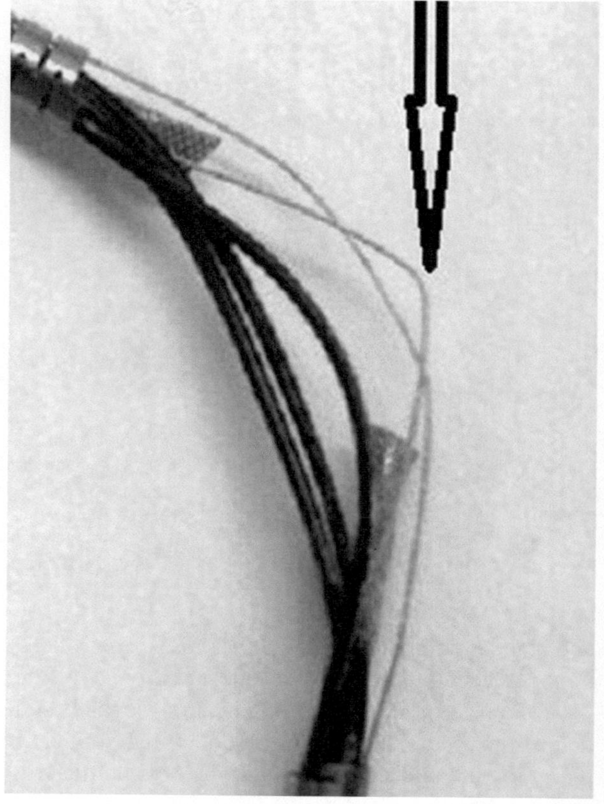

Fig. 10.4 Post-procedure inspection of flexible ureteroscope, which was pulled through a stenotic infundibulum resulting in locked deflection. Note the kink in the deflection cable of the inner bend radius of the flexible ureteroscope (marked by arrow)

Scabbard avulsions involve entrapment of semi-rigid ureteroscopes. The mechanism is believed to involve the gradual advancement of the larger-diameter proximal ureteroscope shaft within a relatively tight intravesical distal ureter. Upon removal, a two-point avulsion involving both the distal and proximal ureteral portions results in the ureter appearing like a scabbard on the semi-rigid ureteroscope. Ordon et al. advise to always make sure ureteral mucosa is visualized moving away while the ureteroscope is being withdrawn, and if not, then the potential for a scabbard avulsion should be recognized [18]. They postulate that placing a second semi-rigid ureteroscope and attempting to incise the intramural ureter with laser may free the entrapped semi-rigid ureteroscope.

Management of ureteral avulsion differs depending on the segment of ureter involved and the thickness of ureter injured. Complete avulsions always require formal surgical repair, which may be done immediately, or as a staged procedure, depending on the particular circumstances of the case. The benefits of delayed repair include a better understanding of the anatomy and the size of the ureteral defect. This can be ascertained by simultaneous antegrade and retrograde contrast studies (Fig. 10.7). A percutaneous nephrostomy is often required in order to maximize drainage and minimize urinoma formation. Delayed repair also gives the

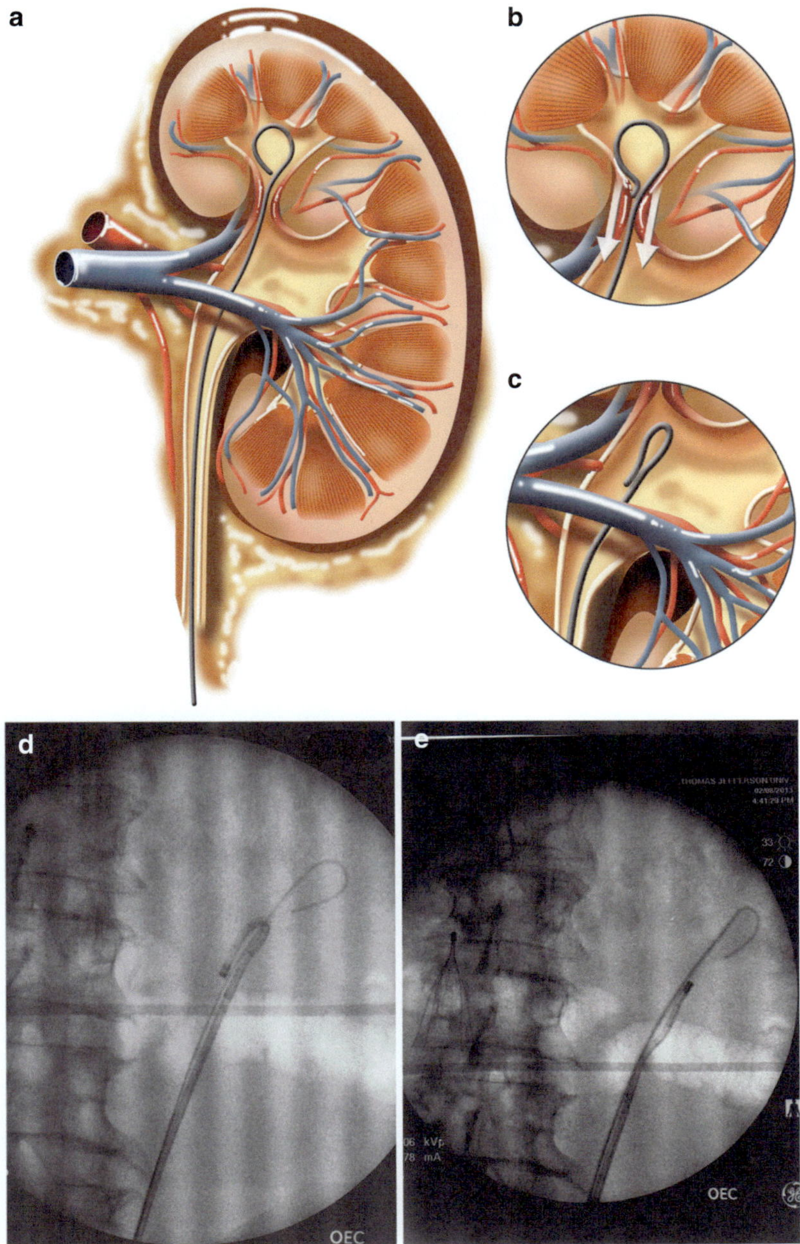

Fig. 10.5 (**a**) Flexible ureteroscope is in maximal deflection in an upper pole calyx, drained by a stenotic infundibulum, which had just been previously opened with balloon dilation. (**b**) Flexible ureteroscope was unknowingly pulled through stenotic infundibulum while in maximal deflection. (**c**) Flexible ureteroscope in locked downward deflection within the renal pelvis, unable to be safely removed. (**d**) Live fluoroscopic image of flexible ureteroscope in locked deflection within the space of the renal pelvis. Note safety wire present. (**e**) Fluoroscopic image of flexible ureteroscope after being straightened with retrograde coaxial dilator, which allowed for safe removal

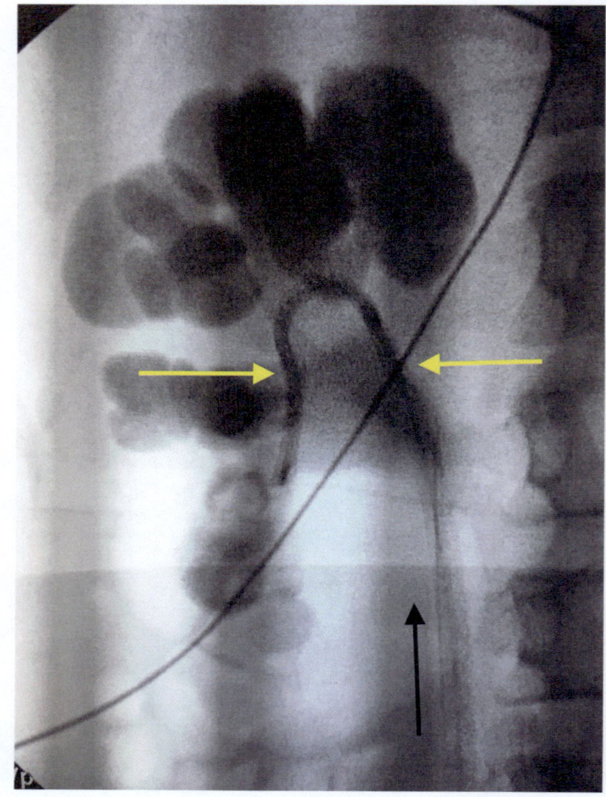

Fig. 10.6 Single-use flexible ureteroscope with extreme passive deflection in attempt to reach a very dependent right lower pole calyx. Continued upward advancement of the ureteroscope (black arrow) against the fixed upper portion of the collecting system can cause pinching or kinking of inner bend radius deflection cable (yellow arrows), resulting in locked deflection

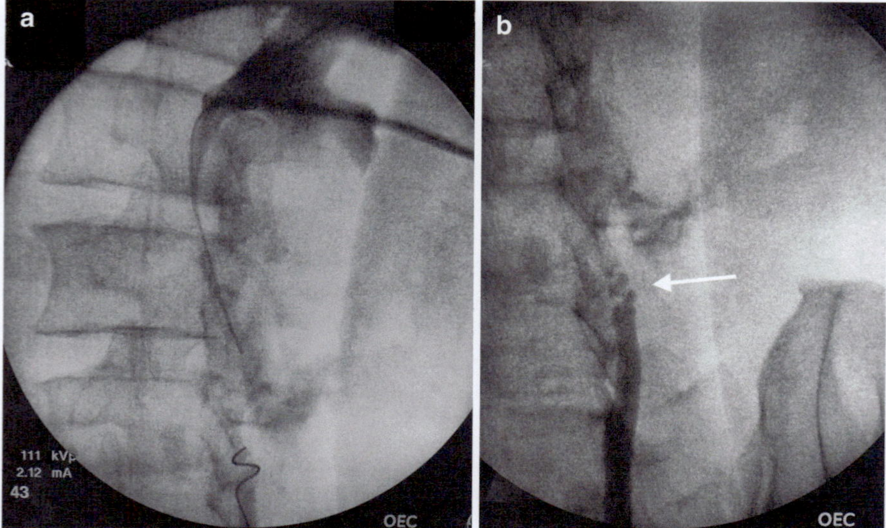

Fig. 10.7 (**a**) Simultaneous antegrade nephrostogram and retrograde pyelogram in a suspected case of ureteral avulsion after attempted basket removal in a referred patient. Note contrast extravasation as well as inability to gain full-length access across the ureter. (**b**) Close-up view of retrograde pyelogram shows accordion-like bunching of the proximal ureter in discontinuity

patient a chance to carefully consider the treatment options. The temptation to perform immediate nephrectomy in this setting should be avoided, as many reconstructive options exist and often allow for renal preservation. Partial ureteral avulsions are significantly less severe and in most cases can be managed with placement of a ureteral stent for 4–6 weeks. Of note there is an elevated risk of ureteral stricture as sequelae of partial avulsions.

Intussusception

Ureteral intussusception is another rare complication of ureteroscopy and can be seen with both retrograde and antegrade manipulation. It is best thought of as an avulsion of the inner mucosal layer of the ureter with subsequent, partial-thickness, and circumferential injury. Much like the case with ureteral avulsions, intussusceptions occur during stone extraction in a ureter that is not sufficiently dilated to accommodate a stone within a retrieval device [19]. In addition to intussusception in the setting of stone removal, there have been case reports describing intussusception caused by biopsy of ureteral polyps and upper tract urothelial carcinomas [20, 21].

Intussusception should be suspected when there is persistent obstruction of the ureter after stone extraction [8]. In such cases, retrograde ureteropyelography reveals what appears to be stripped urothelial mucosal bunched up much like an accordion. Unlike complete ureteral avulsion, cases involving intussusception still maintain integrity of the muscular outer wall of the ureter such that access is still maintained (Fig. 10.8). Definitive treatment for intussusception requires open or laparoscopic excision of the affected portion of the ureter to address the devitalized tissue distal to the injury. Similar to ureteral avulsions, the length and location of the insult will dictate the reconstructive options in cases of benign etiologies. In cases involving upper tract urothelial carcinoma (UTUC), radical nephroureterectomy may be the best option if a normal contralateral kidney exists. If conservative treatment is preferred, ureteral stent placement, if possible, will allow for adequate drainage. Depending on the length of the affected ureter, a stent-dependent ureteral stricture will likely evolve. Much like the strategies recommended for avoidance of ureteral avulsion, avoidance of intussusception is accomplished by retrieving only adequately sized stone fragments under direct vision. In cases involving relatively large intraluminal neoplasms undergoing biopsy and removal with a basket, it is important to first separate any broad-based tumor or polyp from the underlying ureteral mucosa with adequate laser excision.

Hemorrhage

Acute bleeding requiring transfusion during ureteroscopy is rare but also dependent on the procedural indication. A global study on the complications of ureteroscopy coordinated by the CROES group reported that among 11,885 patients undergoing

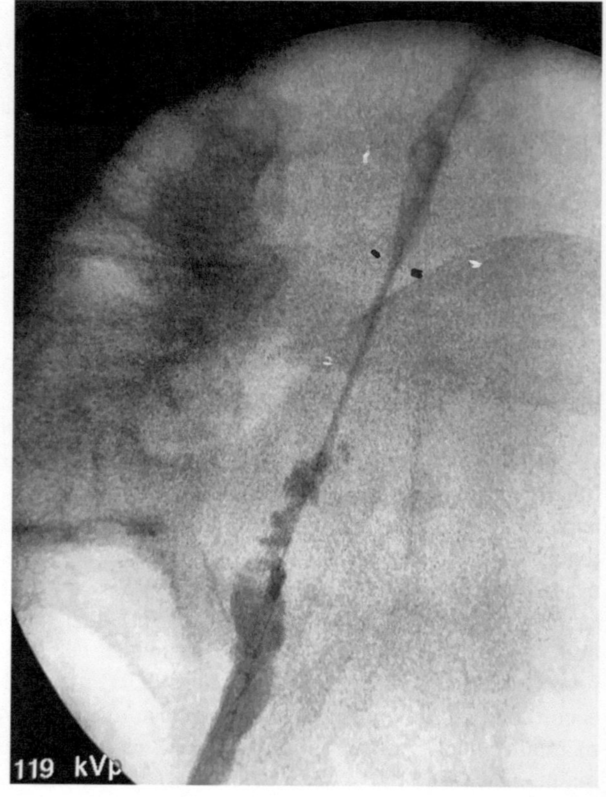

Fig. 10.8 Retrograde pyelogram in a referred patient demonstrates accordion-like bunching of the ureteral mucosa but not full-thickness injury as evidenced by lack of contrast extravasation, preservation of full-length ureteral access, and filling of the upper proximal ureter. These findings are diagnostic of ureteral intussusception, and this case resulted from attempted basket removal of a relatively large ureteral calculus

ureteroscopic stone treatment for renal and/or ureteral stones across 114 international centers, only 0.2% of patients required transfusion [22]. In contrast to stone removal, endopyelotomy and endoureterotomy are the most common procedures in which acute bleeding will be encountered during ureteroscopy with reported transfusion rates ranging from 1% to 16% [23]. The choice of incision location is critical during endopyelotomy to avoid potential violation of vessels adjacent to the ureteropelvic junction (UPJ) or ureter. Significant bleeding as a result of these procedures can be immediate but has also been reported days or even weeks following endourological incision and is postulated to be secondary to delayed arterial thermal injury [24, 25]. Depending on the involved blood vessel, interventions possibly include open vascular surgical repair, endovascular graft placement, or selective embolization. General consensus for incision location during endopyelotomy is the lateral or posterolateral position based on the anatomic studies of Sampaio [26]. In another study of patients with defined UPJ obstructions undergoing endoluminal ultrasound (ELUS), 18.8% had a primarily anterior crossing vessel with a branching lateral component relative to the ureteropelvic junction, and 9.4% had posterior crossing vessels [27]. Therefore, empiric endourological incision without some type of image guidance is a calculated risk. Regular use of intraoperative ELUS or preoperative CT angiogram to define vascular anatomy in the area of interest has been shown to decrease transfusion rates significantly during endopyelotomy [28]. Nevertheless, a high index of suspicion for immediate or delayed bleeding needs to be maintained in these cases with prompt consultation to interventional radiology or vascular surgery, as indicated.

Although not a direct complication, diagnostic ureteroscopy for gross hematuria localized to the upper tract is another possible situation in which significant bleeding might be encountered. This is particularly the case when there is clinical suspicion for a potential uretero-arterial fistula (UAF). This rare entity needs to be on the top of the differential diagnosis in patients with history of pelvic radiation and stent-dependent ureteral strictures, particularly when gross hematuria is significant enough to warrant transfusion [29]. In patients with pre-existing ureteral stents, it is imperative to keep retrograde ureteral access with a guidewire prior to stent removal. If UAF is present, there can be massive amounts of bleeding from the involved ureteral orifice making re-establishment of lost access all but impossible. With access, if bleeding is noted, retrograde catheters or balloon dilators can be inserted which often will tamponade bleeding. Prompt consultation with vascular surgery should be sought, and often definitive treatment involves vascular stent graft placement. Diagnosis of UAF can be challenging. Retrograde pyelogram can, but does not always, demonstrate the fistula due to the unfavorable pressure gradient in the urinary tract relative to the arterial vasculature (Fig. 10.9). Provocative angiography is often required for the diagnosis [30].

Intraoprative Complications (Minor)

Ureteral Wall Insults (Abrasions, False Passages, Perforations)

Histologically, the ureter has an inner mucosal layer composed of urothelial cells backed by the lamina propria, which is further supported by multiple smooth muscle layers, which are outlined in adventitia rich with blood vessels and lymphatics (Fig. 10.10). Minor injuries to the ureteral wall run the spectrum of partial thickness involvement as noted in mucosal abrasions or false passages, to full-thickness involvement as seen in ureteral perforations. Any of these insults can result from placement of a guidewire, coaxial dilator, ureteroscope, or ureteral access sheath.

Mucosal abrasions result from shearing forces against the luminal urothelial layer from either ureteroscope placement or extraction of calculi. Not surprisingly, the reported rate of mucosal abrasion dropped over time, with the introduction of progressively smaller-diameter ureteroscopes. Ureteral access sheath placement can potentially reduce the occurrence of abrasions in cases where repetitive extraction of many stone fragments is anticipated. However, just the mere placement of sheaths sized 12/14Fr, in patients devoid of underlying ureteral pathology, can result in abrasion in up to one third [31]. Practically, abrasions may impair visualization secondary to bleeding but otherwise are well managed with stent placement.

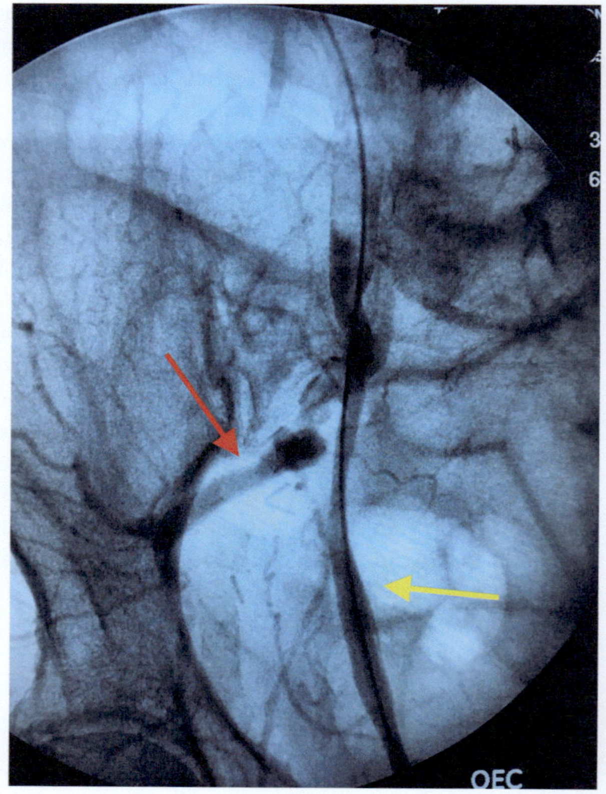

Fig. 10.9 Right retrograde pyelogram performed in a patient with suspected uretero-arterial fistula (UAF). Contrast is injected into the right ureter (yellow arrow) and is seen to opacify the internal iliac artery (red arrow). Diagnosis in this manner may not always be possible secondary to an unfavorable pressure gradient

False passages are usually the product of attempted guidewire placement in the vicinity of obstructing ureteral pathology such as impacted ureteral stones, ureteral neoplasms, or strictures. In these types of cases, the guidewire can move from the true ureteral lumen into a submucosal position while encountering resistance. Relatively small false passage creation by a wire is usually of minimal consequence as long as it is recognized with subsequent removal of the wire and re-establishment of true luminal access, which may require direct ureteroscopic visualization. False passage creation is also not uncommon in relatively narrow distal, intramural ureters while performing semi-rigid ureteroscopy (Fig. 10.11). Depending on the size of the false passage and quality of visualization, either stent placement or redirection of the ureteroscope into the true ureteral lumen should be performed. Cases of avascular necrosis of long segments of ureter have been described when false passages go unrecognized and larger instruments, such as dilators or ureteroscopes, are passed into them and advanced unknowingly. This extension of the false passage, if long enough, serves to severely disrupt blood supply to the inner ureter and can lead to ureteral necrosis [32]. A high index of suspicion should exist in cases of active ureteral obstruction in which guidewire placement is not perfectly smooth or when the wire deviates from its anticipated course on intraoperative fluoroscopic imaging. When this occurs, a relatively small-diameter catheter (4–6 F) should be passed to

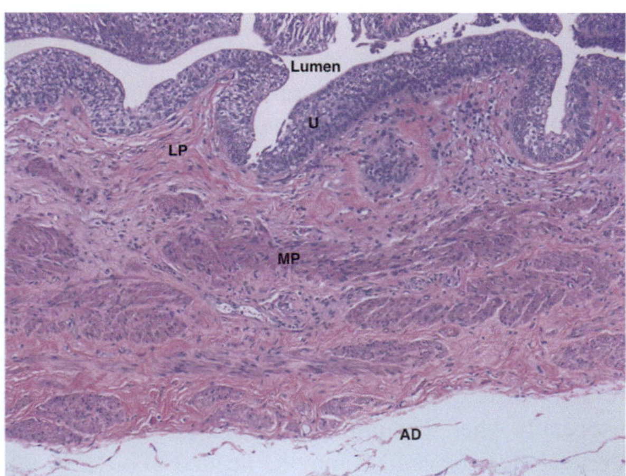

Fig. 10.10 Transverse microscopic cross section of the ureter. U marks the urothelial cell layer. LP denotes the lamina propria, which immediately supports the urothelium. MP shows the inner longitudinal and outer circular muscle layers, while AD marks the adventitia. Ureteral wall insults during ureteroscopy can involve some or all of these layers, resulting in variable degrees of injury and/or ischemia

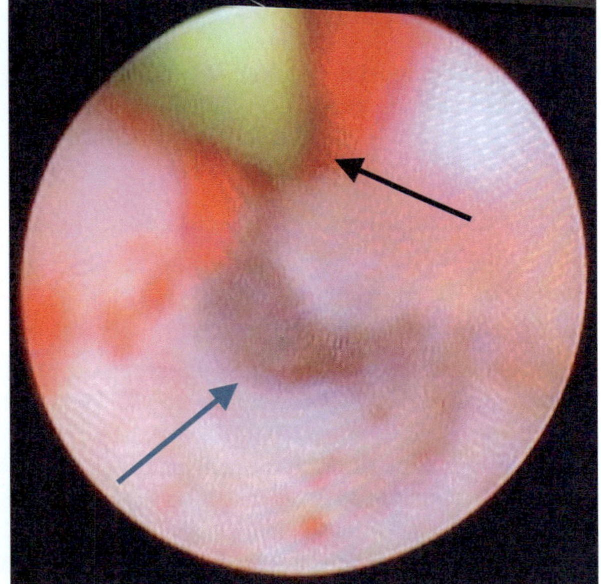

Fig. 10.11 False passage creation (blue arrow) is seen during semi-rigid ureteroscopy in the intramural ureter. Importance of a safety wire is noted, as it marks the true ureteral lumen (black arrow) and secures otherwise tenuous retrograde access

the area of interest and a retrograde pyelogram performed under gentle pressure in order to determine if true access is established prior to the placement of any larger instruments.

A case of an entrapped safety wire has been described in which a guidewire was noted to perforate the ureteral mucosa, enter the submucosal space, and re-enter the luminal space only to exit the ureteral orifice and urethra [33]. This can be thought of conceptually as a two-point false passage creation. This unusual case was reported when the guidewire was blindly being passed through the lumen of a pre-existing stent in a patient with a ureteral calculus. The entrapped wire was ultimately removed with the aid of an 8 F coaxial dilator. No long-term sequelae were noted after temporary stent placement.

Ureteral perforations are full-thickness injuries through the ureteral wall. In large contemporary cohorts of patients undergoing ureteroscopy, the reported incidence is between 0.65% and 1% [22, 34]. Not surprisingly, there has been a trend toward lower incidence of ureteral perforation with smaller-diameter ureteroscopes [35]. Violations of the ureteral wall tend to occur when attempting to advance a ureteroscope, dilator, or access sheath within a relatively narrow ureter. Selective super-stiff wire utilization may reduce perforations since buckling with advancement of the instrument is less likely. Another high-risk situation for encountering perforations is during ureteroscopic laser lithotripsy when a stone is impacted in the ureteral mucosa. Imperfect visualization can lead to perforation during laser lithotripsy especially when the luminal stone cannot clearly be seen. In situations such as these, ureteral stent placement may be needed in order to allow for passive ureteral dilation and a second-stage procedure for definitive stone treatment. Every reasonable attempt should be made to remove calculi within ureteral perforations whenever possible. Three-pronged graspers can be very useful in situations such as these. In the vast majority of cases, ureteral perforations can be managed with transient stent placement. Additional drains are rarely necessary but can be indicated if there is a large fluid collection, especially if infection is present.

Early Postoperative Complications (Major)

Urosepsis

According to a report from the CROES group on 11,885 patients, the rate of fever and severe urosepsis after ureteroscopy is 1.72% and 0.30%, respectively [36]. In the same study, five patients (0.04%) were noted to have died in the 3-month postoperative period, one from urosepsis. In a review of 14 large, contemporary published ureteroscopic series documenting complications in 24,373 patients, Chugh et al. found that infectious complications involved 3.9% of patients [37]. Although not uniformly reported, there were 126 patients with urosepsis, representing 0.51% of those providing data. There were three Clavien V cases (death) reported, but it is not clear how many of these were a result of septic shock. Mortality directly resulting from ureteroscopy is thankfully rare, but urosepsis is the single most likely etiology, especially if other common perioperative sources of mortality such as myocardial infarction, arrhythmia, and pulmonary embolus are excluded [38]. The course of action is clear in patients with upper urinary tract stones and symptomatic infection, especially with concomitant obstruction, as primary surgical stone management should be delayed in favor of immediate drainage and administration of culture-specific antibiotics [39] (Fig. 10.12). The situation is not as clear in patients with asymptomatic colonization of the urine in need of elective surgical stone

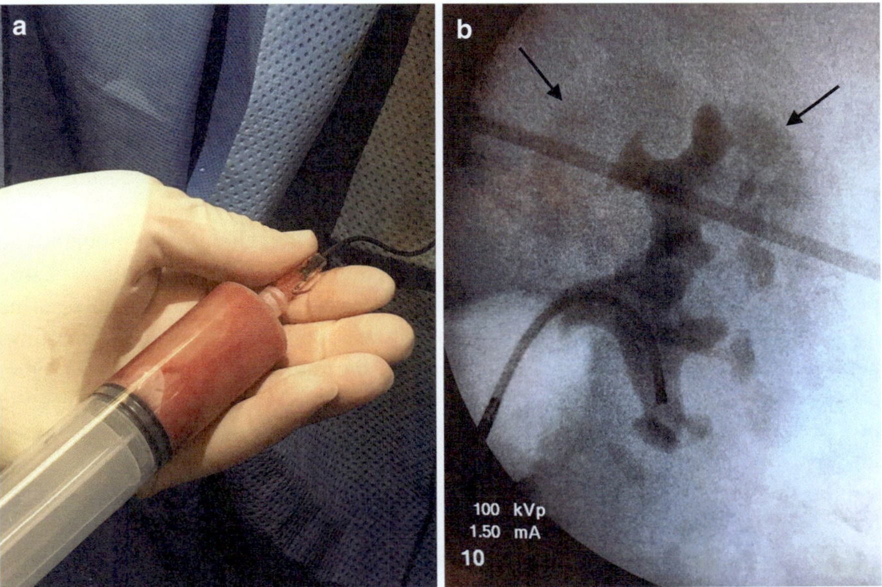

Fig. 10.12 Pyonephrosis (**a**) must be suspected in patients with signs of infection and obstruction, as seen in this purulent renal pelvis aspirate. High-pressure irrigation in this situation can displace organisms from the urine to the blood stream by way of pyelovenous backflow (**b**) and must be avoided in order to avert postoperative urosepsis. The outline of the renal parenchyma with contrast can be seen due to high-pressure contrast irrigation during ureteroscopy (arrows)

treatment. Due to the multifactorial nature of the problem and variable definitions of clinical infection, precise identification of preoperative factors responsible for post-ureteroscopic infections has not been uniform in the existing literature with high-level evidence.

General agreement exists however that it is the combination of colonization of the urine and/or stone(s) with bacteria or fungus, along with high-pressure irrigation, often required for adequate visualization, which is responsible for urosepsis immediately following ureteroscopy [40]. Mitigation strategies have therefore focused on decreasing the amount of viable organisms present and making attempts to keep irrigation pressures low during ureteroscopy.

Careful antibiotic use is essential because it allows for decreasing the quantity of organisms present but can also promote antimicrobial resistance and/or eventual selection of multi-drug-resistant organisms. In terms of preoperative preparation, current guidelines suggest at least a urinalysis be obtained [39] and that a urine culture follow if infection is suspected, followed by culture-specific treatment. The most current version of the American Urologic Association Best Practice Statement on antimicrobial prophylaxis states that a single preoperative dose of antimicrobial prophylaxis should be administered prior to ureteroscopic intervention for stone removal and that the specific agent should be selected in accordance with urine culture results with consideration to the local antibiogram [41]. In addition, these guidelines state that only a single dose of prophylaxis is required even in the presence of asymptomatic bacteriuria for invasive procedures such as ureteroscopy, although intraoperative re-dosing may be appropriate in order to maintain appropriate tissue concentrations. It is also recommended that no further doses of prophylactic agent be prescribed following the procedure in the absence of clinical infection, since this has been shown to promote antibiotic resistance without decreasing surgical site infection.

Despite the best practice policy and guidelines, it is the reliability of preoperative urine cultures in this setting which is concerning. In a prospective study of 462 patients at a single center, Blackmur et al. found that a positive preoperative urine culture, even when treated for 7 days with culture-specific antibiotics in asymptomatic patients, was the only significant variable on multivariate analysis to predict postoperative sepsis with an odds ratio of 4.88 compared to patients with a negative preoperative urine culture [42]. A total of 7.4% of patients in that study developed urosepsis with one mortality. There was imperfect correlation between organisms seen in preoperative urine culture and those identified as the pathogen responsible for urosepsis, with a higher proportion of gram-positive organisms found in the latter. This is a reproducible observation. Eswara et al. found poor correlation (9%) between preoperative urine culture and readmission pathogen in a consecutive series of 328 patients, of which 274 (84%) had ureteroscopic laser lithotripsy and 54 (16%) had PCNL for primary stone treatment [43]. In this series, 3% (11/328) of patients suffered from postoperative sepsis despite either having negative urine cultures or positive cultures treated with preoperative antibiotics. Stone culture performed during surgery for stone removal correctly identified the pathogen in 64% (7/11) of those who went on to develop postoperative sepsis. Interestingly, of those patients with positive preoperative urine cultures, most grew gram-negative organisms, while stone cultures grew predominantly gram-positive organisms or fungal elements, which were the organisms responsible for postoperative sepsis in 80%. Together these studies would suggest that not only are patients with positive preoperative urine cultures at higher risk for urosepsis after ureteroscopy, but that multiple and often, untreated organisms are responsible. This justifies the routine use of stone cultures and strengthens the argument for the further study and development of rapid microbial polymerase chain reaction (PCR) tests to help optimize expeditious postoperative antibiotic choice.

The presence and duration of preoperative ureteral stents have been shown to be a significant risk factor for urosepsis following ureteroscopy [44, 45]. Nevo et al. reported on 1256 consecutive patients undergoing ureteroscopy for stone removal, receiving either routine antibiotic prophylaxis or culture-specific treatment when cultures were positive (16%). Stents were previously placed in 601 (48%). A statistically significant rate of urosepsis was observed in 4.6% of those previously stented compared to only 1.2% of those not stented. Furthermore, the rate of urosepsis was over five times greater in those with stent duration greater than 30 days (6.2%) compared to those with stents less than 30 days (1.1%), again with statistical significance [44]. The recommendation was to attempt to keep stent duration as brief as possible. Moses et al. retrospectively examined 550 patients undergoing ureteroscopy for stone removal and studied factors related to unplanned return to the hospital or admission for infection. The overall rate of infection was 3.4% and was statistically greater in those patients who were previously stented (84.2% vs. 58.6%), in those with operative times greater than 120 minutes (89.5% vs. 32.6%), and interestingly in those in whom AUA best practice policy was followed for antibiotic prophylaxis (78.9% vs. 47.6%). These three factors were significant on multivariate analysis [45]. A very interesting observation was that ciprofloxacin was the prophylactic agent given (in accord with the best practice policy) to 84% of those returning with infection, while almost half of these patients suffered urosepsis with an organism, which was resistant to this agent, typically gram-positive bacteria. The recommendation was for previously stented patients to be given preoperative gram-positive coverage empirically.

Despite the seemingly negative effects of ureteral stents in these studies, it is essential to remember the benefit they provide, namely, the circumvention of obstruction. Blackmur et al. observed this benefit in subgroup analysis of patients with positive preoperative cultures undergoing ureteroscopy for stone removal, in which the rate of postoperative urosepsis was almost four times as high in those patients not previously stented [42]. Therefore, there is a clear advantage in treating previously stented patients, but the advantage diminishes, in terms of post-procedure infection rates, with increased stent dwell time. A practical solution is to prioritize patients with indwelling stents in terms of operating room scheduling.

Ureteral access sheaths have been shown to reduce intrarenal pressures by 57–75% during flexible ureteroscopy [46]. The literature is mixed in terms of infection-related outcomes following ureteroscopy with ureteral access sheath usage. A report from the CROES database on ureteroscopy observed fewer cases of postoperative fever, UTI, and sepsis in those patients in whom a ureteral access sheath was placed (28.6%, 18.6%, 4.3%) compared to those undergoing ureteroscopy without a sheath (39.1%, 23.9%, 15.2%), respectfully [47]. Other groups however have seen no statistically significant advantage with sheath use in terms of reducing post-ureteroscopic infections [42], including those treating patients with cumulative stone burden greater than 2 cm [48]. Zhong et al. examined multiple factors responsible for systemic inflammatory response syndrome (SIRS) in a series of 260 patients undergoing ureteroscopic laser lithotripsy in which all patients were treated with a ureteral access sheath [49]. The rate of SIRS was 8.1%. Both increased stone size and increased irrigation flow rate were noted to correlate with the development of SIRS in both univariate and multivariate analyses. Other significant contributing factors on multivariate analysis were the use of smaller caliber sheaths and the presence of struvite stone composition.

Therefore, not surprisingly, the development of urosepsis following ureteroscopy is a multifactorial process. Special attention should be paid to situations, which may lead to the pyelovenous or pyelolymphatic backflow of organisms from the upper urinary tract. Strategies to circumvent this situation include decreasing the quantity of organisms present during surgical interventions to whatever extent possible and then minimizing intrarenal pressures. Preoperative antibiotics clearly help achieve the former goal but might not treat all organisms present, especially in cases of large stone burden or prolonged operative times. Therefore, extending antimicrobial coverage and performing staged procedures in high-risk patients should be considered. Although necessary for adequate visualization during ureteroscopy, irrigation flow needs to be tempered in high-risk situations, as well. Although not yet formally studied, frequent low-pressure rinsing with small quantities of irrigant, intermittently during ureteroscopic laser lithotripsy, may be a strategy to help keep concentrations of organisms low, minimize pyelovenous backflow, and further diminish the rate of urosepsis following ureteroscopy.

Steinstrasse

The resultant accumulation of pulverized stone fragments in the ureteral lumen following extracorporeal shock wave lithotripsy (ESWL) can have a visual appearance similar to a column of sand or "street of stone" and is known as steinstrasse. This well-known complication of ESWL is directly related to increasing stone size, as well as location, presence of a dilated collecting system, and shock wave energy [50]. It has also been observed that stone composition plays a role, since stones of greater densities tend to break up into relatively larger resultant fragments, less likely to spontaneously pass [51, 52]. With the increasing application of retrograde ureteroscopic laser lithotripsy for larger-sized calculi, it is not surprising that steinstrasse can be encountered. Although not uniformly reported, the rate of steinstrasse in published ureteroscopic series of treated stones measuring at least 2 cm in one dimension lies between 1.6% and 17.4% [53–55]. Approximately half of these patients required additional procedures to clear the stone burden, usually with a second-stage ureteroscopy. Although not formally studied, the authors have anecdotally encountered steinstrasse following ureteroscopic laser lithotripsy of large-volume renal stones with relatively dense composition such as calcium oxalate monohydrate (Fig. 10.13).

Early Postoperative Complications (Minor)

Postoperative Pain

Patients undergoing ureteroscopy are seen unexpectedly in the emergency department (ED) in 6.6–15.6% of cases, while 2.2–5.8% get re-admitted within 30 days of the original procedure [45, 56–58]. In the majority of reports examining unplanned ED visits after ureteroscopy, postoperative pain is reliably the most common reason for patient presentation. Other common reasons include fever, urinary retention, and hematuria. Postoperative stent placement has not been shown to be an independent risk factor for return to the ED after ureteroscopy [50, 57]. Patient perception,

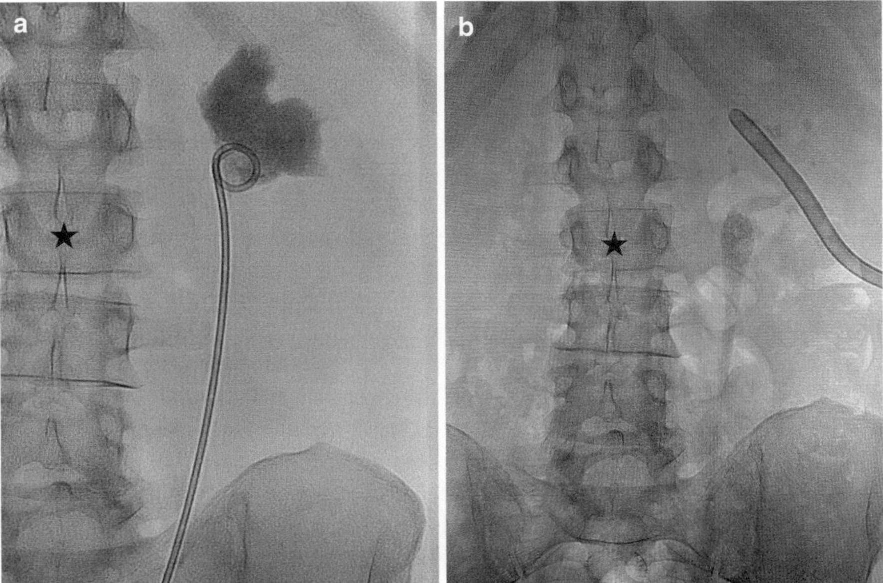

Fig. 10.13 Large-volume left renal stone treated with ureteroscopic laser lithotripsy (**a**) using holmium laser. Resultant massive steinstrasse encountered requiring percutaneous drainage (**b**). Black star marks the L3 vertebral level in both films

education, and experience with previous ureteroscopic surgery likely factor into the decision to seek ED services postoperatively, as "ureteroscopic-naïve" patients have not had the opportunity to acclimate to stent discomfort and other common symptoms following ureteroscopy [58]. This highlights the need for preoperative patient education in order to set realistic expectations and access to urology staff to address postoperative concerns.

Late Postoperative Complications (Major)

Ureteral Stricture Formation

The reported development of ureteral stricture following ureteroscopy in multiple, large contemporary series of patients primarily treated for upper urinary tract calculi is reliably under 1% [8]. Not surprisingly, the rate of stricture formation is higher in patients undergoing ureteroscopy for treatment of upper tract urothelial carcinoma at 8.5–16.7% [59]. This can result from direct ablative treatment of ureteral surface tumors, which can be multifocal, and the need for repetitive ureteroscopic surveillance in these patients in whom local tumor recurrence can be as high as 77% with long-term follow-up [60]. Although the rate of stricture formation differs depending on the indication for ureteroscopy as highlighted above, the threat of irreversible renal cortical loss is the manifestation that needs to be avoided whenever possible.

Traditionally regarded risk factors for ureteral stricture development following ureteroscopy usually have relative ureteral ischemia as a common component (Fig. 10.14). Certain elements of the patient's history are important to consider such as external beam radiation therapy for pelvic malignancies or prior pelvic surgery, both of which can predispose to variable amounts of ureteral ischemia. Impacted ureteral calculi, those that are believed to have been present for extended periods of time, and ureteral perforation at the time of ureteroscopic treatment are considered high-risk features for ureteral stricture formation in up to 24% of cases, although this estimate is likely inflated due to selection bias and a relatively small number of patients [61]. Fam et al. studied ureteral stone impaction prospectively in 77 patients as defined by at least one of the following: difficult wire passage beyond the ureteral stone at the first attempt, moderate or severe hydronephrosis on preoperative CT urogram, or ureteral stone presence at the same location for at least 2 months [62]. Five patients (7.8%) were found to develop strictures within 6 months of ureteroscopic stone treatment. The study analyzed many intraoperative and stone-related risk factors including ureteral perforation, damage to ureteral mucosa, residual stone remaining, stone size, stone location, and duration of impaction. No predictive variables for the development of ureteral stricture were identified. Despite its strength as a prospective study, the authors admit that it was underpowered to detect statistically significant differences among the study groups. Importantly, an additional observation from this study was that all five patients who developed obstructing strictures were asymptomatic. This is in accord with Weizer et al., who found

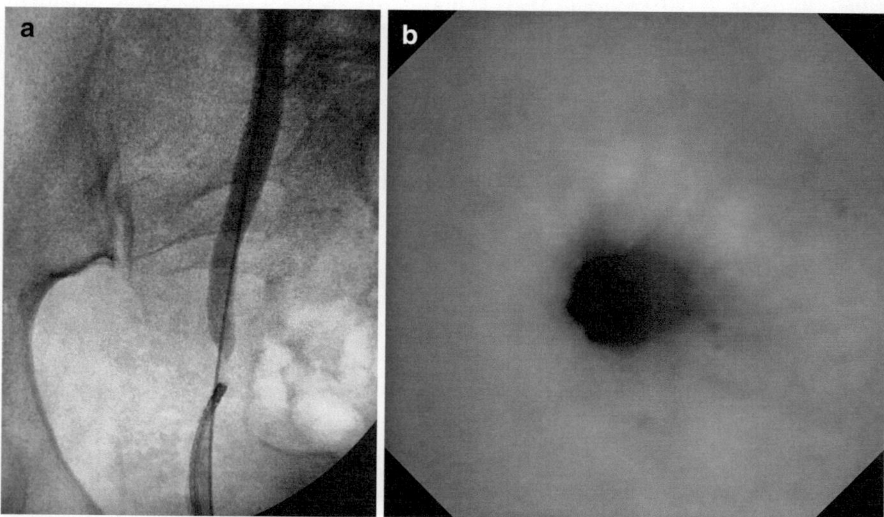

Fig. 10.14 Retrograde pyelogram (**a**) shows short right distal ureteral stricture. (**b**) Ureteroscopic view shows ischemic appearing mucosa with concentric narrowing

silent obstruction present in 23.3% of patients with post-ureteroscopic obstruction following stone treatment [63]. Contemporary imaging guidelines recommend routine renal ultrasound after ureteroscopy for laser lithotripsy to rule out silent obstruction whether due to residual stone fragments or stricture formation [64].

Conclusion

In the majority of cases involving ureteroscopy, complications are generally rare and mostly minor. Unfortunately, major complications still occur in contemporary practice, even when using the most refined endoscopic instruments available. This fact highlights the need for sound surgical judgment, adherence to fundamental practice principles, good patient selection, and a healthy respect for the sophistication of the upper urinary tract.

References

1. Bagley DH, Huffman JL, Lyon ES. Urologic endoscopy: a manual and atlas. Boston: Little, Brown and Company; 1985.
2. DeConinck V, Keller EX, Somani B, Giusti G, Proietti S, Rodriguez-Socarras M, et al. Complications of ureteroscopy: a complete overview. World J Urol. 2019; https://doi.org/10.1007/s00345-019-03012-1.
3. Tanimoto R, Cleary RC, Bagley DH, Hubosky SG. Ureteral avulsion associated with ureteroscopy: insights from the MAUDE database. J Endourol. 2016;30:257–61.
4. Moore EE, Cogbill TH, Jurkovich GJ, McAninch JW, Champion HR, Gennarelli TA, et al. Organ injury scaling. III: chest wall, abdominal vasculature, ureter, bladder, and urethra. J Trauma. 1992;33:337–9.
5. Dindo D, Demartines N, Clavien PA. Classification of surgical complications: a new proposal with evaluation in a cohort of 6336 patients and results of a survey. Ann Surg. 2004;240:205–13.
6. Schoenthaler M, Wilhelm K, Kuehhas FE, Farin E, Bach C, Buchholz N, et al. Postureteroscopic lesion scale: a new management modified organ injury scale–evaluation in 435 ureteroscopic patients. J Endourol. 2012;26:1425–30.
7. May M, Schonthaler M, Gilfrich C, Wolff I, Peter J, Miernik A, et al. Interrater reliability and clinical impact of the Post-Ureteroscopic Lesion Scale (PULS) grading system for ureteral lesions after ureteroscopy: results of the German prospective multicenter BUSTER project. Urologe A. 2018;57:172–80.
8. Johnson DB, Pearle MS. Complications of ureteroscopy. Urol Clin North Am. 2004;31:157–71.
9. Gupta V, Sadasukhi TC, Sharma KK, Yadav RG, Mathur R, Tomar V, et al. Complete ureteral avulsion. ScientificWorldJournal. 2005;5:125–7.
10. de la Rosette JJ, Skrekas T, Segura JW. Handling and prevention of complications in stone basketing. Eur Urol. 2006;50:991–9.
11. Perez Castro E, Osther PJ, Jinga V, Razvi H, Stravodimos KG, Parikh K, et al. Differences in ureteroscopic stone treatment and outcomes for distal, mid-, proximal, or multiple ureteral locations: the Clinical Research Office of the Endourological Society ureteroscopy global study. Eur Urol. 2014;66:102–9.
12. Grasso M. Ureteropyeloscopic treatment of ureteral and intrarenal calculi. Urol Clin North Am. 2000;27:623–31.

13. Hubosky SG, Raval AJ, Bagley DH. Locked deflection during flexible ureteroscopy: incidence and elucidation of the mechanism of an underreported complication. J Endourol. 2015;29:907–12.
14. Anderson JK, Lavers A, Hulbert JC, Monga M. The fractured flexible ureteroscope with locked deflection. J Urol. 2004;171(1):335.
15. Huynh M, Telfer S, Pautler S, Denstedt J, Razvi H. Retained digital flexible ureteroscopes. J Endourol Case Rep. 2017;3(1):24–7.
16. Wallace B, Nham E, Watterson J, Mahoney J, Skinner T. Between a rock and a hard place: a case report of stone fragmentation impaction causing a retained ureteroscope requiring open surgical intervention. J Endourol Case Rep. 6:7–9. https://doi.org/10.1089/cren.2019.0064.
17. Gadzhiev N, Grigoryev V, Okhunov Z, Nguyen N, Pisarev A, Hikmet B, et al. "Valve"-type retainment of flexible ureteroscope in the distal ureter. J Endourol Case Rep. 2017;3(1):108–10.
18. Ordon M, Schuler TD, D'A Honey RJ. Ureteral avulsion during contemporary ureteroscopic stone management: "the scabbard avulsion". J Endourol. 2011;25:1259–62.
19. Sewell J, Blecher G, Tsai K, Bishop C. Calculus-related ureteral intussusception: a case report and literature review. Int J Surg Case Rep. 2015;12:63–6.
20. Gabriel JB, Thomas L, Guarin U, Kondlapoodi P, Chauhan PM. Ureteral intussusception by papillary transitional cell carcinoma. Urology. 1986;28:310–2.
21. Suzuki K, Saito K, Yoshimura N, Ohno Y, Nakashima J, Oshiro H, et al. Ureteral intussusception associated with a fibroepithelial polyp: a case report. Clinical Imaging. 2015;39:901–3.
22. de la Rosette J, Denstedt J, Geavlete P, Keeley F, Matsuda T, Pearle M, et al. The clinical research office of the endourological society ureteroscopy global study: indications, complications, and outcomes in 11,885 patients. J Endourol. 2014;28(2):131–9.
23. Van Cangh PJ, Nesa S, Galeon M, Tombal B, Wese FX, Dardenne AN, et al. Vessels around the ureteropelvic junction: significance and imaging by conventional radiology. J Endourol. 1996;10(2):111–9.
24. Lopes RI, Torricelli FC, Gomes CM, Carnevale F, Bruschini H, Srougi M. Endovascular repair of a nearly fatal iliac artery injury after endoureterotomy. Scan J Urol. 2013;47:437–9.
25. Thomas R, Monga M, Klein EW. Ureteroscopic retrograde endopyelotomy for management of ureteropelvic junction obstruction. J Endourol. 1996;10(2):141–5.
26. Sampaio FJ. Vascular anatomy at the ureteropelvic junction. Urol Clin North Am. 1998;25:251–8.
27. Tawfiek ER, Liu JB, Bagley DH. Ureteroscopic treatment of ureteropelvic junction obstruction. J Urol. 1998;160:1643–7.
28. Hendrikx AJ, Nadorp S, De Beer N, Van Beekum JB, Gravas S. The use of endoluminal ultrasonography for preventing significant bleeding during endopyelotomy: evaluation of helical computed tomography vs endoluminal ultrasonography for detecting crossing vessels. BJU. 2006;97:786–90.
29. Hirsch LM, Amirian MJ, Hubosky SG, Das AK, Abai B, et al. Urologic and endovascular repair of a uretero-iliac artery fistula. Can J Urol. 2015;22(1):7661–5.
30. Vandersteen DR, Saxon RR, Fuchs S, Keller FS, Taylor LM, Barry JM. Diagnosis and management of ureteroiliac artery fistula: value of provocative arteriography followed by common iliac artery embolization and extraanatomic arterial bypass grafting. J Urol. 1997;158:754–8.
31. Traxer O, Thomas A. Prospective evaluation and classification of ureteral wall injuries resulting from insertion of a ureteral access sheath during retrograde intrarenal surgery. J Urol. 2013;189:580–4.
32. Lytton B, Weiss RM, Green DF. Complications of ureteral endoscopy. J Urol. 1987;137:649–53.
33. Efthimiou I, Chousianitis Z, Skrepetis K. Troubleshooting for ureteroscopy complicated by unexpected guidewire looping and entrapment. J Endourol Case Rep. 2017;3(1):84–6.
34. Geavlete P, Georgescu D, Nita G, Mirciulescu V, Cauni V. Complications of 2735 retrograde semirigid ureteroscopy procedures: a single-center experience. J Endourol. 2006;20:179–85.

35. Francesca F, Scattoni V, Nava L, Pompa P, Grasso M, Rigatti P. Failures and complications of transurethral ureteroscopy in 297 cases: conventional rigid instruments vs. small caliber semirigid ureteroscopes. Eur Urol. 1995;28:112–5.
36. Somani BK, Giusti G, Sun Y, Osther PJ, Frank M, De Sio M, et al. Complications associated with ureterorenoscopy (URS) related to treatment of urolithisis: the Clinical Research Office of Endourological Society URS Global Study. World J Urol. 2017;35:675–81.
37. Chugh S, Pietropaolo A, Montanari E, Sarica K, Somani BK. Predictors of urinary infections and urosepsis after ureteroscopy for stone disease: a systematic review from EAU section of urolithiasis (EULIS). Curr Urol Rep. 2020;21:16.
38. Cindolo L, Castellan P, Scoffone CM, Cracco CM, Celia A, Paccaduscio A, et al. Mortality and flexible ureteroscopy: analysis of six cases. World J Urol. 2016;34:305–10.
39. Assimos D, Krambeck A, Miller NL, Monga M, Murad MH, Nelson CP, et al. Surgical management of stones: Amercian Urological Association/Endourological Society Guideline, Part 1. JUrol. 2016;196:1153–60.
40. Osther PJ. Risks of flexible ureteroscopy: pathophysiology and prevention. Urolithiasis. 2018;46:59–67.
41. Lightner DJ, Wymer K, Sanchez J, Kavoussi L. Best Practice Statement on urologic procedures and antimicrobial prophylaxis. J Urol. 2020;203:351–6.
42. Blackmur JP, Maitra NU, Marri RR, Housami F, Malki M, McIlhenny C. Analysis of factors' association with risk of postoperative urosepsis in patients undergoing ureteroscopy for treatment of stone disease. J Endourol. 2016;30:963–9.
43. Eswara JR, Sharif-Tabrizi A, Sacco D. Positive stone culture is associated with a higher rate of urosepsis after endourological procedures. Urolith. 2013;41:411–4.
44. Nevo A, Mano R, Baniel J, Lifshitz DA. Ureteric stent dwelling time: a risk factor for post-ureteroscopy sepsis. BJU. 2017;120:117–22.
45. Moses RA, Ghali FM, Pais VM, Hyams ES. Unplanned hospital return for infection following ureteroscopy: can we identify modifiable risk factors? J Urol. 2016;195:931–6.
46. Auge BK, Pietrow PK, Lallas CD, Raj GV, Santa-Cruz RW, Preminger GM. Ureteral access sheath provides protection against elevated renal presssues during routine flexible ureteroscopic stone manipulation. J Endourol. 2004;18:33–6.
47. Traxer O, Wendt-Nordahl G, Sodha H, Rassweiler J, Meretyk S, Tefekli A, et al. Differences in renal stone treatment and outcomes for patients treated either with or without the support of a ureteral access sheath: the Clinical Research Office of the Endourological Society Ureteroscopy Global Study. World J Urol. 2015;33:2137–44.
48. Geraghty RM, Ishii H, Somani BK. Outcomes of flexible ureteroscopy and laser fragmentation for treatment of large renal stones with and without the use of ureteral access sheaths: Results from a university hospital with a review of the literature. Scan J Urol. 2016;50:216–9.
49. Zhong W, Leto G, Wang L, Zeng G. Systemic Inflammatory Response Syndrome after flexible ureteroscopic lithotripsy: a study of risk factors. J Endourol. 2015;29:25–8.
50. Madbouly K, Sheir KZ, Elsobky E, Eraky I, Kenawy M. Risk factors for the formation of a steinstrasse after extracorporeal shock wave lithotripsy: a statistical model. J Urol. 2002;167:1239–42.
51. Dretler SP. Stone fragility – a new therapeutic distinction. J Urol. 1988;139:1124–7.
52. Newmark JR, Wong MYC, Lingeman JE. Complications of extracorporeal shockwave lithotripsy. In: Smith AD, Badlani GH, Bagley DH, Clayman RV, Jordan GH, Kavoussi LR, Lingeman JE, Preminger GM, Segura JW, editors. Smith's textbook of endourology. St. Louis: Quality Medical Publishing; 1996. p. 680–93.
53. Hyams ES, Munver R, Bird VG, Uberoi J, Shah O. Flexible ureterorenoscopy and Holmium laser lithotripsy for the management of renal stone burdens that measure 2 to 3 cm: a multi-institutional experience. J Endourol. 2010;24:1583–8.
54. Al-Qahtani SM, Gil-deiz-de-Medina S, Traxer O. Predictors of clinical outcomes of flexible ureterorenoscopy with holmium laser for renal stone greater than 2 cm. Advances in Urol. 2012; https://doi.org/10.1155/2012/543537.

55. Mariani AJ. Combined electrohydraulic and holmium: YAG laser ureteroscopic nephrolithotripsy of large (> 2 cm) renal calculi. Indian J Urol. 2008;24:521–5.
56. Mittakanti HR, Conti SL, Pao AC, Chertow GM, Liao JC, Leppert JT, et al. Unplanned emergency department visits and hosptial admission following ureteroscopy: do ureteral stents make a difference? Urology. 2018;117:44–9.
57. Carlos EC, Peters CE, Wollin DA, Winship BB, Davis LG, Li J, et al. Psychiatric diagnoses and other factors associated with emergency department return within 30 days of ureteroscopy. J Urol. 2019;201:556–62.
58. Bloom J, Matthews G, Phillips J. Factors influencing readmission after elective ureteroscopy. J Urol. 2016;195:1487–91.
59. Hubosky SG, Bagley DH. Diagnosis and treatment of upper urinary tract neoplasms. In: Smith AD, Preminger GM, Kavoussi LR, Badlani GH, editors. Smith's textbook of endourology. Oxford: Wiley-Blackwell; 2019. p. 568–83.
60. Grasso M, Fishman AI, Cohen AB. Ureteroscopic and extirpative treatment of upper urinary tract urothelial carcinoma: a 15-year comprehensive review of 160 consecutive patients. BJU. 2012;110:1618–26.
61. Roberts WW, Cadeddu JA, Micali S, Kavoussi LR, Moore RG. Ureteral stricture formation after removal of impacted calcuil. J Urol. 1998;159:723–6.
62. Fam XI, Singam P, Kong Ho CC, Sridharan R, Hod R, Bahadzor B, et al. Ureteral stricture formation after ureteroscope treatment of impacted calculi: a prospective study. Korean J Urol. 2015;56:63–7.
63. Weizer AZ, Auge BK, Silverstein AD, Delvecchio FC, Brizuela RM, Dahm P, et al. Routine postoperative imaging is important after ureteroscopic stone manipulation. J Urol. 2002;168:46–50.
64. Fulgham PF, Assimos DG, Pearle MS, Preminger GM. Clinical effectiveness protocols for Imaging in the management of ureteral calculous disease: AUA technology assessment. J Urol. 2013;189:1203–13.

Index

A

Abdominal plain film, 16, 17
Ablative capacity, 69
Accordion, 64
Adjuvant check point inhibitors, 195
Adjuvant chemotherapy for UTUC, 194, 195
Adjuvant treatment
  bacillus calmette-guérin (BCG), 192
  mitomycin C (MMC), 187–189
  mitomycin gel topical therapy, 189, 191
  systemic treatment, 193
  thiotepa, 192
  topical luminal therapy, 193
  topical treatment, 185, 186
    delivery routes, 186
    instillation techniques, 186, 187
ALARA, *see* As low as reasonably
      achievable (ALARA)
Albarran deflector, 3, 6
Allen stirrup design, 144
Angled hydromer-coated catheter, 7, 10
Antegrade ureteroscopy, 235
  endoscopic access, 242
  indications for, 235
    complete ureteral obstruction, 236
    considerations, 241
    difficulty accessing ureteral orifice,
      238, 240
    proximal ureteral stones, 240, 241
  patient positioning, 241, 242
  post treatment
    antibiotics, 244, 245
    drainage, 242–244
Antibiotic prophylaxis, 110
Antibiotics, 244, 245
Anticoagulation/antiplatelet therapy, 54

Antimicrobial prophylaxis, 265
Antiretropulsion devices, 63, 64
Articulating tipless nitinol basket, 60
"As low as reasonably achievable"
      (ALARA), 95, 99
Autoimmune effects, 196
Avicenna roboflex, 41–44

B

Bacillus calmette-guérin (BCG), 187, 192
  complications and side effects of, 192
Ballistic lithotripsy, 71
Basketing techniques, 64–66
Benign ureteral strictures, 220
Bentson wire, 10
Biomarkers, 158–160
Blood-borne pathogens, 99

C

Calcium oxalate monohydrate, 138
Caliceal diverticula, stones in, 124
Carcinoma-in-situ (CIS), 192
Charge-coupled devices (CCD), 34
CHROMA mode, 168
Chronically dilated ureter with multiple
      tortuosities, 48
Chronic kidney disease (CKD), solitary kidney
      or patients with, 196
Chronic unilateral hematuria (CUH)
  definition of, 225
  diagnosis of, 229, 230
  etiology of, 225, 226, 228
  treatment for, 230–232
CLARA mode, 168

Clavien-Dindo classification system, 250
Clinically insignificant residual fragments
        (CIRF), 118
Coagulopathy, 54
Complementary metal oxide semiconductors
        (CMOS), 34
Complete ureteral obstruction, 236
Computed tomography (CT), 20, 127
    advantages, 20
    CT urogram, 22, 23
    CT urography, 21
    dual energy CT, 21
    limitations, 22–24
    for tumor assessment, 21
Cone-tipped ureteropyelogram, 11
Confocal laser endomicroscopy (CLE), 167,
        170, 171
Conventional radiography, 16, 17
Cystoscope, 2
Cystoscopy with retrograde pyelogram (RGP),
        216, 221
Cytospins, 162

D
Dark ureteroscope, 236
Diagnostic ureterorenoscopy (URS), 166, 175
Difficult urethral access, 1–3
    impacted calculi, 7–10
    modifications for, 92
    occlusive ureteral tumor, 10
    reimplanted ureter, 6, 7
    ureteral narrowing or stricture, 11, 12
    ureteral orifice, 3–6
    ureteropelvic junction obstruction, 12
Distal ureteral stones, 112
Distal ureterectomy, 6
Doppler sonography, 17
Dormia basket, 60
Dorsal lithotomy with Allen stirrups, 143
Dual-energy CT, 21
Dusting technique, 129–131

E
Electrocautery, 176
Electrohydraulic lithotripsy (EHL), 68,
        70, 71, 129
Endoluminal ultrasound (ELUS), 260
Endopyelotomy, 209, 212–214, 261
Endoscope, 92
    treatment, 1
Endoureterotomy, 209, 220, 221

Entrapped basket, 66, 67
Ergonomics, 96, 97
Extracorporeal shock wave lithotripsy
        (ESWL), 94, 107, 127, 268
Eye safety, 97
    fluid splash contamination, 99
    laser injury, 97, 98
    prioritizing eye protection, 99, 100
    radiation-induced eye injury, 99

F
False passages, 262
Fiberoptic technology, 31
Flexible cystoscope, 2
Flexible endoscopy, 142
Flexible ureteroscopes (fURS), 30, 31, 34–37,
        40, 80, 82–84, 87, 88, 90, 94, 97,
        129, 225, 229
    indications/guidelines, 117, 118
    lower-pole stones, 123
    multiple stones, 123
    vs. semi-rigid URS, 113
    stone burden, measurement of, 119, 121
    stone-free rate, 118, 119
    stones > 2cm, 121, 122
    stones in caliceal diverticula, 124
    techniques, 121
Fluid splash contamination, 99
Fluorescence in situ hybridization (FISH), 159
18-Fluorodeoxyglucose (18-FDG) PET/CT, 25
Forward grasping devices, 61

G
GC (Gemcitabine, cisplatin), 193
Gemcitabine, paclitaxel, and doxorubicin
        (GTA), 196
Glomerular filtration rate (GFR), 171
Guidewires, 45
    materials, 47
    placement of, 45
    safety guidewire, 47, 50
    sizes and tip design, 45, 46
Gyrus ACMI Invisio DUR D, 31

H
Hemangiomas, 226, 230
Hemorrhage, 259–261
Hereditary non-polyposis colorectal cancer
        (HNPCC). *See* Lynch syndrome
HistoGel, 162

Holmium (Ho) lasers, 68, 69, 129, 221
    Ho: YAG laser, 68, 98, 129, 134, 177
Holmium laser lithotripsy
    dusting technique, 129–131
    fragmentation and extraction, 131
Holmium: yttrium aluminum garnet (Ho:
        YAG) lasers, 68, 98, 128, 129,
        134, 177
Hounsfield units (HU), 20
Hybrid wires, 47, 49
Hydronephrosis, 17, 192
Hydrophilic polymer, 47
Hydrophilic wires, 49
Hydroureter, 17
Hyperuricosuria, 138
Hypospadias, 2

I
Image 1-S technology, 168
Immune checkpoint inhibitors (CPI), 195
Impacted calculi, 7–10
Instillation technique, 186, 187
Interferon-alpha, 192
Intracorporeal lithotrites for ureteroscopy
    EHL, 70, 71
    laser lithotrites (*see* Laser lithotrites)
    pneumatic/ballistic lithotripsy, 71
Intravenous pyelographic (IVP) techniques,
    15, 18–20, 156
    advantages of, 18
    disadvantages of, 19
Intussusception, 259

J
Jelmyto, 189

K
Kidneys, ureters, and bladder (KUB), 16

L
Laparoscopic pyeloplasty, 213, 214
Large intrarenal lesions, ureteroscopic
    treatment of, 177, 179
Large right proximal ureteral stone with
    complete obstruction, 9
Laser ablation, 178
Laser dosimetry, 69
Laser energy, 176, 177
Laser fibers, 129

Laser injury, 97, 98
Laser lithotripsy, 120, 121
    of ureteral stones, 114
Laser lithotrites
    holmium laser, 68, 69
    moses platform, 69, 70
    thulium fiber laser (TFL), 70
Lateralized "essential" hematuria, 93
Linear erythema, 89
Lithotomy
    with flank roll, 145, 146
    modifications of, 144
    position, 143, 144
    reverse, 145
Lithotomy with Flank Roll, 145, 146
LithoVue empower, 63
Lower-pole stones, 123
Low-grade upper urinary tract index
        lesion, 190
Luer-lock ended tubing, 91
Lynch syndrome, 173, 184, 195, 196

M
Macroscopic technologies, 167
Magnetic resonance imaging (MRI), 24
    stone management, 24
    tumor management, 25
Magnetic resonance urography
        (MRU), 158
Meatal stenosis, 1
Metabolic evaluation, 128, 133
    medical history and physical examination,
        133, 135
    radiology, 135
    selection of, 141
    stone examination, 135, 138
    twenty-four-hour urine collection and early
        morning urine, 138
    urinary and blood analysis, 135
Methemoglobinemia, 4
Microscopic technologies, 167
Mid-ureteral stones, 112
Minute venous ruptures (MVRs), 226
Mitomycin C (MMC), 187–189
Mitomycin-containing reverse thermal gel
        (M-CRTG), 189
Mitomycin gel topical therapy, 189, 191
Moses technology, 69, 70
Mucosal abrasions, 261
Multiple stones, 123
MVAC (Methotrexate, vinblastine,
        adriamycin, and cisplatin), 193

N
Narrow-band imaging (NBI), 167, 168
Narrow-shaft diameter baskets, 65
Neoadjuvant chemotherapy in UTUC, 194
Nephrocalcinosis, 135
Nephrolithiasis, 18
Nephron sparing approaches, rationale for,
        171, 173
Nephroureterectomy (NU), 171, 193
Nitinol, 56, 59, 61, 64
        basket, 59, 65
        hybrid basket/grasper, 59, 62, 65
Non-contrast computed tomography
        (NCCT), 18, 20
Non-retracting instruments, 57
Non-steroidal anti-inflammatory drugs
        (NSAIDS), 228
No-touch ureteroscopy, 89, 90, 175
        indications for, 93
NTrap, 64

O
Obstructing stones, 9
Occlusive ureteral tumor, 10
Opensure handle, 66
Optical coherence tomography (OCT), 166,
        169, 170

P
Pediatric en bloc kidney transplant, 8
Percutaneous/antegrade nephroscopic
        approaches, 179
Percutaneous nephrolithotomy (PCNL), 117,
        121, 240, 241
Photodynamic diagnosis (PDD), 167–169
Physiologic hydronephrosis, 115
Plain film radiographs, 15
Pneumatic lithotripsy, 71
Polytetrafluoroethylene (PTFE), 56
Popcorning, 130
Positron emission tomography (PET), 25
Postoperative pain, 268, 269
Post-ureteroscopic lesion scale (PULS), 250
Pre-stenting, 113
Prioritizing eye protection, 99, 100
Prone split leg position, 145, 147
Proximal ureteral narrowing/stricture, 191
Proximal ureteral stones, 110, 112, 240, 241
Pseudopolyps, 7
PTFE (polytetrafluorethylene or teflon),
        46, 47

Q
Quick SOFA scoring (qSOFA), 126

R
Radiation, 95, 96
Radiation-induced eye injury, 99
Radical cystectomy, 238
Radiology, 135
Randall's plaque, 135
Reimplanted ureter, 6, 7
Renal papillary necrosis (RPN), 228
Renal stones, treatment algorithm for, 118
Residual fragments (RFs), 127
Residual stone disease, assessment and
        management of, 127, 128
Resistive index, 17
Retrieval deployment device, 63
Retrograde flexible ureteroscopy, 117
Retrograde intra-renal surgery (RIRS), 51.
        See also Retrograde flexible
        ureteroscopy
Retrograde pyelogram (RGP), 9, 10, 22, 23, 80
Retrograde ureteropyelography, 90, 157
Reverse lithotomy, 145
Right proximal ureteral upper tract urothelial
        carcinoma, 10
Rigid cystoscope, 3
Rigid ureteroscopes, 31
Robotic platforms for ureteroscopy, 40
        avicenna roboflex, 41, 43, 44
        Sensei Magellan robotic catheter system, 41

S
Safety guidewire (SG), 47, 50
Scabbard avulsions, 256
Semi-rigid ureteroscopes, 31, 80–82, 129
        vs. flexible URS, 113
Sensei Magellan robotic catheter system, 41
Sepsis, 125, 126
Sequential organ failure assessment (SOFA)
        scoring, 126
Single-use ureteroscopes, 38–40
Slip coat, 47
Solitary kidney or patients with chronic kidney
        disease (CKD), 196
Stainless steel flat wire basket, 58
Steinstrasse, 268
Steroid therapy, 196
Stone cone, 64
Stone fragmentation, 69
Stone free rate (SFR), 117–119

Stone management, 24
Stone retrieval devices, 56, 57
   antiretropulsion devices, 63, 64
   basketing techniques, 57, 64–66
      historical development, 57–61
   entrapped basket, 66, 67
   forward grasping devices, 61
   retrieval deployment device, 63
Stones, 16
   burden, measurement of, 119, 121
   in caliceal diverticula, 124
   cone, 64
   examination, 135, 138
   fragmentation, 69
   management, 24
   size, 123
Storz Image 1-S technology, 167
Storz professional image enhancement system
      (SPIES), 167, 168
Surveillance cystoscopy, 183
Surveillance ureteroscopy, 93
Systemic inflammatory response syndrome
      (SIRS), 125, 126

T
Tent sign, 116
Therapeutic ureteroscopy, 93
Thiotepa, 192
Thulium fiber laser (TFL), 35, 70
Topical luminal therapy, 193
Transient vesicoureteral reflux (VUR), 6
Tumor assessment, CT for, 21
Tumor management, 25
Type IVa carbapatite stones, 138

U
Ultrasonography (US), 16
Ultrasound (US), 17, 18, 158
Upper tract carcinoma in situ (UT-CIS), 166
Upper tract urothelial cancers (UTUC), 16, 20,
      21, 24, 89, 219
   adjuvant treatment for (*see* Adjuvant
      treatment)
   diagnosis of
      grading with ureteroscopy, 162–165
      imaging, 156–158
      specimen processing, 162
      ureteroscopic biopsy technique,
         160, 161
      urinary cytology and
         biomarkers, 158–160

   image enhancement techniques
      Image 1-S technology, 168
      NBI, 167, 168
      PDD, 168, 169
   optical diagnostic techniques
      confocal laser endomicroscopy (CLE),
         170, 171
      optical coherence tomography (OCT),
         169, 170
   staging of, 165, 166
   ureteroscopy for
      biopsy and physical removal of tissue,
         174, 175
      complications, 184
      energy sources, ureteroscopic tumor
         ablation, 175, 176
      large intrarenal lesions, ureteroscopic
         treatment of, 177–179
      laser energy, 176, 177
      nephron sparing approaches, rationale
         for, 171, 173
      outcomes and recurrence, 180–184
      patient positioning, 173, 174
      percutaneous/antegrade nephroscopic
         approaches, 179
Upper urinary tract, imaging of, 15
   conventional radiography/abdominal plain
      film, 16, 17
   CT, 20
      advantages, 20
      dual-energy CT, 21
      limitations, 22–24
      for tumor assessment, 21
   intravenous pyelography (IVP), 18–20
   MRI, 24
      stone management, 24
      tumor management, 25
   PET, 25
   ultrasound (US), 17, 18
Upper urinary tract obstruction, 209
Ureteral access sheaths (UAS), 94, 114,
      127, 267
   characteristics/specifications, 51
   in children, 55
   coagulopathy, 54
   complications, 55
   guideline recommendations, 55
   insertion success rate, 54
   irrigation and intrarenal pressure, 53
   multiple instrument reinsertions and
      withdrawals, 53
   stone-free rate, 53
   ureteroscope durability, 54

Ureteral avulsion, 251, 252, 254–256, 259
Ureteral dilation and pre-stenting, 113
Ureteral inflammation, 240
Ureteral narrowing/stricture, 11, 12, 113
Ureteral orifice, 3–6, 238, 240
Ureteral perforations, 264
Ureteral resectoscopes, 175
Ureteral stenosis, 192
Ureteral stones, 106
   indications and treatment alternatives,
      106, 107
    techniques, tips and tricks
      anatomical considerations, 110
      anesthesia, 107, 110
      antibiotic prophylaxis, 110
      basketing, 115
      distal ureteral stones, 112
      flexible versus semi-rigid URS, 113
      laser lithotripsy of ureteral stones, 114
      mid-ureteral stones, 112
      narrow ureteral meatus, 116
      patient positioning and set-up, 110
      pediatrics, 116
      pregnancy, 115, 116
      proximal ureteral stones, 110, 112
      safety guidewire, 113, 114
      ureteral access sheaths (UASs), 114
      ureteral dilation and pre-stenting, 113
Ureteral strictures, 128
   etiology, 219, 220
   formation, 269–271
   outcomes, 221
   patient selection, 220
   surgical techniques, 221
Ureteral wall insults, 261–264
Uretero-arterial fistula (UAF), 261
Ureteroceles, 5
Ureteroneocystotomy, 6
Ureteropelvic junction (UPJ) obstruction, 12
   endopyelotomy, 212, 213
   etiology, 210, 211
   outcomes, 219
   patient selection, 214
   surgical planning, 214, 216
   surgical techniques, 216, 217
Ureteroscope durability, 54
Ureteroscopic biopsy technique, 160, 161
Ureteroscopy, 16, 92, 94, 229, 230, 249
   complications
      classification systems for, 250, 251
      hemorrhage, 259–261
      intussusception, 259
      minor, 249

      postoperative pain, 268, 269
      steinstrasse, 268
      ureteral avulsion, 251, 252,
        254–256, 259
      ureteral stricture formation, 269–271
      ureteral wall insults, 261–264
      urosepsis, 264–268
   flexible ureteroscopes (fURS),
      82–84, 87, 88
   general considerations, 80, 81
   grading with, 162–165
   instrumentation, 90
   long term, post evaluation
      assessment and management of residual
        stone disease, 127, 128
      metabolic evaluation, 128
      ureteral strictures, 128
   need for staged procedure, 92
   positioning for, 142
      lithotomy, modifications of, 144
      lithotomy position, 143, 144
      lithotomy, reverse, 145
      lithotomy with flank roll, 145
      prone split leg position, 145, 147
   robotic platforms for (*see* Robotic
      platforms for ureteroscopy)
   semi-rigid ureteroscopy, 81, 82
   short term, post evaluation
      outpatient clinic or overnight
        stay, 125
      patient positioning, 125
      post-procedural stenting, 126, 127
      SIRS and sepsis, 125, 126
   specifications, 30
      flexible, 31, 34–37
      rigid, 31
      semi-rigid, 31
      single-use, 38–40
   techniques, 90, 91
   for upper tract urothelial carcinoma
      biopsy and physical removal of tissue,
        174, 175
      complications, 184
      energy sources applied for
        ureteroscopic tumor ablation,
        175, 176
      large intrarenal lesions, ureteroscopic
        treatment of, 177–179
      laser energy, 176, 177
      nephron sparing approaches, rationale
        for, 171, 173
      outcomes and recurrence, 180–184
      patient positioning, 173, 174

percutaneous/antegrade nephroscopic
approaches, 179
Ureteroscopy, intracorporeal lithotrites for. *See*
Intracorporeal lithotrites for
ureteroscopy
Ureteroscopy, safety considerations during, 95
for OR staff, 100
for patient, 100, 101
for surgeon
ergonomics, 96, 97
eye safety, 97–100
radiation, 95, 96
Urinary calculi, 7, 136–137
Urinary cytology, 158–160
Urinary obstruction, 16

Urolithiasis, 15, 106
Urosepsis, 264–268
Urothelial cancers, 25
immunotherapeutic drugs for, 197
Urothelial lesions, 21
Urothelial malignancy, 93
UTUC, *see* Upper tract urothelial
cancers (UTUC)

W
Wireless and sheathless ureteroscopy. *See*
No-touch ureteroscopy
Work-related musculoskeletal disorders
(WRMD), 96